CW01497474

ZERO ACCOUNTABILITY IN A FAILED SYSTEM

HOW BIG PHARMA WEAPONIZES VACCINES, PUBLIC HEALTH, AND THE LAW

BY DR. SHERRI TENPENNY

FOREWORD BY DR. SUZANNE HUMPHRIES

Accolades for *Zero Accountability*

I remember well meeting you at NVIC's Second International Public Conference on Vaccination in 2000. I knew then that you would bring a new, important voice to the public debate about vaccine risks that began in the 19th century with parents and doctors protesting the reactivity of smallpox vaccine. In 1982, this debate accelerated with parents and doctors protesting the reactivity of whole-cell pertussis vaccine in DPT shots. Your steadfast advocacy has been instrumental in revealing the truth about the role that one-size-fits-all vaccine policies and laws play in compromising the health of children and adults. Congratulations for staying the course and for writing this book to further educate the public about the need to hold those operating the public health system accountable for the poor health outcomes of so many Americans.

–Barbara Loe Fisher
Author, speaker, writer, activist
Founder of The National Vaccine Information Center

Matthew 5:16 reads, "Let your light shine before men, that they may see your good works, and glorify your Father which is in heaven." The Pharmaceutical Industry blankets humanity in an ever-thickening veil of darkness of deceit, greed, and death… all in the name of greed and profit. For over 20 years, I have considered Dr Sherri Tenpenny a light, guide, and resource for truth. I trust her information to protect me and my family from the pitfalls of this ever-darkening and criminal empire! Read this book!

–Dr. Bryan Ardis
Best Selling Author of Moving Beyond COVID-19 Lies,
Restoring Health and Hope for Humanity
Host of TheDrArdisShow Podcast

Dr. Tenpenny has been on the frontlines of the truth about vaccines and Big Pharma for decades. Her work is the reason my adult children never got the usual childhood poisons…and I will be forever grateful to her. For those who are just waking up to the fraud that has passed for our public health system, welcome to the truth that will set you free and safeguard your health."

–Christiane Northrup, MD
Multiple NY Times bestselling author of Women's Bodies,
Women's Wisdom and The Wisdom of Menopause

Dr. Tenpenny is a medical pioneer and a courageous truthteller. Many of her warnings have been borne out by events and hers is a unique and important voice."

Dr. Tenpenny is one of the few doctors who grew up with the advantage of being completely unvaccinated. Because of the wisdom of her father, she became a physician who questioned why each year children were impaled with more and more shots. Dr. Tenpenny realized that once doctors and nurses were indoctrinated into vaccine religion, it is nearly impossible to wake them up. This is not so true with the public, particularly in the wake of the COVID-19 vaccine debacle. *Zero Accountability in a Failed System* is a shot across the bow to the medical orthodoxy. This incredible work is fortified with the Tenpenny Library--one of the most extensive collections of scientific data and reports on vaccines, their ingredients, and the safety profiles of individual and combination shots. She believes the only way to right the ship is to call out fraud and demand accountability. So get ready for this locked and loaded, explosive masterpiece on what has happened to the medical system."

In a time when deception is the currency of control, truth becomes the most powerful act of resistance. *Zero Accountability in a Failed System* is more than just a revelation—it is a roadmap to reclaiming autonomy, demanding justice, and breaking free from the narratives designed to keep us in fear. Dr. Sherri Tenpenny fearlessly exposes the corruption that has gone unchecked for too long, arming readers with the knowledge to challenge the status quo and protect their families. May this book inspire not just awareness, but action—because when the people awaken, the system can no longer stand on its lies.

Dr. Tenpenny has always been a light in the darkness of the Pharmaceutical Industrial Complex, fearlessly speaking out against corruption in the medical industry. If we had more doctors like Sherri, trust in health care would be much higher."

Dr. Tenpenny has been a trailblazer and frontline warrior in the fight to expose the effects of vaccines on our children. Long before a lot of us physicians woke up to the ills of big pharma, she was sounding the alarm. If you want sound data-based information on what to know about vaccines, you should read her book and listen to her works. Dr. Tenpenny is my go-to for information and I always recommend that people listen to her before deciding to vaccinate or not. I wholeheartedly recommend this book."

–*Stella Immanuel MD*
Physician, Author, international speaker, entrepreneur and minister of the gospel

Zero Accountability in a Failed System is a gut-wrenching exposé that rips the curtain back on the deep-seated corruption within Big Pharma, public health, and the legal system. Dr. Sherri Tenpenny doesn't just reveal the lies—we've all suspected them—she shows how these institutions have been weaponized against us, putting profits ahead of human lives. If you've ever felt betrayed by the medical system or questioned the relentless push for pharmaceuticals, this book will shake you to your core. It's not just a read—it's a wake-up call, a battle cry, and a roadmap to reclaiming medical freedom. You need to read this book before it's too late.

–*Eric Nepute D.C, DNM*
Author, international speaker and biotech entrepreneur

Dr. Sherri Tenpenny's *Zero Accountability in a Failed System* is a clarion call for transparency, challenging the sanctity of a system where profit trumps public health. It's not just a book; it's a revolution in print, arming readers with the truth to fight against a narrative designed to control and deceive. How very proud I am to have been named with her as one of the so-called Disinformation Dozen, when in fact, all she shares is the truth to millions for decades.

–*Erin Elizabeth*
Writer, Activist and Founder of Health Nut News

Dr. Sherri Tenpenny is an incredible friend and true giant in the world of health freedom. The health freedom movement was the army that ended the COVID tyranny and much of that movement finds its roots in Dr. Tenpenny's meticulous work. I'm honored to call Dr. T a friend and to support her work on another incredible book.

Attorney Tom Renz
The Tom Renz Show & TomRenz.com

If we are to restore the promise of a healthy America, the MAHA movement needs to learn the causal connection to the chronic disease epidemic under which we currently suffer. Dr. Sherri Tenpenny knows that we did not get here by accident as she reveals, in her extensive and exhaustive research, precisely how it happened.

Zero Accountability in a Failed System is the comprehensive book we need right now to make the MAHA dream a reality. There are few physicians in my 25-plus years of broadcasting messages of health freedom that have exhibited the tenacity, integrity and spiritual energy to withstand the negative forces allied against anyone revealing the dark secrets that enslave us to a pharmaceutical-only construct. If we are to break free from the United States of DRUGMERICA and restore the promise that is a HEALTHY America, this book provides the roadmap to make it possible (and even likely!). Thank you Dr. Sherri Tenpenny, you are a true healing hero for our age!"

–Robert Scott Bell, D.A. Hom.
The Robert Scott Bell Show

Dr. Tenpenny spoke out about the real healthcare truths long before many woke up. I respect Dr. Tenpenny, and her book is one that will shine further light on how humanity can heal. Dr. Tenpenny believes as I do, that health does not come through a needle and freedom does not come from compliance. Thank you, Dr. Tenpenny, for standing up for the patient's right to make informed medical choices.

–Priscilla Romans
Founder & CEO Graith Care

Dr. Sherri Tenpenny's analysis exposes the origin and impact of the corruption entrenched in the medical establishment, pharmaceutical industry, and government. Her work helps us understand how fear of illness was used to deprive people of their civil rights.

With this knowledge, we can break the vicious circle of corrupt medicine, restore the ethical principles of medicine, and build virtuous cycles of continuous health improvement.

-Warner Mendenhall
Mendenhall Law Group

Dr. Sherri Tenpenny has been a heroic presence from the beginning of COVID, warning about the dangers of the jabs and then identifying the specific adverse effects that were so horrific that no one else wanted to face them. She deserves the gratitude of the nation for her courage and honesty as a physician and a scientist.

-Peter Breggin MD, Psychiatrist
Author of COVID-19 and the Global
Predators: We Are the Prey

We've been living in a broken, corrupt health system that ensures no one is healthy by accident, while making disease and poor health the norm. Dr. Tenpenny has been at the front lines courageously shining the light of truth on the dirty secrets of corruption while empowering individuals with the knowledge they need to choose a path of deliberate wellness for them and their families. The broken system of corruption is now on its deathbed and *Zero Accountability in a Failed System* will make sure it has a nail in its coffin while ushering in the new paradigm where being healthy is normal again! Thank you Dr. Tenpenny!

– JP Sears, Author and Comedian

"Dr. Tenpenny is pretty much the ideal family doctor you imagine before you found out about the toils and troubles of Big Pharma medicine. She's one of the only doctors who has consistently stood up against the medical institutions when obvious harm to innocent people was being done by them. She has principles, a healing touch and countenance, and cares from the deepest part of her heart. Her words will touch you and assist with nourishing your healthy lifestyle."

-David 'Avocado Wolfe'
Author, Medical Freedom Fighter, Adventurer,
Orator, Biodynamic Farmer, Meme Lord

For decades, the medical establishment turned a deaf ear to concerns about vaccine harms. Dr. Sherri Tenpenny, once a lone voice in the wilderness, has become a leading authority on medical corruption. In *"Zero Accountability in a Failed System,"* Dr. Tenpenny's 20+ years of research come to fruition in a sweeping exposé of corruption in the medical establishment, pharmaceutical industry, and government. This book empowers readers with actionable insights to navigate a system designed to suppress dissent. If you're ready to ditch the Kool-Aid and embrace the truth, this book is your essential guide to navigating a system that prioritizes profit over people.

-Reinette Senum
Political Activist

Disclaimer

DEDICATION

This book is dedicated to:

The millions worldwide who have died from
an experimental COVID-19 jab.

Those whose lives have been forever changed
by a COVID-19 countermeasure.

Those who lost loved ones to COVID-19
due to mismanaged medical care.

The nearly 2 million individuals who have
filed injury compensation claims.

Your stories and struggles will not be forgotten.

Your voices matter.

OTHER BOOKS

by Dr. Sherri Tenpenny

FOWL! Bird Flu: It's Not What You Think

Saying No To Vaccines: A Resource Guide For All Ages

Challenging the Vaccination Dogma

The MMR Vaccine: The Loss of Future Generations
Over An Unrealistic Fear of the Measles

40 Mechanisms of Injury

Medical Essentials for Emergencies

The Truth About Colonoscopies

Vaccine Epidemic (Chapter Contributor)

Contents

FOREWORD

by Dr. Suzanne Humphries

Before writing Dissolving Illusions, I believed the story about interspecies viral transmission. During childhood, we all heard about the dreadful 1918 Spanish flu, which was supposedly a type of bird flu. Anyone over the age of 50 would have memories of the hysteria evoked by the 1976 swine flu scare and the consequences of that vaccine.

In medical school, our class was informed that HIV/AIDS came from monkeys in Africa, and the disease had mysteriously jumped into a gay male flight attendant, only to later spread to infants and heterosexuals, becoming a worldwide "pandemic" managed with lifelong pharmaceutical drugs, much like other diseases such as diabetes and hypothyroidism. In the second year of residency, in the middle of the AIDS pandemic in the Bronx, New York, lots of doctors made careers by becoming HIV/AIDS specialists. Then came the day when it dawned on me that if there ever were a cure for AIDS, lots of doctors would have to find new niches. Would they feel let down if there was actually a cure?

During my medical internship, I discovered a book titled *Inventing the AIDS Virus* by noted geneticist and cell biologist Dr.[1] Duesberg. The information was fascinating. When I shared my thoughts on the subject, my colleagues told me to shut up and stop talking about what they referred to as foolish conspiracy theories – as if it were simply a theory that lifestyle choices, accompanying comorbidities, and risky sexual behaviors could lead to infections or diseases.

Being young and early in my career, I shut up, forgot about it, and soldiered on. From 1993 to 2011, while I ascended the golden stairway in the ivory medical tower, I continued to have even more questions regarding the implementation of today's medical tools, which are supposed to be the best the world has ever seen.

There were questions like, "How come science is so advanced, yet we can't cure autoimmune thyroiditis, arthritis, and glomerulonephritis?" and "Why are children so sick?" and "How could it be that the world's best 20th-century medicine had such a limited repertoire?" and "Why are doctors around me seemingly quite happy just to keep giving drugs that began with "anti" and never striving for cures?" and "Why are doctors and their children sick so often and taking so many drugs?"

In 2008, it wasn't a bird flu vaccine that cracked the windshield of my cognitive dissonance. It was the swine flu vaccine against the H1N1 flu that we were told came from pigs. Patient after patient told me they were fine until they had "that vaccine." As a nephrologist, I was duty-bound to consider all possible exposures that could have influenced the health of the souls sitting in front of me. I had no idea that considering a vaccine as a potential culprit in renal failure was off-limits. Hospital administration personnel insisted that what I observed in my medical office and in my hospitalized patients wasn't happening. They also demanded that I just drop it.

"Vaccines are safe and effective."
"Vaccine injury is one in a million."
"Correlation doesn't equal causation."
"Anti-vaxxers are ruining herd immunity."
"Standing orders for flu vaccination upon hospital admission are to become a universal measure."

Other rote mantras, spewed from their desperately bankrupt understanding of vaccination and immunity, included lines like, "Vaccines saved us from smallpox," along with the declaration of post-vaccine kidney failure: "They just got the flu because the vaccine didn't have time to work. Flu can cause kidney failure." Nice try . . . flu hardly ever caused the severity of kidney failure I was suddenly witnessing.

In 2008, not many licensed medical doctors publicly discussed the downsides to vaccination, but after doing some internet searches, the name Dr. Sherri Tenpenny kept popping up. I began reading everything she had written.

I recall one of the podcasts where she was interviewed. The interviewer asked her something I was just beginning to ponder, "So, are any vaccines worth giving?" She immediately responded with a very confident "no, not a one." I knew in every cell of my body that she was right.

Years later, after doing my due diligence, I now stand shoulder-to-shoulder with her as an anti-vaxxer. The only exception I make for human vaccines is autologous tumor vaccines for advanced cancer situations.

After the podcast finished, I emailed Dr. Tenpenny, not expecting a response. To my pleasant surprise, a thoughtful reply landed in my inbox within a day. It didn't take long to realize that Dr. T is one of the brightest, hardest-working people among us today. Additionally, she possesses a level of endurance that most of us only dream of having. She juggled numerous projects, including a busy holistic medical practice and a Facebook page that was just getting started, which later grew to a massive social media following. Amazingly, she responded almost daily to every issue on that page. Dr. T was fighting against ruthless harassers while also addressing the concerns of parents and individuals just awakening to the corruption. Despite everything happening in her world, including the mysterious burning of her medical office to ashes, she took the time to respond to a letter from a doctor—me—who didn't know where to turn after the backlash from the hospital's vaccine policy had erupted in my face. Her reply during such a busy and chaotic time marked the beginning of a lasting 16-year friendship, which started during the Gates Foundation's promise to make 2010-2020 "The Decade of Vaccines."

Regarding my vaccine-injured kidney patients, most doctors understand how frequently drugs are responsible for acute kidney failure situations. One of the first lessons we learn as nephrologists is to review the patient's medication list because, most of the time, the source of acute kidney failure can be found there. Fortunately, kidneys can often recover if the harmful agent is removed in time. Why would a vaccine issue be any different? I naively believed that by utilizing the medical and scientific literature on this matter, I could swiftly change the discussion about the problems I observed in-house. I never anticipated the arrogant, forceful ignorance and cowardice I encountered from my colleagues, CDC gatekeepers, and hospital officials.

Dr. Tenpenny assisted me in refining a written position paper to the CEO and governing body of Eastern Maine Medical Center. It was met with prideful, indignant egos and willfully deaf ears. Suddenly, instead of being an honored nephrologist, they saw me as a quack and a villain for suggesting that vaccine injections caused issues for my patients, even though no other explanation made sense.

It wasn't until I'd known Sherri for about a year that I learned she had written a book called *"Fowl! Bird Flu: It's Not What You Think."* I eagerly purchased a copy and devoured it, with a growing realization about how many wrong ideas had been fed to physicians about the bird flu. I realized how easy it was to ignorantly absorb the daily hospital dogma regarding the flu's origins, dangers, and pathophysiology, and then confidently parrot out the same mainstream drivel to patients.

Like most doctors, I was also naïve to the political systems that shaped many policies that affected me as a child and even as a doctor. For example, in 2003, the smallpox vaccine was "offered" to me to help treat other people who were expected to develop general complications or infectious smallpox...from the vaccine!

Dr. Tenpenny's book, *Fowl,* written in 2005, was a very needed piece of the puzzle, and at the time, one of the best books I'd ever read. The pages turned like a mystery being revealed, artfully and colorfully, until the very last word. That time in my career was an exciting period of eye-opening discovery. I suggested to her that the book was too good to sit on a back shelf, virtually unrecognized. She said that at some point, she would edit and update it, filling in some of the gaps. Being a woman of her word, she has just done what she promised, and has she ever delivered!

I took my first private nephrology job in 2001, the year of the Twin Towers debacle, which ushered in the preconceived Patriot Act. Before that, I could drive 10 minutes to the airport in Bangor, Maine, and board my flight immediately. Everything changed after the Patriot Act was passed. Airports continue to be a nightmare to navigate, and our taxes are paid to the abusive TSA agents who push us around. We can now see that the long-term goal was to restrict human movement, and place conditions on who could move. And who could earn COVID-19 vaccine passes to gain a few lockdown privileges. . .over an infection that has 1.4% mortality. Dr. Tenpenny elaborates on the Patriot Act, supposedly drafted to protect us from terrorist planes with the capacity to fly straight into steel-framed buildings.

By 2008, our private medical office was being pushed to convert our handwritten charts to electronic health records (EHRs). I hated reading the long, redundant, and confusing reports from other providers who had already adopted the EHRs, and I fought not to convert our office to their use. But by the time I left the practice in 2011, EHRs had become a way of life, supposedly to prevent medical errors and to make sharing information with other providers easier. Dr. Tenpenny includes meticulous detail on just how nefarious the EHR conversion was and why my instincts were correct. It was a necessary step taken to control doctors and the public.

In her new book, *Zero Accountability in a Failed System,* she covers the basics of vaccine components and manufacture, and clearly defines the politically driven medico-legal landscape that continues to allow and encourage pharmaceutical skullduggery. She also elaborates in great detail on how the PREP Act threw the doors wide open to enable the COVID-19 fiasco. The political deals, the dangerous drugs, and the "treatment" methods were forced onto the public with zero liability.

Though I was awake to much of the COVID fiasco, I still learned a lot from her new book, such as the impotent legislation that is supposed to protect those whose lives were wrecked by "taking one for the team." Did you know that the statute of limitations has run out for most of the COVID-19 vaccine-injured to file a claim? To add insult to misery, most people applied to the wrong government department to even be considered for injury compensation. I won't spoil the shock value of Dr. T's revelations beyond that. People fall for vaccine trickery because they don't know history, and they don't want to learn about legislation quietly inserted into unrelated bills late at night. They fear disease due to a lack of knowledge about how to support or enhance the immune system, already designed to combat environmental allergens, toxins, and circulating infections.

They watch Big Pharma ads on television, and believe that toxic drugs and vaccines are the keys to alleviating their fears and keeping them alive. They are unaware of the many lies surrounding the true origins of feared diseases. They also do not know how doctors, both in the past and present, treat illnesses with untested and dangerous interventions, making morbidity and mortality appear far worse, which further fuels mass fear.

In both books, Dr. Tenpenny chronicles the case of an Asian boy whose death in 1997 lit the spark of publicity over bird flu. Once that hype hit the news, there was no turning back, even though none of the boys' contacts, who also tested positive, even developed symptoms. Later, it was recognized that he probably died because doctors treated his viral illness with high doses of aspirin. Despite strong efforts, scientists found no bird flu in his blood or body until three months after his death.

Hunting down viruses is no easy task. Everyone should be reminded how difficult it was to identify the cancer-causing SV40 (Simian

Virus 40, a monkey virus) in laboratory samples because of potential contamination from laboratory sources or the humans working in the lab. Contaminants in the cultures made it almost impossible for SV40 expert Dr. Michele Carbone and his colleagues, the most skilled and advanced scientists working with SV40, to identify the virus with certainty, even using ultra-sensitive testing. Eventually, using painstaking techniques to prevent contamination, they found SV40 numerous times but only in tumor samples, not in the surrounding tissue. The Institute of Medicine, the National Cancer Institute, and the CDC all published letters negating Carbone and other scientists' research that reported SV40 in human tumors. They cited the work of inexperienced Dr. Keerti Shah, who did not isolate SV40 in tissue samples. Veteran scientists found Shah's techniques to be highly flawed. The whole story can be read in the amazing book, *The Virus and The Vaccine,* by Debbie Bookchin and Jim Schumacher.[2]

My point is that if so much effort was needed to demonstrate the presence of SV40 in human tumors and to establish that it was NOT a contaminant, why did the scientific community accept that H5N1 was not found in any tracheal aspirates from the boy until *three months* after his death? Was that a contaminant or merely an artifact enhanced by the news narratives?

Deadly treatments, like that of the boy from Hong Kong who died after experiencing a flu-like illness and receiving aspirin therapy, are not new. In the 1800s and early 1900s, during periods of poverty, poor living conditions, food shortages, and the coincident occurrence of rickets, and economic depression all contributed to high death rates from measles. But even after many environmental conditions had been addressed, doctors persisted with bizarre treatments for measles, such as "serum therapy." This method involved taking several milliliters of blood from a parent who had measles and injecting it into the child's buttock muscles. The results were disastrous. Thankfully, by the 1960s, measles had become a relatively benign infection in the developed world, with a decline in the death rate of over 99%.

Polio is the poster child for vaccine belief. Many people are unaware that treatments for paralysis were just as, if not more, brutal than measles serum therapy. Surgeons lanced tendons and confined children in casts for up to two years. The debilitating effects imposed by physicians set the stage for the March of Dimes Campaign, which funded one of the most corrupt national vaccine trials in history. The sensational publicity surrounding the Francis Trial led to the licensing of a dangerous polio vaccine before doctors had the opportunity to review any research results. In just eight hours, and with almost no information, a licensing board was pressured into approving the Salk polio vaccine. The public was so gullible and frightened that very little coercion was necessary to compel parents to line up their children for multiple doses of the new (and experimental) polio vaccine. Later, due to numerous adverse vaccine reactions, including paralysis and death, manufacturers were successfully sued. The result? They teetered on the brink of bankruptcy from the payouts.

Francis didn't release his full trial data and evaluation until 1957, two years after the vaccine had been approved and administered to millions. Had doctors seen the Francis Trial results, with its poor study design and misleading data interpretation, none would have given the jab to a single child. When Dr. Fred Klenner examined a portion of the publicized data from the flawed trial, he wrote a scathing article published in the Tristate Medical Journal in June 1955. By 1984, doctors were instructed not to discuss any doubts as to the safety of the polio vaccines with their patients or colleagues:

> "...any possible doubts, whether or not well founded, about the safety of the vaccine cannot be allowed to exist in view of the need to assure that the vaccine will continue to be used to the maximum extent consistent with the nation's public health objectives."[3]

In the period between the adverse events linked to polio vaccines and the rushed-to-market swine flu shots in 1976, manufacturers were understandably concerned for their own welfare.

Instead of improving the safety of vaccines, the 1986 National Child Vaccine Injury Act was signed into law, giving blanket protection to manufacturers. From there, the situation went from bad to horrid. Dr. Tenpenny meticulously lists and describes every step taken to bring us to today. That path was paved with separate vaccine, quarantine, and pandemic legislation, made possible by corrupt Congressmen, the WHO, and significant conflicts of interest.

I have continuously stated that the vaccine situation is the same today as it was 200 years ago. Dissenting voices from the past have been hidden, humiliated, retracted, de-licensed, and buried beneath a tombstone that reads, "Don't go where these quacks have gone."

The world continues to be gripped by fear over a virus that is said to have evolved from a bat and an anteater, both of which live in separate parts of the globe, yet somehow must have shared intimate space. Along the way, the virus acquired Rabies G8 protein, HIV GP120 sequences, a staph toxin (which has been used as a bioweapon in warfare), krait and cobra toxin codes, and a furin cleavage site (considered a detonator by geneticists). It appears that it was perfectly designed to wipe out humanity. This troubling concoction is now part of the childhood vaccine schedule, complete with instructions to jab it into the legs of a baby three times before their sixth month of life. Dr. Tenpenny meticulously reveals, through research and documents, exactly how this debacle occurred.

If you were deceived by the bird flu hoax in 2004, if you fell for the swine flu in 2009, and if you were tricked into compliance by COVID-19 fear tactics in 2020, you want to avoid being misled any further regarding alleged novel pathogen threats and their associated vaccines. Dr. Tenpenny's book will clarify many misleading facts, revealing patterns that have been repeated over and over. She explores the psychology behind pandemic initiation, propagation, and the consistently profitable attempts at contagion termination. She presented the facts in meticulous detail, and this book will satisfy readers of all levels.

The next time Fauci, Hotez or any other politician's mouthpiece tells you that another warp speed vaccine for bird flu or monkeypox or dengue fever or sloth fever or "disease X" is "safe and effective with no side effects," don't listen. These jabs will not stop you from getting sick, and they will certainly not stop the transmission of the disease. Next time, what will your response be?

The details in Dr. Tenpenny's new book will show you why caution and due diligence are crucial skills you MUST possess. You will see how the term "health" has been hijacked and completely transformed away from anything a rational person would deem as "wellness." Healthy people initiatives are a misnomer, instead creating dangerous environments that the fearful and uninformed masses eagerly follow.

This book will help you discuss political issues with ease. It will encourage you to make a difference that could change the course of events. Dr. T has done all the work for you. Knowledge is power, especially in these times of propaganda and lies. If you want to counterbalance the corporate-fueled insistence on dangerous policies and vaccines, read the book and share what you learn.

Dr. Suzanne Humphries, 2024
Internist, Nephrologist
Co-Author of *Dissolving Illusions* and the *Dissolving Illusions* companion book.

ACKNOWLEDGEMENTS

They say it takes a village to raise a child, and it takes an entire city to launch a book. When I first agreed – at everyone's urging – to take on this book project, I knew how much effort it would require; I've been through it several times before. But this book turned out to be bigger and more important than I had originally conceived.

A heartfelt thank you to my devoted core team – Michelle, Dianne, and Patricia – who managed all the expansive day-to-day operations while I focused on writing. You led the way while the rest of the team – Amanda, Cookie, and Heather – helped keep the wheels turning smoothly.

A special shout-out to Jackie: Thank you for tirelessly reading and re-reading every chapter, handling the extensive references, creating the index, and formatting the book. This book is in print because of your dedication and teamwork. "Thank you" seems inadequate for what you have helped to launch.

Once again, a huge thank you to LFA for your meticulous, eagle-eyed editing. Your work made this book stronger and clearer.

Special thanks to Melissa and the entire TIMC team, who have expertly and effortlessly kept Tenpenny Integrative Medical Center running smoothly in my absence.

Thank you to Allison and SelfPublishing.com for your invaluable help in naming this book – months of trial and error paid off, given its breadth and scope. Your willingness to take on the challenge made all the difference.

And lastly, a special thank you to Jeremy for your training and guidance with the marketing. Your expertise helped put this book into the hands of many.

"Fight for your opinions, but do not believe that they contain the whole truth, or the only truth."

Charles A. Dana, US newspaper editor (1819-1897)

PROLOGUE

On May 2, 2024, while waiting backstage at Del Bigtree's *The HighWire* show for my interview, investigative reporter Jefferey Jaxen delivered a segment just before I went live, discussing the latest H5N1 avian flu scare.

Jaxen's report focused on the detection of high concentrations of the H5N1 bird flu virus in raw, unpasteurized milk from infected mammals, a finding recently highlighted by the World Health Organization (WHO) in a press release dated April 26, 2024. As I listened to Jaxen, I couldn't help but think, "The WHO is clearly trying to stir up another panic." This kind of fear-mongering isn't new – it's a familiar pattern we saw during the COVID-19 panic and many times before that. In fact, it's the same type of hysteria I wrote about nearly two decades ago when I published *FOWL: Bird Flu Is Not What You Think.*

In the early 2000s, bird flu captured both national and international attention. Even back then, and especially now, it was hard to understand why such an uproar was being created over so few reported cases. When the bird flu scare began in 2003, I questioned: What was the motive, and who was behind this? I find myself asking the same questions today:

Why would governments and global authorities abandon a rational, commonsense approach to a situation involving a handful of infections in chickens and cows and only a few "suspected" deaths in humans?

I've long been skeptical of government interventions, particularly those driven by the vaccine industry. After decades of research and tens of thousands of hours investigating the problems associated with vaccines, my stance remains unchanged. Having lived through the COVID debacle over the last few years, my disdain and suspicion toward global governments and Big Pharma have only deepened. It has become more evident than ever that these entities are consumed with a lust for power, aiming for ownership and control over every living thing, especially humans and their DNA.

When I wrote *FOWL* in 2004, I questioned the motivation of government agencies and the multinational conglomerates. I put together a list of questions and began to search for plausible answers to this pandemic push. The questions are as relevant for the bird flu threats today as they were then:

1. Why were farm chickens becoming sick? Since birds have long been known to be carriers of hundreds of influenza virus strains, what made them more susceptible to the effects of the H5N1 virus?
2. Who wanted to cull millions of chickens and *why*, when the vast majority of birds were not tested? Or if tested, were *not positive* for the H5N1 virus and were not ill? Whose interests did it serve to eliminate independent farmers and then impact the global food supply?
3. Why were the human cases clustered in Southeast Asia during the 2003-4 outbreak?
4. The vaccine manufacturers always win, but the stakes surrounding the first bird flu outbreak were higher than usual.

What was behind the nearly blank check handed to vaccine manufacturers, *then* and *now*?

5. What are the similarities between the bird flu outbreak in 2004 and what seemed to be unfolding in 2024?

After nearly 20 years, it is sobering how much further they've pushed their agenda. Now that we've gone through the COVID-19 fiasco, a whole new light has been shed on the globalist shenanigans.

FOWL stirred up considerable controversy, and similarly, this book will spark discussion and raise concerns. While many of you may be familiar with parts of this story, you'll be shocked by the sheer scale of the plan that has been put in place that began two decades ago. For many, the COVID-19 crisis was a major "wake-up" call. Unpacking how the legal framework was built will undoubtedly provide even more clarity and reveal the deeper layers of this orchestrated effort. This exploration will leave you questioning not only what happened, but what could happen next.

The current H5N1 scare is merely the latest installment in a long line of recycled pandemic narratives, all designed to advance control, manipulation, and, most critically, profit. While the media fuels the drama and fear-driven policies, the real beneficiaries aren't just Big Pharma, but the powerful global organizations – the WHO, the UN, and the WEF – that aim to establish a framework for total global governance. These entities thrive on fear, pushing through legislation that solidifies their power while diverting vast sums of money into the healthcare and vaccine industries. Each new "threat" is just another chapter in this rehearsed cycle of global control.

My book, *FOWL*, delved into the often-overlooked connection between influenza A viruses found in wild and domestic birds – particularly migratory waterfowl, geese, ducks, chickens, and turkeys – and how environmental factors, particularly dioxins, played a significant role in the impact of these viruses. But over the last 20 years what is more important is how the bird flu scare of 2003 to 2005 shaped the legislative landscape, setting the stage for future pandemic responses. The tactics, policies, and legislative actions taken during that time became a template that was not only used for COVID-19 but will no doubt be used in future health crises, all while promoting a global agenda of centralized control and profit-driven motives.

"Be fast, have no regrets...if you need to be right before you move, you will never win."

~Mike Ryan, WHO epidemiologist in March, 2020

CHAPTER 1
Same Playbook, Different Era

Here's how they created a pandemic fear-frenzy in 2003-4. You will see the similarities with 2024.

- The narrative started with an obscure case of H5N1 on a small rural farm in an Asian country. It's an isolated case, but it circulates in the global media.
- Next, H5N1 was found in backyard poultry, but it soon spread to commercial poultry.
- Next, the pathogen was found in dead migratory birds who were then blamed for spreading the virus beyond the original outbreak borders.[9]

Next came a flurry of scientific papers burst on the scene, declaring that more dead wild birds were found. The birds were tested and an aggressive influenza type A viral subtype was found. The authors of the early identification papers used scary wording like "viral endemic disease" and "highly pathogenic avian influenza (HPAI)," as well as "major worldwide problem," "major public health risk," "unpredictable mutations," and "significant economic losses." They reported that "high mortalities will follow" without specifying whether the anticipated mortality was going to be high in birds or high in humans.

At some point during the growing rhetoric leading to the 2003 pandemic, the narrative began to use the ominous buzz phrase "will it jump to humans?" After all, a bridge between infected birds and infected humans had to be fashioned. Researchers began describing detailed interactions between wild migratory ducks and domestic poultry.

FAST FORWARD

The first H5N1 infection in humans was reported in July 2022 in Ecuador. The following year, in May 2023, a single H5N1 bird flu case was identified in Chile in a man who presented with severe influenza-like symptoms.[10] In the US, the stories started with two dead mountain lions found dead in northern California. For some reason, H5N1 was suspected in both cases, and authorities tested for co-infections even before H5N1 was identified.

> "The main pathological finding for these two mountain lions was encephalitis, which is inflammation of the brain. Additionally, there were lesions in the lungs causing pulmonary edema. The lesions in the brain and lungs were associated with the virus, but additional testing is being performed to rule out the possibility of co-infection," said Dr. Jaime Rudd, a specialist who investigates the association between pesticide and disease in CDFW's." Wildlife Health Lab.[11]

The government's article in *Wildlife California* went on to say that H5N1 infections in wild carnivores across the US and Canada were rare and unusual. In 2023, the total number of infected animals found was only about 54. Was this a large enough number to spike a concern or was this just sensationalizing? Identifying the H5N1 virus in only 54 animals out of the millions of wild mammalian species in the US equates to looking for a problem, not identifying one. To further emphasize the point, a study from 2022 documented that H5N1 has been found in domestic poultry or wild birds in 61 countries since it was first isolated from a domestic goose in China in 2006.[12]

Since H5N1 was first identified in 1996, highly pathogenic avian influenza (HPAI) has mostly been limited to wild birds, especially ducks. But that changed on March 25, 2024, when US health officials announced the first-ever detection of HPAI in dairy cows. By May 22, 2024, H5N1 had spread to 52 dairy herds across nine states: Colorado, Idaho, Kansas, Michigan, New Mexico, North Carolina, Ohio, South Dakota, and Texas. Symptoms in cows were vague, including decreased milk production, loss of appetite, and a thicker milk consistency, with some cows showing clear nasal discharge. Illness typically lasted two to four weeks, but it was unclear how long infected cows shed the virus.

This boils down to something we are familiar with: The Hegelian dialectic: Problem. Reaction. Solution.

This is how the hype began two decades ago. It appears they are using the same playbook again.

"Those who cannot remember the past are condemned to repeat it."

~George Santayana, The Life of Reason, 1905

CHAPTER 2

Identifying a Problem or Creating One?

The 2003 bird flu scare marked a significant turning point in global health policy and the development of surveillance systems that would expand the scope of public health measures. As the fear of a pandemic grew, governments and organizations such as the World Health Organization (WHO) began massive stockpiling of drugs and vaccines, setting the stage for the mandatory vaccination policies that would later become a fixture in global health strategy. It also laid the groundwork for what are now known as "covered countermeasures," which involve the use of medical products – like vaccines and antiviral drugs – that can be deployed during public health emergencies, with legal protections for manufacturers and distributors.

The bird flu hysteria began with a seemingly innocent incident in 1997 at a Hong Kong preschool, where a small petting zoo housed chickens and ducks. After several days, a three-year-old boy from the class developed severe respiratory symptoms, progressing rapidly to pneumonia and organ failure. Despite medical intervention, the child passed away within six days. This incident marked the first case of human infection with the H5N1 strain of avian influenza, a virus that would later become the focal point of the bird flu panic. Ironically, the child had been treated with aspirin, which some physicians speculated could have exacerbated the severity of the illness. This incident, however tragic, served as a catalyst for the global health system's push to prepare for a pandemic, and the WHO began laying out plans for future global vaccination strategies and emergency measures.

Doctors requested an autopsy to determine why the boy had died, but the results were perplexing. Pathologists found no underlying immunodeficiency or cardiopulmonary disease that would have contributed to the boy's death. Even more confusing was that a virus isolated from a tracheal aspirate could not be identified.

Highlight

Reye's syndrome is a rare disorder that can affect all body organs, but most often it is associated with brain swelling (encephalopathy) and liver failure. It is primarily a children's disease, although it can occur at any age. The syndrome often begins during the recovery stage of a viral illness during which aspirin was given. The CDC's surveillance data between 1980 and 1997 found that cases of Reye's syndrome were preceded by influenza infection 73%, varicella infection 21%, and gastroenteritis infections 14% of the time. This data led to a recommendation in 1980 to not give children aspirin for a fever. The number of reported cases of Reye's syndrome fell dramatically following the implementation of this widespread warning.[12]

It wasn't until three months later (in August) that a virus was confirmed by a reference laboratory in the Netherlands and by the CDC in the United States (US) to be an avian influenza A virus, H5N1, subsequently named A/Hong Kong/156/97.[13] In a report published later, researchers held that this particular bird flu virus had not previously caused infection in humans.

In the days following the identification, there was no shortage of tension as officials scrambled to determine whether the virus had been contracted by others who had been exposed to the ill child. Teams from the WHO and the CDC descended on Hong Kong to determine how the boy had been exposed to the virus and to assess the subsequent potential public health impact. According to investigators, one of the chickens in the petting zoo had died several days before the child's symptoms had appeared. It was postulated that the exposure to the ill bird or its feces provided a means for the virus to "jump species" and infect the boy. Sweeping investigations of the birds in the surrounding area revealed that three outbreaks of H5N1 had occurred in poultry farms in the Hong Kong New Territory earlier in 1997. Approximately 2,000 human samples were collected from those who had been in contact with the boy, the school's petting zoo, or the birds from the rural areas.

Significantly, none of the dead child's four closest relatives tested positive for antibodies that would indicate the presence of the H5N1 virus. However, a few others who had been in contact with the child had positive tests. Nearly two percent of health care workers who cared for him, one percent of his classmates, and two percent of the family's neighbors showed evidence of having contact with the "new virus." Despite the presence of H5N1 antibodies in their blood, all of these people were symptom-free.[14]

Does this sound familiar?

A second case of H5N1 infection was confirmed in Hong Kong on November 26, 1997, and more cases appeared throughout December. The samples taken from birds during this outbreak were identical matches to the virus collected from the deceased child. There were a total of 18 confirmed cases affecting eight males and ten females, ranging in age from one to 60.

The news of the direct bird-to-human transmission sent a chill throughout the medical and scientific community: This was reported to be the first documented isolation of H5N1 in humans and was all public health officials around the globe needed to hear, even though there was no evidence of human-to-human transmission and no further human infections occurred. They believed the next pandemic had arrived. Today, instead of reflecting worry at the presence of an H5N1 infection, the WHO, CDC, and vaccine manufacturers would be rubbing their hands together and jumping up and down with glee.

CONTINUED OUTBREAKS

A few sporadic outbreaks of highly pathogenic avian influenza occurred throughout the world between 1997 and late 2002. However, beginning late in 2003 and throughout early 2004, outbreaks of H5N1 were reported among poultry concentrated in a few countries in Southeast Asia: Loas, Cambodia, Indonesia, but primarily in Thailand, and Vietnam. Approximately 45 people tested positive for the H5N1 virus and a handful had died. The finger pointing began as to the cause of the problem and family farmers throughout the region were in the crosshairs. Although 20 years apart, it's amazing how similar these two stories are. In the first go-around, it started with a boy in a petting zoo. Today's hype centers around a single suspected case in a Texas farmer.

Today, as in 2003, it is difficult to redirect people away from what they have been told and what they have come to believe is true about the "coming bird flu." We were told then, literally on a daily basis, that the next global pandemic was about to arrive and that it would be "the end of Western civilization as we know it," wreaking economic havoc on the world, leaving "no person untouched." Both television and print media chronicled daily reports to keep us worried and in a state of impending doom. Seventeen years later, we went through a similar but heightened experience at the beginning of COVID-19.

But what if the proclamations about bird flu, monkeypox, and others are false? What if nearly everything you've been hearing about the "coming pandemic" is incorrect? What if you were presented with an overwhelming amount of information that shows what the media is hyping about the "next pandemic" is not true? After the experience of COVID-19, would you question what you have been hearing on the airwaves? As I have said many times: "Fool me once, shame on you. Fool me twice? It isn't going to happen."

Even though the COVID-19 pandemic is officially over, to this very day, the masses are encouraged to rush out and get tested to see if they have "the COVID" whenever they have a cough, a fever, and some malaise. We were trained to anticipate getting COVID-19 boosters in the same way we have been long-conditioned to get an annual flu shot, even though the death and injury rates from the COVID-19 jabs continue to grow all around us.

When the nationwide "get your flu shot" campaigns begin each fall, few are aware that this flurry of attention is not due to spontaneous reporting of a few cases of the flu, but due to a coordinated plan, highly funded by the vaccine manufacturers, in conjunction with the CDC and local health departments, using the media as a mouthpiece. The core message is: *"Influenza vaccination is the primary method for preventing influenza and its severe complications. Flu shots save lives."* The same is now being said about getting annual COVID-19 injections.

DO FLU SHOTS SAVE LIVES?

At the CDC, the Health Communication Science Office (HCSO) is under the umbrella of the National Center for Immunization and Respiratory Diseases (NCIRD). This agency is responsible for developing influenza vaccination-related communications, messages, and materials. Those efforts are designed to educate healthcare providers to remind their patients how "serious the flu can be." The materials are written to persuade people, especially the elderly and the immunocompromised, to get their annual flu shot. The information also changes every year, ranging from reports of low efficacy due to "weak strain match" to different forms of the vaccine: nasal spray, intradermal, high-dose, and quadrivalent formulas.

The CDC devotes an enormous amount of time, energy, and money towards getting everyone, from babies six months of age to end of life seniors, vaccinated with the influenza vaccine. Their approach is straight from Marketing Central – from cute Facebook graphics, such as the Wild to Mild campaign, to cartoonish infographics with animated images, to pre-recorded public service announcements.[15] The same messaging tactics are being used to push healthcare providers, veterinarians, and public health officials to get and give vaccines for bird flu, monkeypox, dengue fever, and COVID-19 boosters. The marketing ploy is used to manipulate the psyche of the general public into believing flu shots are good for them and as safe as eating an apple. It's amazing how they amassed, organized, then published such a large amount of information regarding bird flu in a matter of a few months. Take a good look at the bird flu pages on the CDC.gov/bird-flu website. You'll be amazed.[16]

How many times have these messages been used to hammer the "necessity" of the flu vaccine into our collective consciousness? In 2004, Glenn Nowak, PhD, the Associate Director for Communications at the CDC, presented a 7-step strategy at the National Immunization Program to manipulate public perception about the flu shot. The presentation revealed just how extensively the media is used to influence consumers into believing the flu vaccine is crucial. During the week of September 21 to 28, 2004, a staggering 1,056 messages, roughly one every fifteen minutes, were broadcast, urging viewers and listeners to get their flu shot. The most intense promotion typically starts in early October and continues through mid-February, with an average of 200 stories per week for 20 weeks. That's at least 4,000 messages per season, constantly reinforcing the narrative.

In 2004, the cost of a 30-second prime time advertisement on a major national television network varied significantly, with some shows commanding much higher prices than others. The average price was reported to be around $150,000. But the most expensive 30-second ad slots were during the popular reality show "American Idol" on FOX, which cost $658,333. The scripted drama "ER" on NBC also had high-priced 30-second ads at $479,250. Primetime TV advertising in 2023 was even more expensive. A local commercial cost a few thousand dollars, and the cost range extended to millions of dollars for national exposure during a primetime program, such as during the Superbowl. While these costs are almost pocket change for Big Pharma, our tax dollars are used by the CDC to buy these ads, with the costs most likely buried into the CDC's "influenza planning and response" budget, a line item set at $251M for FY2023.[17]

Network stories on the evening news regarding influenza outbreaks and where to get your "free flu shot" equate to millions of dollars of free advertising for Big Pharma. Convenient locations where flu shots can be obtained – such as churches, pharmacies, urgent care clinics, retail chains such as Walgreens and DrugMart, grocery stores, and health departments – are promoted on the local evening news and during radio broadcasts. This is a free publicity bonanza for flu vaccine manufacturers, among the wealthiest companies on earth.

What types of messages? Here is a partial list from Nowak's presentation in 2004, including statistics regarding the number of times the message went out on the airwaves.[18]

Message	Number of messages per week
Doctors recommend/urge flu shot	(285)
The flu kills 36,000 per year	(221)
This could be a bad/serious flu year	(174)
Flu vaccine is the best defense against the flu	(149)
Oct./Nov./Dec. is the best time to get the vaccine	(117)
Now is a good time to get the flu vaccine	(106)

The fear-mongering tactics were first trialed during the bird flu hype of 2003 and were exponentially compounded during the COVID-19 fiasco. Governments and pharmaceutical companies began practicing their pitch in 2003, learning just how well fear can be used to sell their agenda. Over time, they refined and ramped up the fear-based messages, using them as a powerful weapon. What people often fail to realize is that every move by governments and drug companies is a market test. They push an agenda hard until they receive enough pushback. Then, they step back to analyze the data: What worked? What didn't? What should be pushed harder next time? What should be dropped? The same tactics that were used to market flu shots each fall were applied during COVID-19. And then as suddenly and as intensely as the push for the shots starts, the media hawking subsides, fading away as quickly as snow melting in the spring.

Given the level of indoctrination, it's no surprise that the average person viewed the COVID-19 jab in the same way they've been taught to view the flu vaccine – as the most important, even the only way, to avoid getting sick. The media's constant messaging, combined with years of fear-driven promotion, has ingrained the idea that vaccines are the sole defense against illness. With these tactics already tested and refined, there's little doubt that the media will use similar strategies to promote mass vaccination for future pandemics or even for a vaccine against "Disease X" once it becomes available. The challenge in convincing people to reconsider their stance on vaccines and to recognize that what they are injecting into their bodies can not only be ineffective but also harmful, is immense. The constant barrage of information has created an almost unshakable belief in the safety and necessity of vaccines, making it difficult for individuals to critically evaluate the true risks involved.

THE BELIEF IN VACCINES

Research into the way people process media reports sheds light on the reasons it is difficult for people to change their "beliefs," even in light of new, compelling information. A study, from 2003 by psychologist Professor Stephan Lewandowsky from the University of Western Australia, is as important today and as applicable as it was when it was written twenty years ago.

Lewandowsky investigated the effects of retractions and disconfirmations on people's memories of and beliefs about events relating to the war in Iraq. More than 800 people from three countries – Germany, Australia, and the US – were shown a list of events reported in the media. Some of the events were completely true, some were reported as true and then retracted, and some were complete fabrications. Each study participant indicated whether or not he or she had heard of the event and rated the likelihood of it being true. Then, for each report the individuals had recalled hearing, they were asked to note whether it had subsequently been retracted and if the recall changed their feeling about the original report.

The results of the study were both fascinating and telling. The more clearly the Germans and the Australians recalled that an event had been retracted, the less they believed that the original claim had been true. However, if Americans recalled hearing the report, *even once*, they tended to believe it was true *even if it had been retracted or was a lie.*[19]

An interview reported in *The Wall Street Journal* with Dr. Lewandowsky explained that people build "mental models" of what they believe is true. He went on to say, "By the time they receive a retraction, the original misinformation has already become integrated into their mental model, or world view, and disregarding it would leave their world (as they know it) in shambles." In other words, Americans will continue to believe something is the truth even after they have been shown the information is false.[20]

The study also supports the formation of what is referred to as "false memories." False memories are constructed by combining actual memories, or information, with new content that is *suggested* by others. Over time, the individual may forget the source of the original information, but with constant repetition, he or she will come to believe the added suggestions are completely true. The more comfortable a person becomes with a particular version of the truth – for example, that vaccines are safe, effective, and cause little harm – the less likely he or she is to question the premise. It appears that people will not trust corrected information – for example, showing proof that a vaccine has not been tested for long term safety – unless they are already suspicious about the original premise, or something substantial occurs, such as a vaccine injury, to cause them to take another look at their perceived "truth." This explains why today, nearly five years since the beginning of COVID-19, so many people are still unwilling to accept that the unstudied, experimental injection caused a very large uptick in all-cause mortality and a large drop in global fertility.

According to Lewandowsky's study on Iraqi news events, Americans are the most difficult group to convince that what they initially believed is indeed false, even when presented with irrefutable evidence. For example, although no weapons of mass destruction were ever discovered, nearly 30 percent of US respondents continued to believe they existed somewhere. Another example are masks. Even though there have been at least 150 published studies confirming irrefutably that masks offer no protection against infection, Americans can still be seen wearing them, even when driving alone in their car. Given that a fact is not true, those responses are built on a belief in a false memory. Lewandowsky said in multiple different interviews that "it appears Americans accept what they hear at face value, especially if they hear it reported on television's evening news."

THINKING FOR YOURSELF

In much the same way, it is difficult to redirect people away from what they have been told and what they have come to believe was true about the next pandemic. Many people were so incredibly frightened by the COVID-19 hysteria that they have never recovered, and they are already experiencing anxiety over what's coming next. We are told the next global pandemic is about to arrive and (again) it will be "the end of Western civilization as we know it, wreaking economic havoc around the world so pervasively that no person will be untouched." Television, the internet, and print media continually release reports to keep us worried and in a state of anxiety. We've lived through two episodes of this fear-mongering, in 2005 and in 2020; can we resist the next round of fear mongering? When you start to hear the hype this time, will you pause and question what you are hearing or reading? Or, will you be part of the 30 percent who will not be convinced, no matter how convincing the argument?

The idea of another pandemic exposes the insidious and perverse agendas of the multinational conglomerates and the globalist goals promoted by the WHO and the WEF. They have nothing to do with health or with living well. These unelected, self-appointed "leaders" are determined to remove your right to bodily autonomy, your right to refuse injections and microchips, your right to free speech, your freedom to travel, and much more. Hopefully, the information in this book will open your eyes to the truth about the agendas that have been in the making for decades. Although they are not new, they are in full implementation mode right now. They have built a working model and created a reproducible, fear-based template.

Knowing the truth, especially about influenza and what is coming through that needle will give you the strength to resist the lies and propaganda as they unfold.

"From the bitterness of disease, man learns the sweetness of health."

~Catalan Proverb

CHAPTER 3

Microbes, the Flu, and Current Controversies

A strong argument can be made that germs are rulers of the world. Epidemics, inextricably intertwined with the agricultural and industrial revolution, have left their mark on history in cultures around the world. For thousands of years the effects of germs have played a significant role in the evolution of modern civilization, from the shaping of public policy to the outcome of wars.

In 1586, the Holy Roman Emperor Maximillian II and an army of 80,000 prepared to invade Hungary, which was under Turkish domination. The invasion was unsuccessful, not because the Turks were militarily superior, but rather that the Roman ranks were decimated due to a typhus epidemic. Similarly, the Swedes lost control of Russia in 1708 because of the bubonic plague.

In the late 18th and early 19th centuries, Napoleon's greatest adversary was not the British navy. It was microbes. His Russian campaign stands out as a classic example of strategic blundering. Students of history know that the Russian winter proved to be a more implacable enemy than the Czar's forces, yet few know that the size of the army had already been whittled down by typhus, a group of bacterial illnesses that cause similar symptoms, including high fever, chills, rash, body aches, cough, digestive issues and confusion. Types include murine (endemic) typhus, epidemic typhus, and scrub typhus, all of which are spread by fleas, lice or chiggers. Of the 320,000 to 600,000 soldiers (accounts vary dramatically) who left France, 70 percent succumbed to typhus before they reached Moscow. Russians used delaying tactics that allowed typhus to ravage the remainder of Napoleon's troops even more. Only 50,000 soldiers were left to occupy Russia and after the winter, a mere 3,000 returned home to France.

The 19th century saw several other wars where the outcomes were determined as much by diseases as by weapons. During the Crimean War (1854-1856), as an example, ten times as many British soldiers died from dysentery as from Russian bullets.[21]

In the modern history of disease and warfare, World War I particularly stands out. On the heels of the "war to end all wars" came a pandemic – a worldwide outbreak of the relatively benign infection called "influenza." History reports that the virus originated in the US and was carried by soldiers to France. When the war ended and the troops returned home, the "Spanish Flu" returned home with them. In an effort to halt the spread of the disease, many cities, states, and countries placed restrictions on gatherings and travel. Restaurants, dance halls, and theaters were closed for up to a year. Some communities even outlawed the shaking of hands.

Sound familiar?

But as quickly as it appeared, the Great Influenza Pandemic retreated, leaving deaths and questions in its wake.[22]

WHAT WE CALL "THE FLU" TODAY

The flu is conventionally defined as a "highly contagious illness caused by viruses that infect the respiratory tract." Adenovirus causes the common cold, and by comparison, influenza viruses are associated with more severe symptoms. Influenza is thought to spread from person-to-person via respiratory droplets released by coughing and sneezing. The particles bind to mucous present on the surface of the respiratory tract and then bury themselves into the epithelial cells that line the lungs. Following an incubation period of about 48 hours, symptoms abruptly appear.

Of course, a textbook list of symptoms does not quite capture the angst endured by those who contract the flu in any given year. There's an old joke about the "24-hour bug" that goes something like this: the first twelve hours you're afraid you're going to die, and then for the next twelve hours, you feel so miserable you're afraid you might not. As the body goes through the complex physiological process of expelling the contaminated mucus in the sinuses and the lungs, the symptoms can be wretched.

While no one wants to get the flu – even with the quasi-perk of a couple of days off from work or school – the fact remains that most adults and children recover completely within two weeks. Most overtly healthy individuals, *whether living in 1566 or 2005 or 2024*, will not contract the flu at all.

THE CONTROVERSY

At the beginning of the worldwide COVID lockdown, masks, and social distancing rules, a small but very vocal group of very bold doctors and lay-researchers began to investigate the reality of viruses and question the whole scientific field of virology, adopting what has become the "no virus" theory. The majority of their assertions are based on four basic arguments:

Argument #1: Viral "infections" do not follow Koch's postulates for causing infectious disease.

Argument #2: Viruses have not been isolated and identified, therefore they do not exist.

Argument #3: Pictures of what is called a virus are similar or the same as pictures that have no virus. No picture, no proof.

Argument #4: Contagion is a myth, meaning, an infection such as the flu or chickenpox or measles cannot be spread from one person to the next.

Let's take a look at these four arguments.

ARGUMENT #1: KOCH'S POSTULATES

First published in 1890, Robert Koch established the criteria used to assess whether a microorganism is the cause of a disease. As originally stated, the four criteria are:

1. The microorganism must be found in diseased but not healthy individuals;
2. The microorganism must be cultured from the diseased individual;
3. Inoculation of a healthy individual with the cultured microorganism must reproduce the disease; and
4. The microorganism must be re-isolated from the inoculated, diseased individual and be matched to the original microorganism.

Koch's postulates have long been the cornerstone for establishing the criteria used by the scientific community to come to agreement about whether a microorganism is the cause of an infectious disease. However, from the beginning, Koch had to modify the first postulate when it was discovered that an asymptomatic person could be positive for cholera or typhoid; i.e., the organism was found in healthy people without manifesting the illness.

Thomas M. Rivers (1888–1962), the twentieth president of the American Association of Immunologists, spent more than 30 years at the Rockefeller Institute Hospital, where he served as director from 1937 to 1955. He was on the board of editors for *The Journal of Immunology* from 1936 to 1942, and then was an Associate Editor from 1943 to 1951. In 1937, Rivers laid out a critique of Koch's postulates as being only partially correct and that the postulates were meant to be *"guidelines, not absolutes."*

In an article published in the *Journal of Bacteriology* in 1937 and titled "Viruses and Koch's Postulates," Rivers stated:

> "Koch's postulates have had a profound influence on workers investigating infectious maladies. For many years, an infectious agent was not accepted as the cause of a disease unless the postulates had been satisfied. With the development of the science of immunology, however, immunological reactions added much to the knowledge of the specific relation of microbes to disease. It is possible to bring excellent evidence that an organism is the cause of a malady without the complete satisfaction of the postulates. "In spite of this fact, there are certain workers who still refuse to agree that the cause of an infectious disease has been discovered unless all the conditions originally laid down by Koch have been met. This is particularly true regarding the viral maladies..."[23]

He went on to say:

> "At the time when they were formulated, Koch's postulates were essential for the progress of knowledge of infectious

diseases; but progress having left behind old rules requires new ones which some day, without doubt, will also be declared obsolete. ***Thus, in regard to certain diseases, particularly those caused by viruses, the blind adherence to Koch's postulates may act as a hindrance instead of an aid...***" [23]

A separate, more recent article, "Koch's Postulates and Infectious Proteins," published in 2006 in the journal *Acta Neuropathologica*, discusses how the rules of the postulates have been problematic to apply to infectious prions. The authors stated:

"The unorthodox mechanism by which prion diseases are transmitted, involving specific physicochemical characteristics of the protein as well as susceptibility traits of the host, has made these disorders refractory to analysis within the context of the original Koch's postulates."

Because there are a growing list of conditions and diseases that are causally related to transmissible proteins (prions), the authors have suggested an updated version of Koch's postulates, concluding:

"The postulates have proven their mettle over time in the bacterial domain, so while they do have relevance, ***they must be adapted to accommodate etiological causes by atypical pathogens and viruses.***"[24]

ARGUMENT #2: VIRUSES HAVE NOT BEEN ISOLATED AND IDENTIFIED, THEREFORE THEY DO NOT EXIST.

In the textbook, *Infectious Disease, Third Edition,* published by Mosby Press, (2010), Chapter 161, pg. 1590 is about influenza viruses. This is a small excerpt from the chapter:[25]

Influenza viruses are enveloped, single-stranded, RNA viruses of the family *Orthomyxoviridae*. There are three major antigenic types: A, B and C. The virus (virion) has an irregular spherical shape with a lipid envelope, approximately 80–120 nanometers in diameter. The surface is covered with spike-like projections composed of the two primary viral glycoproteins, HA and NA, which are involved in host cell attachment and host cell exit, respectively. Influenza A is currently classified with 16 different HA (H1-H16) and 9 different NA (N1-N9) molecules are known to exist.

The influenza A genome encodes 11 viral proteins:

- haemagglutinin (HA), which is divided into two domains or subunits (HA1 and HA2);
- neuraminidase (NA);
- two matrix proteins (M1 and M2); M1 is found within the lipid bilayer, which surrounds the virus core. M2 (a transmembrane ion channel) is also present on the external surface of the virus;
- nucleoprotein (NP); and
- two nonstructural proteins (NS1 and NS2, also known as NEP, or nuclear export protein).

Dr. Vincent Racaniello, a professor and podcaster on the topic of virology for more than 40 years, teaches and writes from his website *Virology Blog*.[26] In 2021, he wrote an article entitled "Understanding virus isolates, variants, and strains." In the post, he talked about the importance of accurate viral naming and nomenclature, stating this:

> "Isolates of other viruses are also precisely named. I'm a big fan of the very detailed influenza virus nomenclature, which is as follows: Virus name/antigenic type/host

of origin (if other than human)/geographical origin/ serial number/last two digits (or all four digits) of year of isolation/hemagglutinin subtype neuraminidase subtype. Examples include:

1. influenza A virus A/duck/Germany/1868/68 (H6N1)
2. influenza A virus A/chicken/Vietnam/ NCVD-404/2010 (H5N1)."

A peer-reviewed article published by Jens Kuhn in 2021 for the *Encyclopedia of Virology* starts out by saying:

"Whereas virus taxonomy has been a niche subspecialty over many decades, the field has recently gained importance due to the exponentially increasing number of new viruses discovered by next-generation sequencing methods." [27]

Kuhn goes into great detail cataloging, identifying, and explaining the details of viral classification, dating from the 1960s to the present. That's an enormous amount of work and detail over something that doesn't exist.

ARGUMENT #3: PICTURES OF WHAT ARE CALLED VIRUSES ARE SIMILAR TO PICTURES THAT HAVE NO VIRUS. NO PICTURE, NO PROOF.

This is rather easy to counterpoint. After all, we have no pictures of laser beams, ultrasound waves, X-rays, EMFs, or 5G frequencies, but they obviously exist and we can see the results of their use.

ARGUMENT #4: CONTAGION IS A MYTH

Contagion, by definition, is the spread of a disease or infection from one person to another through close personal contact. Two of the oldest diseases associated with contagion are leprosy, from the Bible, and smallpox, historically from around the world.

Many arguments have been made using sputum from a sick animal or human, inserting it into the nose, throat, or arm of a healthy animal or human, and nothing happens, meaning the person does not become ill. But what if the pathogen's virulence had already been neutralized by the white blood cells and cytokines in the mucus, and the mucus was merely expelling a non-contagious, "dead" pathogen, one that has lost its ability to replicate?

I have yet to hear an adequate explanation for how chickenpox parties work, why measles can spread quickly through a community, or why rabies from the bite of a sick and infected animal can be deadly if there is no such thing as a virus. And what about plants? Two examples of major epidemic diseases that wiped out entire crops are the wheat streak mosaic virus and the potato tuber necrotic ringspot virus. There are other epidemics caused by plant viruses that wiped out entire industries, such as the papaya industry in Hawaii in 1994. Most examples involve long-distance virus dispersal via the international trade routes and transportation of infected seeds or planting material.[28]

And what about massive betanodavirus outbreaks in fish, known to infect over 40 marine fish species worldwide, including populations in Australia, Asia, Europe, North America, Africa, and the South Pacific? This viral infection mostly damages the central nervous system of younger fish (larvae, fry, fingerlings), but older fish can be affected too, with school losses ranging from 15 to 100%.[29] Though the germ theory brought many fundamental changes to the understanding of diseases and epidemics, society has continued to experience contagious diseases that have a much longer history. Personal susceptibilities, sexual choices, dietary preferences, the availability of food and its cleanliness, social environments including war and politics have long played a role in explaining contagion and epidemics. Not every illness is caused solely by EMFs, 5G, poor sanitation, contaminated food, or polluted water. I will continue to read, listen, and learn from researchers in both camps. I'm open to having my mind changed, and open to accepting a new perspective. But at this point, I am not convinced that there is "no such thing as a virus."

For the rest of this book, the material is positioned from the perspective that viruses exist, including H5N1, but viruses are not as "deadly" as the global planners would have us believe. My purpose for writing this book, which includes some material from my book, *FOWL*, is to dispel the fear mongering, expose the details of the horrible, injectable concoctions they want to mandate us to take, and to lay out the details of how long this disaster has been in development within our own government.

Knowledge is power; my hope is this book will give you both, especially with the start-stop frenzied reports of another pandemic about to materialize in January 2025, as hyped recently by COVID-19 promoter, Peter Hotez MD, PhD from Baylor College of Medicine. What was bird flu about twenty years ago? Is it any different today?

"We are watching very closely to see how the disease associated with bird flu, when it hits humans, is evolving."

~David Nabarro, WHO, (1999-2005), UN (2005-2014)

CHAPTER 4

H5N1: What You Need to Know

All influenza viruses are not created equal. Or, taking from Orwell's novel, *Animal House* (1945), "all influenza viruses are equal, but some influenza viruses are more equal than others."

Influenza viruses are identified as three distinct immunogenic types – A, B, and C – and a large number of subtypes. Type C viruses are associated with either a very mild respiratory illness or no symptoms at all. They are not associated with epidemics and do not carry with them a public health impact. Influenza Type B viruses also tend to be part of minor illnesses. Having a propensity for older people, influenza type B viruses are most often identified in nursing home outbreaks. Influenza types C and B have not been identified in any species except humans.

Influenza viruses in category "A" are known to infect many different species. They are divided into subtypes based on different combinations of two surface proteins called antigens. Any foreign substance that enters the bloodstream and stimulates the immune system to produce antibodies is defined as an antigen.

The outer shell of influenza A viruses is covered with two types of antigens: one is called "hemagglutinin," signified by the abbreviation (H) or (HA); the other is called "neuraminidase," identified as (N) or (NA). The differences between the "H" and the "N" antigens provide the basis for classifying and naming all the many subtypes of influenza type A viruses. Sixteen different H antigens (referred to as H1 to H16) and nine different N proteins (referred as to N1 to N9) are commonly known to exist. The various combinations of these antigens are the basis for sub-typing and naming, such as H1N1 and H7N3. Notably, every possible combination of H and N can be found in wild and domestic birds, primarily waterfowl.

A virus is not a living organism, but when its environment is optimized, it can unfold and make copies of itself that can then be passed on to other hosts. This is rather similar to a tetanus spore that can remain dormant for years but can germinate and release the potent toxin, tetanospasmin, under optimized anaerobic conditions. The ability to replicate is what gives the impression that a virus is "alive." There are only five groups in which influenza A viruses can replicate: large land mammals, sea mammals, wild birds, domestic birds, and humans. Land mammals associated with influenza viruses include swine and horses; sea mammals encompass seals, dolphins, and whales.

Since 1977, only a few influenza A viruses, specifically H1N1, H1N2, H7N3, and H3N2, have been associated with humans.

Even though the official nomenclature for identifying individual viruses is cumbersome and long, the naming system serves as "code" for virologists and other researchers to identify different characteristics. For example, the official name of one H5N1 viral subtype is A/chicken/ Vietnam/ HauGiang/178/2004 (H5N1). Breaking it down, the code identifies the virus as an influenza type A virus, isolated from a chicken in Vietnam, in the city of HauGiang. It was the 178th virus isolated in 2004 of serotype H5N1.[30]

The number of different serotypes for H5N1 alone is in the hundreds; the number of antigenically distinct influenza A viruses is in the tens of thousands. The fact that hundreds of subtypes exist for H5N1 influenza virus is more than just a scientific curiosity. As stated by Nancy Cox, PhD, Chief of the Influenza Branch, National Center for Infectious Diseases, at the CDC back in 2005, "If we don't get a good match, the vaccine will be less effective, producing illness, hospitalizations and death." For those who purport the importance of getting a vaccine to "protect," how can a "close match" be good enough?

Just because a virus is present doesn't mean that it is causing a problem. Just like there are several microbiomes of bacteria on living creatures, there is also a fungome as well as a virome. All three have normal inhabitants, symbionts, and colonizers that do not cause disease. In fact, influenza A viruses are completely benign, silent passengers in the intestinal tracts of waterfowl, part of the bird's symbiont virome. During transglobal seasonal migration, thousands of ducks and geese congregate in available lakes and ponds along their journey. An examination of the lake water after the flocks have converged would reveal tens of billions of influenza A particles. As many as 130 viral subtypes have been identified in the viral soup. It is this free exchange of genetic material between viruses that scientists watch closely.

Influenza A subtypes have been delineated as either "mildly pathogenic," meaning they cause minimal or no disease, or "highly pathogenic," meaning their presence has been associated with widespread death among all types of birds and mammals. All outbreaks of "Highly Pathogenic Avian Influenza" (HPAI) viruses since the 1980s have been caused by antigen subtypes H5, H7, and H9. For this discussion, these three antigenic types are important to remember – 5, 7, and 9. The bird flu virus is a highly pathogenic subtype referred to as H5N1. Unlike what is being portrayed by the media, outbreaks of highly pathogenic viruses are not new; these viruses have been causing problems in bird populations for a very long time.

OLD PLAYER IN A NEW GAME

The first highly pathogenic avian influenza virus was isolated on the Italian peninsula in 1878. Like many human immigrants of the Ellis Island era, Fowl Plague as it became known, reached the shores of the US via New York City sometime in 1924. The initial outbreak, along with another that occurred five years later, was contained through the destruction of the poultry in the entire area.

Culling, the widespread killing of an entire population of infected animals, is based on a long-held assumption that once a viral outbreak occurs, the only way to eliminate transmission is to massacre every possible host, even if the animal is completely healthy, because the virus is thought to be transmitted indefinitely through the stool. For bird flu, when *one* chicken becomes sick and tests positive for the HPAI virus, culling the entire flock is the first course of action recommended by the Food and Agriculture Organization of the United Nations (FAO), the World Organization for Animal Health (formerly Office International des Epizooties, or OIE), and the WHO, to get outbreaks under control. Even vaccination of a herd or flock is of no value if "disease-free status" must be proven, because it is not possible to distinguish between vaccinated and infected animals.[31]

As a result, between 1997 and 2003, the H5N1 outbreak in Hong Kong and the H7N7 outbreak in the Netherlands resulted in the brutal destruction of more than 31.5 million chickens. I will spare you the details of the gruesome and horrifying ways these family birds were killed in the name of "public health."

LEARN MORE

Culling has been accepted as a legitimate public health measure since it was first used in the UK in 1714 to contain an outbreak of rinderpest, a diarrheal disease in cattle. Both wild and domestic animals have been targeted, in an attempt to manage or curb outbreaks of zoonotic disease, an infectious illness that can be transmitted between animals or from animals to humans.

KILLING THE CHICKENS, DESTROYING THE ECONOMY

Records show that since 1959, there have been 21 reported outbreaks of highly pathogenic avian influenza worldwide. The majority of these have occurred in Europe, with a few emerging in Mexico and Canada. Of the 21 incidents, five resulted in significant losses to regional economies. Minor outbreaks occurred sporadically throughout the US and abroad until 1983, when a major epidemic of highly pathogenic H5N2 appeared on farms in rural Pennsylvania. Two years and $70 million later, the outbreak had been controlled. Nearly 17 million birds – mostly chickens and domestic ducks – had been destroyed, leading to escalated consumer costs of approximately $350 million, mostly due to a 30 percent jump in retail egg prices.[31]

In another part of the world and nearly ten years later (2001), H5N1 viruses were isolated at the Western Wholesale Food Market in Hong Kong from geese imported into the central slaughterhouse. Widespread testing was undertaken and many birds throughout the province were found to be positive, prompting authorities to order the slaughter of virtually all poultry – chickens, ducks, geese, and quail – in the territory. The slaughter cost the farms and markets across the region more than $10 million.[32]

In February 2004, an outbreak of H5N2 viruses afflicted poultry on a single farm in Gonzales County, located in south-central Texas. This was the first outbreak of a highly pathogenic strain in the US in more than 20 years. Detected through routine monitoring for the presence of pathogenic influenza viruses, the affected birds were quarantined and the area was disinfected. The quarantine was lifted March 26, 2004, and, after five days, the US Department of Agriculture announced that the Texas outbreak had been completely eradicated.[33]

Less than a month later, an outbreak of highly pathogenic H7N2 was identified in a flock of chickens in Pocomoke City, Maryland. On Sunday, March 7, 2004 a total of 118,000 farm birds were culled and 210,000 birds on a second farm under the same ownership were destroyed the following day. Later that week, another 40,000 chickens from a third farm owned by the same farmer were also destroyed. Officials also included another 71 farms within the quarantine area. They killed 328,000 chickens at its center, containing the outbreak to 12 large chicken houses.[34]

And now, twenty years later in 2024, the media is recycling the fear-factor about H5N1 and governments are culling millions of chickens and thousands of cows. In fact, between 2020 and 2024, more than 250 million chickens and other birds have been culled globally due to outbreaks of the highly pathogenic avian influenza. Officials have been poking around farms for the last year, checking to see if the H5N1 virus has landed on any other farm animals. And even though most cows have no signs of illness, inspectors have unnecessarily slaughtered them with some farms losing up to 10% of their herd.

What is disturbing, and has apparently been overlooked by public health and agriculture offices around the world, is a study done in 2016 by an independent expert panel in the UK. Researchers concluded that culling was ineffective in reducing infection in a herd of cattle. The panel also concluded that proactive culling was also ineffective because it is "resource intensive" in terms of manpower, time, and financial loss. Another immediate argument against culling is that animals suffer both emotional and physical pain between the moment they are grabbed to be culled (shot, poisoned, strangled, suffocated, etc.) and put to death.[35]

The preceding chronology documents that avian influenza outbreaks have occurred in the US with varying degrees of severity for many years. In fact, since 2022, Animal and Plant Health Inspection Service (APHIS), a part of the USDA, has detected and reported H5N1 virus in more than 23 species mammals.[29] Looking at the list of tested animals which were tested in many states across the US, which includes black bears and bottle-nosed dolphins, it make me shake my head: Don't the officials at the Animal and Plant Health Inspection Service, part of the USDA, have more important things to do?[36]

Taken in context, there is very real concern for economic losses to the poultry industry. Keep in mind past experiences with H5N1 and other HPAI outbreaks in various parts of the world over the last few decades have a striking similarity to the current bird flu outbreak that is generating global attention.

The importance of this chart is that there have only been 462 bird flu-associated deaths worldwide *since 2003*. Further, there have only been eight deaths in the last four years. Sometime in the last few years, bird flu (H5N1) has mutated to a mild disease only causing conjunctivitis, commonly known as "pink eye."

Why all the hysteria and fear-mongering?

Cumulative number of confirmed human cases† for avian influenza A(H5N1) reported to WHO, 2003-2024

Country	2003-2009* cases	deaths	2010-2014* cases	deaths	2015-2019* cases	deaths	2020 cases	deaths	2021 cases	deaths	2022 cases	deaths	2023 cases	deaths	2024 cases	deaths	Total cases	deaths
Azerbaijan	8	5															8	5
Bangladesh	1		6	1	1												8	1
Cambodia	9	7	47	30									6	4	5	1	67	42
Canada			1	1													1	1
Chile													1				1	
China	38	25	9	5	6	1					2	1					55	32
Djibouti	1																1	
Ecuador													1				1	
Egypt	90	27	120	50	149	43											359	120
India									1	1							1	1
Indonesia	162	134	35	31	3	3											200	168
Iraq	3	2															3	2
Lao People's Democratic Republic	2	2					1										3	2
Myanmar	1																1	
Nepal					1	1											1	1
Nigeria	1	1															1	1
Pakistan	3	1															3	1
Spain											2						2	
Thailand	25	17															25	17
Turkey	12	4															12	4
United Kingdom									1				4				5	
United States of America											1						1	
Viet Nam	112	57	15	7							1						128	64
Total	**468**	**282**	**233**	**125**	**160**	**48**	**1**		**2**	**1**	**6**	**1**	**12**	**4**	**5**	**1**	**887**	**462**

*2003, 2009, 2010-2014 and 2015-2019 total figures. Breakdown by year available on subsequent table.
†This count includes reported detections in asymptomatic individuals. In some cases, the confirmation of infection versus transient contamination of the nasopharynx/oropharynx with virus particles after exposure to infected birds or contaminated environment remains inconclusive. Total number of cases includes number of deaths.
WHO reports only laboratory confirmed cases. All dates refer to onset of illness.
Source: WHO/GIP, data in HQ as of 26 February 2024

World Health Organization

Source:https://cdn.who.int/media/docs/default-source/influenza/
h5n1-human-case-cumulative-table/2024_feb_tableh5n1.pdf

HIGHLIGHT

As of June, 2024, bird flu had been detected in approximately 85 herds across 12 states but only three farm workers had been sickened, two of them with an eye infection (conjunctivitis). While public health officials say "the risk to humans is low, the ominous threat continues," with whispers of "concerns are growing." Officials started to request that people working with or around farm animals wear protective clothing and masks, and calls for testing began. The ranchers and workers complied. They've trained us well, haven't they?

DRIFTING AND SHIFTING: HOW VIRUSES CHANGE

For symptoms to occur, a virus must undergo replication. Only when a virus bypasses the body's several layers of immunological protection can it proliferate, triggering the cascade of symptoms associated with the flu.

Viral replication is a complex task and defects often occur during the process, resulting in an "offspring" that is not the exact copy of its parent. If a small alteration in the genetic makeup of an influenza virus is repeated, it is said to become a permanent change, creating a brand-new strain. Even though the new strain is related to the parent virus, the subtle differences make it "antigenically distinct," meaning that it seems like a brand-new virus to the immune system. This change, called an antigenic "drift," accounts for the differences in each year's influenza viruses. The CDC takes advantage of this drift, using it to justify the production of a new flu shot each season.

Each influenza virus is made up of eight gene segments that can manufacture, or "code" for, at least ten proteins. The proteins can "reassort," or exchange, when two viruses cohabitate in the same cell. For example, if the human influenza virus H3N2 is in a pig that is simultaneously harboring an avian influenza virus (say, H6N4 from a chicken), the two viruses have an opportunity to exchange genes, resulting in a new "recombinant" virus. This process – the blending of two different viruses – is called *"reassortment."* Reassortment is what virologists and public health officials are vigilant about. They have concerns that a new "super influenza virus" could emerge and be particularly dangerous to humans, depending on which gene or genes are acquired during the swap.

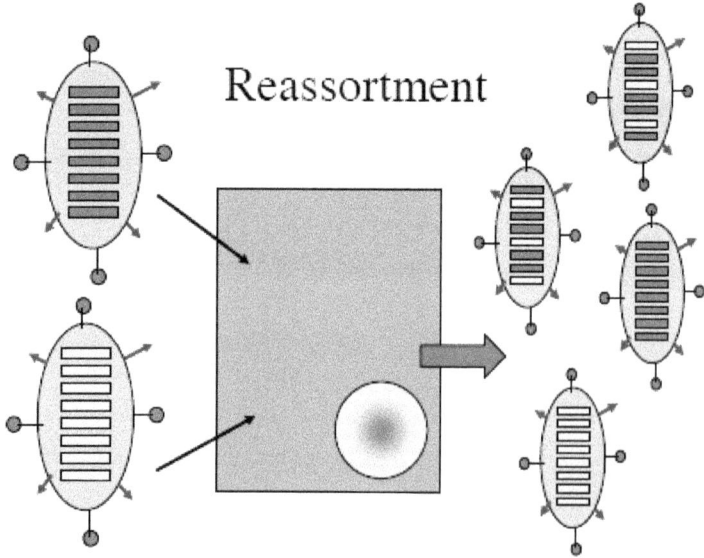

Diagram reproduced with permission from Dr. Vikram Misra, Professor and Head of the Department of Microbiology, Western College of Veterinary Medicine, University of Saskatchewan. (Slide #15 of the presentation.)

ANTIGENIC SHIFT: PANDEMIC CONCERNS

Monitoring the tendency of influenza viruses to undergo antigenic drifts and shifts has been the work of the WHO Global Influenza Program since its inception in 1947. The concern is that a major change in the (H) and/or (N) viral surface proteins will occur, igniting the next global pandemic, which by definition is an infectious outbreak occurring over a very wide area, crossing international boundaries, and usually affecting a large number of people. There is much dispute over the cause of the Influenza Pandemic of 1918. It has been long held that the pandemic virus emerged when an influenza virus from a bird reassorted with an influenza virus from a pig, resulting in a virus that could infect humans. Other theories for the massive number of deaths have included:

- It was the most virulent influenza strain ever to occur across the world, thus it killed millions.
- Aspirin toxicity: troops were given **up to 30 grams** per day (*the typical adult dose for fever is 325 to 650 mg every four hours with a maximum of 4,000 mg (**4 grams**) in 24 hours*).
- Widespread typhoid vaccination of the troops prior to deployment caused immunosuppression and death from influenza.
- Massive sunspot emissions adversely affected the immune system.
- Widespread use of global radar launched at the beginning of World War I (WWI) was really the killer, not a virus.

In 2004 government scientists released what, at the time, was called the "definitive evidence" identifying the 1918 virus as an avian virus that had "jumped species" and infected humans. The work involved the recreation of viruses extracted from lung tissue of two soldiers and an Alaskan woman who died during the 1918 pandemic. The soldiers' tissue samples had been saved in an army pathology warehouse, and the woman's remains had been preserved in a mass grave in the permanently frozen ground. "We now think that the 1918 virus was an entirely avian-like virus that adapted to humans," said Mr. Jeffrey Taubenberger, researcher from the Armed Forces Pathology Institute. The report, a culmination of ten years of work, was published in two respected journals, *Nature* and *Science,* in October 2005.[37,38]

The publication date was timely. It legitimized worries that bird flu could be transmitted directly to humans. It played into the hands of those in the Bush Administration who were preparing to spend billions of dollars to prepare for a bird flu outbreak. It was the first of many cycles; watch still today as they recycle the fear for massive effectiveness.

From my rotting body, flowers shall grow and
I am in them and that is eternity."

~Edvard Munch, artist

CHAPTER 5

Perspective on Past Pandemics

The CDC and WHO continually warn us that we are primed for the next pandemic. Forecasters are calling for the next global pandemic to be similar to COVID-19 in which up to 17 million died and perhaps as many as two billion have been injured by the jab, and more boosters are on the way.

But we've been through this before – more than once. That is why their ability to cause massive fear and manipulate the entire world into obedience has been so perplexing. Three major pandemic outbreaks have occurred in the recent past. They have used the patterns of the outbreaks to repeatedly flame the fire of fear and worry. They have found a template that works.

SPANISH FLU (1918–1919)

The most highly discussed outbreak is the global influenza pandemic of 1918. Called the "Spanish Flu," it gained its name from the press in politically neutral Spain. Some of the earliest printed reports of the flu's impact originated from Spain, which were not censored during World War I. Reportedly, more than 200 million people fell ill and death estimates ranged from 30 to 100 million, an ever changing and escalating number. Adjusting for today's population, a similar pandemic would yield a modern death toll of 175 to 350 million. In retrospect, the Great Influenza pandemic was small compared to the Great COVID-19 pandemic deception.

Ten influenza pandemics, defined by clinical and epidemiological records, have occurred in the last 300 years. The serotypes of the six outbreaks have been identified.

H2N2 (1889)	**H2N2 (1957)**
H3N8 (1900)	**H3N2 (1968)**
H1N1 (1918)	**H1N1 (1977)**

Thoughts about the evolution of the pandemic virus were previously discussed but the official narrative remains interesting. In the spring of 1918, many flu-like symptoms were recorded, with typical sore throat, headache, fever, and loss of appetite. Even though the geographic origin of the epidemic is still debated, the most widely accepted location for the first reported illness was at Fort Riley Army Camp, located in Haskell County, Kansas. The story goes like this: on the morning of March 4, 1918, the company cook, Albert Gitchell, reported to duty with a temperature of 103°F (39.5°C). Similar symptoms were soon reported from two more recruits: Corporal Lee Drake and Sergeant Adolph Hurby. Within two days, 522 men in the camp were reportedly sick with a flu-like illness. Throughout the summer, infections became increasingly more severe. By mid-August, three additional and significant outbreaks had been reported that seemed to be completely unrelated because they occurred in such disparate locations: Brest, France; Freetown, Sierra Leone; and Boston, Massachusetts.

Among US military personnel, death rates reportedly ranged from 5 to 10 percent among those afflicted. While it is clear that most who were ill were soldiers, the illness also spread quickly throughout the local civilian populations. People without symptoms could be struck suddenly and rendered too feeble to walk within hours; many would die the next day. A key symptom was the presence of cyanosis, a blue discoloration to the face due to rapid accumulation of fluid in the lungs. Not surprisingly, even with the best available care of the day, nearly one-third of those with the Spanish flu reportedly died.

The highest mortality rate occurred among those who developed rapidly progressing pneumonia. Because penicillin was not discovered until 1928, many deaths were likely due to secondary bacterial infections, and would have been prevented today. As pointed out in a letter published in *The Wall Street Journal* on November 1, 2005, by Dr. Edward H. Livingston, chairman of Gastrointestinal and Endocrine Surgery at the University of Texas Southwestern School of Medicine, hospitalization at the turn of the century didn't have much to offer. Even the use of intravenous therapy, routine today, was nonexistent in 1918. His astute comments included, "In 1918, care of the flu patient was limited to rest, **providing aspirin,** oxygen, and other supportive measures. The primary cause of death was pneumonia from bacterial infection as a result of the flu. Lacking antibiotics, there was no effective way of treating the pneumonia."

Therefore, a significant proportion of the deaths may be attributable to aspirin toxicity. Livingston's article went on to say:

> "A confluence of events created a 'perfect storm' for widespread salicylate toxicity. The loss of Bayer's patent on aspirin in February 1917 allowed many manufacturers into the lucrative aspirin market. In fact, the sale of aspirin more than doubled between 1918 and 1920. Tins and bottles of aspirin contained few instructions and no warnings. There was a great *fear of the Spanish influenza*, an illness that had been spreading like wildfire."[39] (*emphasis added*)

Apparently the level at which salicylate toxicity occurs can vary among individuals, explaining why some appeared to tolerate a high dose of the medication and others died from it. A study of 177 adults who had aspirin toxicity (a 15% mortality rate) found the most common presentations were depressed consciousness (61%) and respiratory failure (47%), which could occur even at therapeutic, non-toxic aspirin levels. The US army camps with the highest mortality rate found that the doctors had used the standard treatment recommendations, which included 100,000 tablets of aspirin.

The Spanish Flu remains a topic of historical uncertainty and debate. Questions surrounding the illness's origins, its exceptionally high mortality rate, and even the total number of deaths remain unresolved. Despite this ambiguity, in 2020 the media tried to draw parallels between deaths from the Spanish Flu and deaths CAUSED by the impending COVID-19 infection. However, COVID deaths never really materialized, and were actually found to be about 0.2% of all infections.

LEARN MORE

As mentioned previously, when aspirin (a salicylate) is given during a viral infection it can cause Reye's Syndrome, mostly experienced in children but it has also been seen in adults. The reason the case-fatality rate was especially high among young adults during the 1918-1919 influenza pandemic is not completely understood. The use of high doses of aspirin as a contributing factor to the severity of illness and excessive deaths is not unfounded. Physicians used extremely high doses of salicylates, as much as **30 grams per day**. Today, the typical adult aspirin dose for fever is 325 mg to 650 mg every four hours with a maximum of 4,000 mg per day (**4 grams per day**) in 24 hours. An excessively high salicylate level can act as a poison, leading to pulmonary edema, hyperventilation, and impaired ability to clear mucus from the lungs. According to a research article published in *Clinical Infectious Diseases* (2009), the US Surgeon General, the US Navy, and the *Journal of the American Medical Association* recommended use of aspirin just *before* a spike in deaths in October 1918. Notably, a test to measure the salicylate level in the blood was not developed until the 1940s. The unusual, nonlinear kinetics of salicylate accumulation which predisposed to toxicity were unknown until the 1960s.[39]

The media also frequently overlooked the societal and medical advancements of the last century. Early 20th-century conditions complicate the accuracy of any morbidity and mortality estimates: rudimentary medical infrastructure, inconsistent record-keeping, and a non-existent public health system made global mortality statistics inherently unreliable. For instance, in 1999, the CDC estimated the death toll of the Spanish Flu at 20 million, ignoring the possible role of aspirin toxicity in increasing fatalities. By 2005, this estimate expanded significantly to a range of 20 to 100 million – a disparity that underscores the speculative nature of the figures. During a CDC press briefing teleconference on November 2, 2005, John Wellerman of Bloomberg News asked a direct question of the CDC panel regarding the bird flu pandemic, "I want to find out why the **estimates of [anticipated] deaths** from the current outbreak have increased so much. I believe last year the studies said 200,000 people might die during the pandemic. This iteration you're now 1.9 million." (*emphasis added*)

The Director of the National Vaccine Program, Dr. Bruce Gelling, fielded the question and responded, "We actually provided two estimates [last year]. One of them was based on the 1957-1958 pandemic which, when reviewing past pandemics, was relatively mild. We don't know what the H5N1 virus will do, we don't know what any virus will do, but we felt that it would be best suited to have our preparations **based on the worst case,** which in modern memory, would be the **influenza of 1918.**" (*emphasis added*)

After the initial severe outbreaks in 1918, the subsequent outbreaks occurred in waves during 1919 and 1920 and were not as severe as the initial rounds. Within 18 months after its onset, the 1918 flu epidemic disappeared as rapidly as it began. No one knows why.

How similar does this sound to COVID-19?

HIGHLIGHT

As time goes on, it is becoming increasingly clear that most people who died between 2021 and 2024 did not die from a COVID-19 infection. Instead, they died from medical neglect in hospitals, medical malpractice without appropriate medications (ivermectin, hydroxychloroquine, budesonide, and others), and from a complication of the COVID-19 injections -- two shots and a booster. The actual death rate from the infection itself was -- and remains -- around 0.2%.

ASIAN FLU (1957-1958)

A new influenza virus, H2N2, was isolated in Singapore in February 1957 and was found in Hong Kong later that same year. The new flu strain circulated throughout the southern hemisphere and was identified in the US in June 1957. Ultimately blamed for the deaths of nearly 70,000 Americans, H2N2 was thought to have originated by the reassortment of genes in wild ducks. Notably different from the 1918 pandemic, the highest mortality rates occurred among the elderly. Worldwide, one million people reportedly died during the 1957 flu pandemic.

HONG KONG FLU (1968-1969)

When the novel subtype virus H3N2 was first identified in Hong Kong in August 1968, the WHO was quick to issue a shrill warning: Another worldwide pandemic was looming. The outbreak pattern was predicted to be similar to that seen in 1957, but this global outbreak was different. Nearly everywhere, the clinical symptoms were mild and the mortality was low. The disease seemed to spread slowly rather than explosively. In some countries, absentee rates and increased deaths rates were slight or absent altogether.

Canada, for example, experienced practically no deaths from the novel strain of influenza. In the UK, deaths from influenza-like illness and pneumonia were actually lower than in the preceding year. A similar picture was seen in most of Europe where symptoms were mild and excessive deaths were negligible. In contrast, the US was the notable exception. Nearly 34,000 deaths were attributed to the H3N2 influenza, mostly in the elderly.

LESSONS FROM PAST PANDEMICS

The WHO has created a 12-point list of "lessons learned" from previous pandemics. However, a critical view of the three historical global influenza outbreaks can lead to different lessons than those deduced by the WHO.

Summary of WHO "Lessons Learned"
from Previous Pandemics

1. Pandemics behave as unpredictably as the viruses that cause them.
2. The severity of the illness cannot be known in advance.
3. The pandemic may cause severe disease in young adults, a major determinant of overall impact.
4. The epidemiological potential of a virus tends to unfold in waves.
5. Viral surveillance by WHO laboratories is critically important.
6. Most pandemics have originated in parts of Asia where dense populations of humans live in close proximity to ducks and pigs.
7. Quarantine and travel restrictions have shown little effect.
8. Delaying spread is desirable so that fewer people at a time will require healthcare.
9. The impact of vaccines on a pandemic remains to be demonstrated.
10. Countries with domestic manufacturing capacity will be the first to receive vaccines.
11. The interval between successive outbreak waves is unpredictable.
12. In the best-case scenario, a pandemic will cause excess mortality only at the extremes of life and in persons with underlying chronic disease, the same high-risk groups as the season influenza.

Here are a few alternate lessons learned from previous outbreaks:

1. Malnutrition played a role in the 1918 pandemic.

Whereas a fit and healthy person, under ordinary circumstances, is resistant to infections, situations like war, chemical exposures, and natural disasters lead to increased susceptibility. During wartime, shortages of fresh food lead to malnutrition and lack of clean water can lead to widespread immunocompromise.

In 1985, the Director of National Institute of Allergy and Infectious Disease (NIAID), Dr. Anthony Fauci, declared that malnutrition was the most prevalent cause of human immune deficiency diseases throughout the world. That is equally true today. On May 24, 2018, the United Nations Security Council unanimously passed a resolution condemning the use of food insecurity, defined as conditions that result in not having enough food to meet basic needs, and starvation as a tactic of war. According to the WHO, around 2.33 billion people globally faced moderate or severe food insecurity in 2023. Among those, over 864 million people experienced severe food shortages, going without food for days at a time. Were these people more susceptible to COVID-19 infection and were they also more likely to suffer an injury after the jab?

2. Two of the three worldwide influenza outbreaks were directly associated with war.

Global outbreaks of influenza occurred around the time of American-involved wars: World War I and Vietnam. In fact, the WHO attributed the 1968 outbreak to the return of US troops to California from Southeast Asia (Vietnam). Poor hygiene, emotional stress, pre-deployment vaccines, and chemical exposures to horrific toxins such as napalm and Agent Orange contributed to the weakening of immune systems, and no doubt contributed to the outbreak of influenza.

3. The general health of those who contracted influenza is unknown.

During a widespread outbreak, the underlying health conditions of those who became ill and/or died are unknown. Influenza could have been blamed for the cause of death when the person actually died from something else such as congestive heart failure, bacterial pneumonia, or even from the medical treatments rendered, from mega doses of aspirin to remdesivir.

4. Mass vaccination of soldiers may have weakened their immune systems and contributed to influenza deaths.

What vaccines were given to soldiers prior to deploying to the battlefield in 1918? The historical article by Shanks, "Legacy of the 1914-18 War" explains many details of the vaccines given at the time.[40]

- **Typhoid:** Typhoid was one of the most pervasive diseases among soldiers. It is a bacterial infection caused by *Salmonella typhi* and primarily spreads through contaminated food and water or close contact with an infected person. Symptoms include prolonged fever, weakness, abdominal pain, and sometimes rash. Without proper treatment, it can lead to serious complications, including intestinal perforation, which can be fatal. During the early 1900s, soldiers were constantly exposed to fecal-contaminated environments; if infected, the illness carried a 10% case-fatality rate and a three to six month hospital stay.

  Developed by Almroth Wright in 1896, the typhoid vaccine was first used on British soldiers during the Boer War (1899-1902). A whole-cell vaccine made from *Salmonella typhi* bacteria inactivated by heat or with phenol, the vaccines were contaminated with bacterial endotoxin, residual phenol, and bacterial cell wall proteins, leading to severe local and autoimmune reactions.

  Even though it was still under investigation, the US army ordered all soldiers in the WWI theater to receive the typhoid vaccine. This compulsion was eventually instituted in the French and Italian armies too. While it reduced the incidence of typhoid fever, its impact was not overwhelmingly positive. Most soldiers became very sick after being vaccinated; some became completely incapacitated for days to weeks. More than 35,000 of roughly 4 million vaccinated US soldiers were admitted to hospital after vaccination. The vaccine was thought to reduce the rate of severe infection by about 70%.

- **Tetanus:** WWI predated vaccination with tetanus toxoid as we know it today. Therefore, the only prevention or treatment available was anti-tetanus toxin made from horse serum, which was not a benign product. Many people experienced anaphylaxis after being injected with the foreign proteins from a horse.

A large study was undertaken by the British Army Medical Core in which two million men were vaccinated as soon as possible after they had been wounded. The resulting data showed a lowered mortality rate among the vaccinated, which was difficult to interpret. When large-scale vaccination campaigns are undertaken for an uncommon infection such as tetanus, the results of the clinical trial can make the vaccine look overly beneficial.

For example, the CDC posts a review article every two to four years on the number of reported cases of tetanus. From 1995 to 2000, there were 254 cases reported with 34 deaths. Similarly, from 2009 to 2017, 264 cases were reported, with 19 deaths. In all surveys, on average, 17% of infected people had four *or more* tetanus shots and still contracted the disease.

- **Smallpox:** Routine smallpox vaccination had been going on in the military for nearly one hundred years by the time of WWI. Historically, this vaccination was introduced using a method called *variolation*, where material from a smallpox pustule of one person was introduced into the skin of a second person to induce a milder form of the disease and confer immunity. This practice carried a risk of transmitting smallpox or other infections. During WWI, soldiers were routinely vaccinated with the vaccinia-based (cowpox) smallpox vaccine.

- **Yellow fever:** The development of the yellow fever vaccine began in the late 19th century from the work of the Panama Canal Commission led by Walter Reed, an influential American army physician. Reed's team proved that yellow fever was transmitted by mosquitoes, not by direct human contact. The vaccine was first made by attenuating the yellow fever virus by passing it through multiple animal hosts. It was first tested in humans in 1937.

During World War I, minimal efforts were made to vaccinate troops with an early, undeveloped vaccine if they were heading to regions where yellow fever was endemic, especially parts of Africa and South America. But wide use of the yellow fever vaccine on military recruits did not begin until the 1940s.

The impact of mass vaccination on the troops and within the civilian population could have led to immune system disruption and an increased susceptibility to the effects of influenza viruses. They could have also received other injections during that period of time, including crude versions of cholera, plague, and whole cell pertussis vaccines, weakening their immune system. Near the turn of the century, many new drugs and vaccines were trialed on soldiers, a large and captive set of test subjects. The results were reported frequently in medical journals. Some interventions showed efficacy and became part of the medical armamentarium; others did not and were abandoned. Some non-pharmaceutical solutions worked exceedingly well, such as the report of the successful elimination of the symptoms of the Spanish flu on board the naval ship, Susquehanna, with colloidal silver. Unfortunately, this marvelous, non-toxic solution was set aside for "real medicine" – prescription antibiotics.

As the 1968-69 pandemic fizzled out, global pharma companies had learned that mass vaccination campaigns were good for business. Governments learned that an entire population could be manipulated by creating fear around a theoretically deadly boogieman called a virus. But they also learned that creating outbreak stories in far away, third-world countries had lost its impact. Few cared about what was happening in southeast Asia. A new tactic was needed.

What began to take shape was a new fear-based idea -- one that could not be controlled, and one that was random and ever-present.

The idea?

Create the threat of a virus leaking "accidentally" from a lab.

"Power concedes nothing without a demand. Find out just what people will submit to and you have found out the exact amount of injustice and wrong which will be imposed upon them…"

~Frederick Douglas, Human Rights Activist (1818-1895)

CHAPTER 6
The Swine Flu Fiasco and The 9/11 Smallpox Scare

Pharmaceutical companies quickly recognized the opportunity for vast profits by fast-tracking vaccines, with governments serving as their primary customers. These companies understood that those injured by vaccines would become long-term consumers of medical care and drugs, perpetuating a cycle of dependence. However, as the fear of distant pandemics began to lose its grip on the public, the pharmaceutical industry needed a new narrative, so they created one: a virus that could be leaked from a secret lab – the threat could come from anywhere, be deadlier than anything previously encountered, and have no known cure. This theory had all the elements needed to stoke widespread panic. The catch? There was a vaccine, offering the only hope for survival.

The first test for the new premise came in 2021, when several vials labeled as "smallpox" were discovered at a Merck & Co. vaccine research facility near Philadelphia. The media was activated and hundreds of reports erupted across social media and online print publications to whip the public into a frenzy. Then, two days later, it was reported that the vials did not contain the smallpox virus after all. After the CDC and the FBI concluded their investigations, according to the Department of Homeland Security (DHS), the vials were found to contain vaccinia, a relatively benign virus used to make an attenuated form of the smallpox vaccine and many other vaccines, but not live smallpox viruses.[41]

Since the onset of COVID-19 hysteria, the debate over whether the virus was intentionally or accidentally released from a lab remains unresolved in many circles. Regardless of the origins, Frederick Douglass' 1800s quote, which opens this chapter, has gained a new, eerie relevance. Reflecting on what people believed during the COVID-19 crisis is almost unbelievable: the idea that a flimsy mask could prevent infection, the blind compliance with fabricated social distancing rules, and the acceptance of repeated, even dangerous PCR tests, including the bizarre drive-by testing setups. Now, we're left to come to grips with the ongoing tragedies brought about by what some have determined to be a bioweapon.

All of these measures took a serious toll on families as members disagreed loudly about the necessity of the jab for participating in various family outings. Confused and frightened seniors died alone in hospitals and nursing homes because family and friends were not allowed to visit. People couldn't say goodbye or grieve with their relatives because funeral gatherings were not allowed. Businesses were divided, with many being labeled "non-essential." Churches were closed. Gatherings were prohibited, even in private homes. As we moved away from the totalitarian lockdowns, disrespect toward each other and towards our children has remained for years.

In an interview with Neil Cavuto on FOX News July 22, 2022, Dr. Deborah Birx, White House Coronavirus Response Coordinator under

President Donald Trump said, *"I knew these vaccines were not going to protect against infection. And I think we overplayed the vaccines…"*

Really? Blood is on your hands, Dr. Birx.[42]

They will always try to scare us. It's part of the template they created. In recent memory, they've used fear to hype smallpox (2001), SARS (2002), bird flu (2005), and H1N1 (2009). During COVID-19, they perfected a tool twenty years in the making: **weaponized fear.** In fact, they really lit up the cannons during COVID-19. The whole world trembled and obeyed for long months that rolled into years. But have they overplayed their hand? Let's go back in time and review their way of thinking.

Since the 1970s, epidemiologists have theorized that major antigenic shifts in influenza viruses seem to occur in 11-year cycles. The 11-year model appeared to function well, since there were exactly 11 years between the pandemics of 1946, 1957, and 1968. Also, historical comparisons showed that the 1957 disease was similar to the 1889 disease, and the 1968 disease was similar to that of 1900.

However, the convenient construct of an 11-year cycle fell apart when no pandemic appeared in 1979, although they thought one was about to occur in 1976. That would-be pandemic became the fiasco called the swine flu.

FORT DIX: ANOTHER STORY BEGINS

Even though April 30, 1975 marked the end of the US presence in Vietnam, young men across the country continued to sign up for the all-volunteer army. Just after the Christmas holiday in 1975, thousands of enthusiastic new army recruits reported to the barracks at Fort Dix, New Jersey, to begin basic training. However, by mid-January, many were complaining of flu-like symptoms; a few were even hospitalized.

One recruit reported to his drill instructor that he felt tired and weak. Given the option to rest, he opted instead to participate in a five-mile training march on a cold February night. Twenty-four hours later, on February 6, 1976, 19-year-old Private David Lewis of Ashley Falls, Massachusetts, was dead. Word arrived the following week from the CDC laboratory that his death was caused by an influenza type A virus. What was worrisome was that four additional samples taken from ill recruits at Fort Dix had also tested positive for influenza A virus – a viral type that had previously been detected only in pigs. Alarms started to sound throughout the public health community. Had a pig virus "jumped species" and directly infected a human? Was this the start of another pandemic?

On February 20, 1976, the New York Times ran a story titled: "US Calls Flu Alert On Possible Return of Epidemic Virus." The article read, "Experts said that there was little danger of any 'wildfire' epidemic on the newly found virus," and that the flu cluster at Fort Dix may be nothing more than a "curiosity." However, what started as a possible fluke quickly ramped up to a national emergency.[43]

Within three weeks of Lewis' death, researchers and public health officials converged on Washington, D.C. with two goals: (1) to persuade members of Congress to implement a costly new program involving the rapid development of a novel vaccine; and (2) to implement an expanded program of mass vaccination.

A nationwide campaign was launched by the CDC with the urgency of a five-alarm fire; they were in search of other cases of what had been dubbed "swine flu." In addition to a few earlier cases reported in Minnesota and Wisconsin, already known to the CDC, the investigation turned up a few isolated occurrences throughout Pennsylvania, Virginia, and Mississippi. Every case, except for one questionable instance in Virginia, involved human-to-pig contact.

By March 15, word reached President Ford by way of the CDC that the country was on the verge of a major influenza pandemic. Calling an urgent meeting with his top advisors including, among others, Richard Cheney and Donald Rumsfeld, the President was unanimously urged to begin preparing for a massive vaccination program. As a point of caution, Ford postponed his decision until he had the assurances of scientists on how to proceed.

COMMENTARY

The swine flu fiasco was in 1976. How similar to COVID-19 is this already sounding? Here's a comparison: 1) only a few cases had been reported; 2) advisors to the president, the CDC, and the National Institutes of Health (NIH) immediately began reporting ominous warnings; 3) a vaccine, already on its way, was ready in less than a year, long before cell line technologies and mRNA platforms had been created to fast-track vaccine development; and 4) money was almost instantly available...lots of money.

The following week, Ford met with a "blue-ribbon" panel of experts from the CDC and the NIH, including renowned polio vaccine experts Drs. Jonas Salk and Albert Sabin. Hearing the consensus of opinions from his team that the massive program was not only necessary but also critically important, the president presented his case to the American people on March 24, 1976. During the nationally televised address, he announced the formation of the "National Influenza Immunization Program" and a plan for the mass vaccination of all Americans. At the same time, the President appealed to Congress for the funds to make it happen.

With unparalleled haste, Rep. Paul G. Rogers (D-FL), chairman of the Health and the Environment Committee, rushed bill HR 13012 through his subcommittee and sent it directly to the House floor on

April 5, 1976. Even though most members of the House had neither seen nor read the legislation, the bill passed that same day by a vote of 354-12. With only minor modifications, the Senate approved the appropriations for the bill, 61-7, a mere four days later. Now that the money was in place – funded by taxpayers – all that was needed was a vaccine. Of note, after leaving Congress in 1979, Rep. Rogers became a member of the Board of Directors for Merck & Co. and for the Mutual Life Insurance of New York.

RECENT PAINFUL MEMORIES FOR PHARMA

Almost immediately, liability protection emerged as an issue for the vaccine makers. Vaccine injury lawsuits were a recent memory in the minds of the insurance underwriters, having weathered the storms of litigation with Cutter Laboratories during the implementation of the polio vaccine program. In 1955, Cutter was one of several pharmaceutical companies licensed to produce Salk's killed-virus polio vaccine. Through a series of errors, thousands of vaccine lots containing the live virus had been released to the general public, causing polio and severe illness in more than 40,000 children; 200 became permanently paralyzed and 10 had died.

The ensuing 28-day jury trial took place in Oakland, California's Alameda County Superior Court. In the end, the jury found that Cutter was not negligent in the production of the vaccine but nonetheless awarded one victim $147,300, equivalent to $1.726M in today's dollars. The Court reasoned Cutter had met production standards of the day, but was liable for marketing a vaccine it claimed was safe when clearly it was not. The verdict, which was upheld on appeal, not only opened the door for more lawsuits against makers of defective vaccines, it drove Cutter out of the vaccine business.

The damage award to the Cutter vaccines was not monumental, even by 1955 standards, but the problems and risks associated with the polio vaccines were enough to get the attention of the vaccine manufacturers' insurance companies. If the liability was too high, insurance companies would not issue coverage to protect the vaccine manufacturers from future suits arising from side effects associated with their products. If lawsuits were associated with the polio vaccine, they could certainly happen with any other vaccine as well, including the new, fast-tracked swine flu vaccine.

Once Congress announced it was willing to fund the production of the new swine flu vaccine, the insurance companies made their positions known. On April 8,1976, the Federal Insurance Company advised Merck pharmaceuticals that all liability and defense costs that might be associated with claims arising from their fast-tracked swine flu vaccine would not be covered by the insurance plan. Within days, the other three vaccine manufacturers – Merrell, Parke-Davis, and Wyeth – received similar notices from their insurance providers. About that same time, T. Lawrence Jones, president of the American Insurance Association, had a meeting with government officials, letting them know that the insurance industry had no plans to ensure any of the manufacturers for liability that could arise with rapid production and the massive campaign intended for the swine flu vaccine.

The pressure was on from all sides to get government money into the game. If the swine flu program was going to get off the ground, the federal government would have to put up the money – our tax dollars – to protect a private industry. The government would need to assume liability for any and all problems that could arise from potential vaccine injuries.

Some legislators argued that passing protective legislation would lead to careless manufacturing on the part of the drug companies. Others continued to argue that without the vaccine a raging epidemic could occur with millions of deaths and production must continue at all costs.

In the middle of the heated debate, a strange outbreak was reported that shifted public opinion and secured all the benefits sought by the drug companies and their underwriters. In early July 1976, an unusually deadly respiratory infection occurred among guests attending a bicentennial celebration at the Bellevue-Stratford Hotel in Philadelphia. Two days after the start of the annual American Legion Convention, one veteran after another became ill. Ultimately, 221 were stricken and 34 eventually died. Fearing the worst, pandemonium broke out. Even though the disease did not clinically resemble influenza, the Secretary of Health, Education, and Welfare (HEW) David Mathews suggested there was a "possibility" that the swine flu virus was causing the illnesses. Congress was forced -- by the press and a panicked public -- to halt the debate with pharma over money and take action.

On August 12, 1976 President Ford signed the National Swine Flu Immunization Program and Tort Claim Bill of 1976 into law.[46] With the funding in place for the manufacturers to make the vaccine, and with liability protection also in place to satisfy the insurance providers, both parties had a green light to proceed. The national program was launched with the intent of vaccinating every man, woman, and child in America with an untested, fast-tracked swine flu vaccine.

LEARN MORE

It wasn't until six months later, on January 18, 1977, that the causative agent for the outbreak in Philadelphia was determined to be a bacteria that was ultimately named *Legionella* and the infection became known as Legionnaires Disease. Analysis revealed that the source of the organism was the hotel's water tower that circulated through its air conditioning system. Since that time, water-pumped air conditioning systems in the Bellevue-Stratford Hotel have been changed and federal agencies have tightened regulations for public buildings that still have water cooling towers as part of their air conditioning systems.

A Gallup Poll conducted in late August 1976 showed that 93 percent of Americans were aware of the mass vaccination program, but only 52 percent intended to get the shot. A bigger push was needed to ensure the success of the lofty goals of the nationwide vaccination plan. Based on the results of the August poll, an unprecedented national media campaign was launched to convince the wary public to participate in the program. The government's unwavering message, sent out through every form of media, was that the vaccine was both "safe and necessary."

But not everyone was convinced, and the campaign had a few outspoken opponents.

Dr. Russell Alexander of the Public Health School at the University of Washington emerged as the principal voice of reason calling for more evidence before proceeding with the massive roll out plan. His general view was that *"you should be conservative about putting foreign material into the human body." (emphasis added)* That's always true… but especially when you are talking about injecting 200 million bodies. The need should be estimated conservatively. If you don't need to give it, don't."[47]

His views were strongly supported by Director of the New Jersey Public Health Laboratories, Dr. Martin Goldfield, who had first identified the virus at Fort Dix as a swine virus. He challenged the decision – made primarily by politicians – to mass vaccinate the general public. Ignoring the bureaucratic hierarchy, Goldfield repeatedly expressed his fierce opposition at CDC meetings, and he was repeatedly ignored. Out of frustration and serious concern for the public, he released his opinions to the rapacious press. A transcript of his interview on "The CBS Evening News" clearly documented Goldfield's position: "There are as many dangers to going ahead with vaccinating the population as there are withholding it. We can soberly estimate that approximately 15 percent of the entire population will suffer a disabling reaction [from the vaccine]."[47]

LEARN MORE

The FDA and the vaccine manufacturers thought they had all their protections in place by releasing the jabs under an EUA (Emergency Use Authorization). But on June 7, 2024 the 9th Circuit Court ruled 2-1 that the vaccine doesn't prevent transmission (spread) of COVID-19 infection and, because the shot is not given for the benefit of others, the recipient has a right to refuse the injection as a medical treatment. The vaccine does not prevent COVID-19 nor does it stop the spread. It's just a matter of time before an avalanche of lawsuits erupts by people who were not allowed the right to refuse.[44] According to Dr. David Martin, CEO of M·CAM Inc. (the international leader in intellectual property-based financial risk management) during an interview on the Maria Zee Show:

> "The 9th Circuit has determined that Jacobson vs. Massachusetts was misapplied and the illusion that public health interest was being served by this mass vaccination fiasco has been pierced by an appellate Court. We can now legitimately say that the manufacturers willfully misled the public by mislabeling these jabs and calling them a 'vaccine,' which is a violation of Federal Trade Commission Act and a violation of the Deceptive Medical Practice Act internationally. More importantly, when this is applied, all the liability shields for manufacturers, doctors, pharmacists, nurses, hospitals, employers, and anyone who enforced pseudo-mandates falls away. We actually now have the ability to say that the 9th Circuit has held that Jacobson was misapplied, that this did not stop infection, did not stop transmission, and as such, the public was willfully misled, which is a crime. Pfizer, Moderna and other vaccine companies are criminally and financially liable for deceiving the public."[45]

This was not what the administration or public health stalwarts wanted the people to hear. Goldfield was soon after relieved of his duties, inferring that his outspoken opposition to mass vaccination had cost him his job.

There was another outspoken opponent, this time FDA Virus Bureau Director, Dr. Anthony Morris (formerly of HEW). Dr. Morris announced early on that a swine influenza vaccine could not be made because there had never been any cases of swine flu in humans to test its effectiveness. Dr. Morris warned his superiors in the federal government that the vaccine would *"be dangerous and most likely ineffective,"* but they had no interest in his admonishments. (*emphasis added*) Bypassing his superiors, he too went directly to the press, warning the public that the vaccine was going to be unsafe and that a massive epidemic was unlikely to occur. As a result, he was fired from his position at the FDA, his experimental animals were destroyed, and the publication of his findings was blocked. And the vaccine program moved forward unopposed.

On October 1, 1976, the national vaccination campaign began, with the first shot given in Indianapolis, Indiana at the State Fair. Thousands of doctors, nurses, and paramedics across the country volunteered to give shots at medical centers, schools, and firehouses. Between the program's inception and its demise a few weeks later, 40 million Americans – approximately one-third of the adult population of the United States – were vaccinated. This made the program the largest vaccination program ever undertaken in the history of the US up to that time.

1976 SWINE FLU AROUND THE WORLD

The impact of the 1976 swine flu outbreak in South America varied by country. Brazil, Argentina, and Chile reported cases, although historical data on the number of cases, number of vaccines administered, and mortality outcomes remain unknown. Nonetheless, vaccine production began swiftly, and vaccination campaigns were initiated in many countries throughout the South American continent. While the scale and intensity of these vaccination campaigns varied by country, the swine flu vaccines were widely dispersed as a preventive measure.

In Europe, the number of swine flu vaccines administered during the 1976 outbreak also varied by country. Vaccine distribution was coordinated by national health authorities and international organizations. The exact number of vaccines administered remains unknown and varied by country. In total, millions of doses of swine flu vaccine were administered globally during the 1976 outbreak threats.

In America, almost as soon as the program began, reports of injuries started to pour in. Three senior citizens in Pittsburgh who had been vaccinated at the same clinic died within several days of receiving the shot. Officials from the CDC were sent to investigate the deaths, concluding that with "no evidence to suggest" the deaths were caused by the vaccine, the program was encouraged to continue.

COMMENTARY

How similar does the 1976 run-up to mass vaccination sound to the launch of the COVID-19 jab? Those who spoke out, arguing that the jab was unsafe, untested, and had no long term studies were severely censored. In 2021, many lost their jobs, pensions, and reputations, similar to Drs. Alexander, Goldfield, and Morris. Cautious minds could not prevail. Public health officials from coast to coast felt they had an opportunity to do in 1976 what they had not been able to do during the influenza outbreaks in 1957 or 1968. Most importantly, they could accomplish their goals using federal funds and liability protection, with Congress and the President taking ultimate responsibility.

Reports of deaths continued to flow in, and within two weeks after the launch of the program, 33 people who had been vaccinated had died. Most foreboding were the dozens of reports of Guillain-Barré syndrome. Despite widespread reports of paralysis and deaths, the barrage of publicity continued undaunted, culminating on October 14, 1976, with the appearance of President Ford and his family receiving swine flu shots on national television, encouraging all those who had not yet received the vaccine to do so as soon as possible.

However, dissent was growing louder by the week because the facts could not be ignored. The CDC's epidemiologists were clearly stating there was no evidence of human-to-human transmission of the swine flu virus and that no further cases of the swine flu virus had occurred in humans. Local doctors were having second thoughts about administering the vaccine and patients were mostly refusing it. A mere six weeks after his dramatic vaccination and appeal to the general public, the president once again appeared on national television, this time to concur with the CDC's decision to suspend the program. But as can only happen in Washington, he simultaneously defended the original decision to vaccinate the entire country to protect its citizens against a non-existent swine flu pandemic. When the CDC issued a press release on December 14, 1976 stating that cases of GBS had been reported in ten states, enough was enough – the program was officially suspended ten weeks after it began.[47]

According to a report in *Newsweek,* posted July 18, 1977, claims totaling more than $1.3 billion were filed by the 532 people who contracted GBS after the swine flu vaccination. While many recovered in the ensuing months, 32 died and up to ten percent remained paralyzed to varying degrees for the rest of their lives.

Because the drug companies had been protected by The Swine Flu Act, claims for injury compensation had to be filed with the federal government. The new Secretary of HEW, Joseph A. Califano Jr., responded to the difficulties experienced when the program erupted into litigation. He declared that, with respect to those alleging GBS, the policy of the government was "to provide compensation to all who contracted GBS from the swine flu vaccine **without having to prove negligence.**" *(emphasis added)*

Instead, claimants only needed to show they had been vaccinated with the swine flu vaccine, had developed Guillain-Barré as a result of a swine flu vaccine, and had suffered damages as a result of that condition.

The Secretary gave two reasons for this policy:

> "First, the informed consent form did not adequately warn individuals that there was a one in 100,000 risk that a person receiving the swine flu shot could contract Guillain-Barré and that one in every two million would die from the condition. Second, with the swine flu program, the Federal Government, in an unprecedented effort, actively urged millions of Americans to get the vaccination and funded the nationwide campaign. Thus we have decided to provide **just compensation** for those who contracted Guillain-Barré as a result of the swine flu program rather than force many individuals to prove government negligence in protracted proceedings."[48]

Although Califano's statement was affirmed and upheld by the Tenth Circuit Court, and it appeared to be a straightforward way to collect damages from the government, it was many years before the victims received their settlements.

Skeptics argued that the Ford administration, already grappling with a stagnant economy and weakened public trust from the highly contentious pardon of former President Richard Nixon, was desperate for a rallying point. The swine flu crisis provided just what was needed. But whatever the motivations, less than 30 percent of adults bothered to get vaccinated. In a belated postscript in *Time Magazine* (1999) ranked the swine flu vaccine 85th on its list of the "100 Worst Ideas of the Century."[49]

LEARN MORE

Guillain-Barré syndrome (GBS) an inflammatory disorder of the peripheral nerves (those outside the brain and spinal cord). Called an "ascending paralysis," GBS starts in the feet and moves up the body, quickly involving the diaphragm and other muscles that aid in breathing. If not treated emergently, GBS can result in respiratory failure. Maximal muscle weakness typically occurs two weeks after the onset of GBS. Treatment often involves long-term hospitalization in the ICU with many patients remaining on a ventilator for many months. Neurorehab can take months to years. GBS can also be triggered by a seasonal influenza vaccine with an estimated 40 cases of GBS occurring each year related to seasonal flu shots.

And what came of the killer epidemic? It never emerged.

It is thought that the total number of cases attributed to swine flu was six and perhaps it was really just one. With all the money spent and the many lives ruined, no outbreaks occurred following the initial few cases at Fort Dix. During the height of the swine flu hype, antibody testing suggested that as many as 500 asymptomatic recruits had been exposed to the swine flu virus. None of the civilians or pigs on any of the farms in the surrounding area tested positive for the specific swine flu virus seen in the army recruits. Even the WHO stated it never detected any signs of the virus internationally, even though millions were tested and vaccinated worldwide. In addition, the swine flu virus was only detected at Fort Dix and no other military bases. A question comes to mind regarding the swine flu "outbreak" that needs to be asked:

Could the Fort Dix recruits have been exposed to something either intentionally or unintentionally that led to an outbreak of illness that was blamed on a virus? We will never know.[47]

HIGHLIGHT

The rollout of the experimental, non-tested COVID-19 jabs produced by Pfizer, Moderna, AstraZeneca, and Johnson & Johnson had begun. Even though a large number of deaths were reported within the first few weeks of January 2021, there were no recalls and no cancellations. The fear-based plan for pushing the jab into the arms of every adult around the world continued for nearly three years, with boosters that are still being advocated. Even now, the COVID-19 bioweapon is treated by government officials as though it is no different than the annual flu shot, advising the shots should be given to everyone six months and older, including pregnant women. And yet, with all the irrefutable evidence that has come out about the illnesses, disabilities, and deaths caused by the COVID-19 shots, the US government has still not removed them from the market nor has it assumed any responsibility.

SMALLPOX: DIFFERENT SCARE, SAME HYPE

The swine flu fiasco took place in 1976. Fast forward 20 years.

The nation's Department of Defense (DoD) and national security divisions were quietly rumbling about the possibility of an act of bioterrorism occurring on US soil. Concerns were discussed with the public health sector about how to protect the country in the event of an attack with a biological weapon. As early as 1999, twenty-one representatives from major medical and research centers, government, military, public health, and emergency management institutions and agencies met to develop a plan to protect the civilian population in the event of a terrorist attack.[50]

Then, the events of September 11, 2001 occurred, commonly referred to as 9/11.

Soon after that eventful day, white powder, thought to be anthrax spores, was discovered in Congressional quarters. Then the Iraqi president, Saddam Hussein, was thought to be harboring massive canisters of anthrax and smallpox; the prevailing sentiment was that he could be planning an "immediate attack" on the American people. Something needed to be done.

Just like the discovery of the isolated swine flu case, government officials bolted off to form a vaccination plan, develop a whole new vaccine, and pass legislation to change public policy. Only this time, there was not even one case of smallpox. The flurry of activity was based only on a *presumption*. But the CDC was one step ahead of the game. In what can be described as a somewhat eerie move, the new recommendations for using the smallpox vaccine had just been issued three months before the attack, in *June 2001*, an update of a policy that had not been reviewed for more than ten years. With the resolutions in place, the government began throwing billions of dollars toward its preferred public health solution: massive vaccination.[50]

However, there was a significant shift in the design of the smallpox mass vaccination plan for 2002. The planning went beyond bureaucratic meetings and opening the government's financial coffers as they did during the swine flu campaign. The CDC held unprecedented town meetings in select locations across the country to solicit feedback from local public health officials and to listen to the concerns of citizens about the possibility of mandatory smallpox vaccination. In parallel with the town meetings, the media ramped up the dire predictions of massive death rates from the scourge of smallpox. The specter of mandatory vaccination erupted on the front page of newspapers and rode the radio airwaves all across the country. Experts on the subject were guests on television talk shows from Oprah to Bill O'Reilly. I was able to attend and participate in two of the CDC town meetings, one in St. Louis and one in Atlanta, to stand against the ramp up of the campaign to reintroduce mass vaccination of the general public with the smallpox vaccine.

In the midst of the drama, factual discrepancies about smallpox infections began to appear. What was being propagated by the government and parroted by the media as the "generally accepted facts" about smallpox simply weren't the "real facts" at all. Refuting those myths was an important step to calm the public's fears; understanding that the same hyperbole had been used to fan the flames of fear about swine flu and smallpox will quell today's fears about smallpox and all future pandemics. Note the similarities between swine flu (1976), smallpox (2002), bird flu (2005), COVID-19, and in 2024, bird flu and monkeypox.

Myth #1: Smallpox is highly contagious.
Fact #1: No, it is not.

During the Town Meeting held in St. Louis on June 8, 2002, Dr. Joel Kuritsky, director of the National Immunization Program and the Early Smallpox Response and Planning task force at the CDC stated clearly, *"Smallpox has a slow transmission and is not highly contagious."* That is a direct contradiction to nearly everything that was being said, or being written, about smallpox throughout the mainstream media.

Correspondingly, bird flu in 2005 was not highly contagious either. There had been no sustained person-to-person transmission and humans seemed to be highly resistant to developing problems thought to be associated with the H5N1 virus. The September 29, 2005, issue of the *New England Journal of Medicine* reported the following:

"The relatively low frequency of influenza A (H5N1) illness in humans despite widespread exposure to infected poultry indicates that the species barrier to acquisition of this avian virus is substantial. Clusters of cases in few family members may be caused by common exposures, although the genetic factors that may affect a host's susceptibility to disease warrant study."[51]

In plain language this means that even with constant exposure to the virus, most people are immune and do not develop symptoms of the flu. Keep in mind that the H5N1 has been around for many years. It hasn't "jumped species" in decades.

A similar plea to "do your part" and "protect grandma" was a loud cry during COVID-19 when the survival rate in all age groups, babies to grandparents was known to be 98.2% or better.

Myth #2: Smallpox is easily spread by casual contact with an infected person.

Fact #2: No, it is not.

Smallpox will not rapidly disseminate throughout a community. "The infection is spread by droplet contamination; coughing or sneezing is not generally part of the infection. Smallpox will not spread like wildfire," said Dr. Walter A. Orenstein, Director of the CDC's National Immunization Program (NIP), at the town meeting held in Atlanta on June 20, 2002.

At the national Town Meetings, CDC officials set the record straight about the spread of smallpox. At the Atlanta town meeting Dr. Kuritsky stated:

> "Given the slow transmission rate and that **people need to be in close contact for nearly a week** to spread the infection, the scenario in which a terrorist could infect himself with smallpox and contaminate an entire city by walking through the streets touching people is purely fiction." *(emphasis added)*

He went on to describe that 37 percent of smallpox cases in Africa and India had a transmission of only one generation, meaning that if a second person contracted smallpox, he did not pass it onto a third person. This explanation, offered by one of the heads of the CDC and an expert on smallpox epidemiology, definitively contradicted models reported on the news that predicted a fast, exponential spread from a few to millions.

Similar to the media myth that smallpox spreads rapidly, there was no meaningful person-to-person transmission from either the 2005 nor the 2024 bird flu scares. Further substantiating the lack of person-to-person transmission, there were essentially no transmissions from COVID-infected patients to healthcare workers in hospital settings, **even when generally accepted isolation measures were not used.** In fact, there was only one confirmed case – in the whole world – of a person-to-person transmission between a critically ill adult woman to her unprotected aunt. Without person-to-person transmission there is no pandemic. As with smallpox, the bird flu pandemic hype turned out to be "purely fiction."[52]

Myth #3: There is no treatment for smallpox.
Fact #3: More accurately, "there were no pharmaceutical drugs for the treatment of smallpox."

Smallpox infections occurred with varying degrees of severity. The most common, called "ordinary discrete smallpox," occurred in more than 40 percent of cases. Manifesting as a small scattering of pustules distributed across the body; the person was marginally ill and required minimal medical care. For mild cases, adequate hydration and fever control for comfort, and to maintain a temperature below 102°F (38.8°C), was the only necessary care. Keeping the skin clean to prevent secondary bacterial infections was also important. The 1927 edition of the *Textbook of Medicine* recommended the use of carbolic acid-soaked gauze to reduce itching and minimize scarring of the skin. Carbolic acid, known for its antiseptic properties, was also commonly applied to manage acute skin ulcerations, helping to alleviate the sharp, pricking pain associated with such conditions.

Myth #4: The death rate from smallpox was 30%.
Fact #4: No, it was not.

Even though nearly every newspaper, magazine article, and television report before and after 2002 has quoted the CDC-generated statistic of a 30 percent death rate from smallpox, the actual death rate was somewhere between 4.2 and 15%.

Tom Mack, MD, MPH, retired from both the University of Southern California (USC) and the CDC, reported at the Atlanta town meeting that the 30 percent fatality rate came from skewed data. Mack claimed to have seen more than 120 smallpox outbreaks in Pakistan during his CDC career in the 1970s. His observation was that villages would have "an importation" every five to ten years, regardless of vaccination status, and the outbreak was always predicated by living conditions and close living arrangements. There were many small outbreaks and individual cases that never came to the attention of the local authorities because *the infection was so mild the person did not seek medical attention.*

Dr. Mack stated that even with a lack of medical care, the case fatality rate in adults was "much lower than is generally advertised" and was really much closer to 10 or 15 percent. His observation was that the statistics were "loaded with children that had a much higher fatality," making the death rate appear much higher than it actually was. Amazingly, he revealed his opinion that "even without mass vaccination, smallpox would have died out anyway. It just would have taken longer."

> NOTE: *The information in quotation marks was taken verbatim from the transcript of the CDC town meeting held in Atlanta on June 19 and 20, 2002. This document, which I have in my possession, is no longer available online. The CDC has replaced the transcript of the town meeting with a summary.*

In an article published in the New England Journal of Medicine on January 30, 2003 entitled, "A Different View of Smallpox and Vaccination," Dr. Mack wrote, "Smallpox is not as infectious as its reputation would suggest...variola major was almost always transmitted at the bedside of the source, not at an external location... None of the 945 cases [of] disease was contracted on an airplane, train, or bus. Any spread into the community from an introduction would thus be limited."[54]

Similarly, the actual death rate from bird flu in 2005, reported by the media to be nearly 50 percent, was completely unknown. Only the deaths of very ill people who died in hospitals and had tested positive for H5N1 were reported. Given how many people in Southeast Asia and across the globe live with and handle poultry, many had uneventful contact with the H5N1 virus. Farmers in Southeast Asia literally sleep with their birds and there was no transmission from birds to humans.

Hundreds, perhaps thousands, of individuals with H5N1 influenza were not sick enough to require medical care, as confirmed by Dick Thompson, spokesperson for the WHO. In an interview with Center for Infectious Disease Research and Policy (CIDRAP) News in March 2005, Thompson stated,

> "The obvious assumption is that others are infected, and either not getting sick, or are not getting sick enough to seek treatment at a hospital. Factoring those patients into the death rate [makes it] impossible to determine, because the denominator is unknown."[55]

Dr. John Allen Paulos, professor of mathematics at Temple University, concurred with Thompson's observation. Based only on cases of severely ill people, Paulos asserts that the reported death rate was an "almost textbook case" of sample bias. He explained that asymptomatic people and those who recovered uneventfully, weren't part of the mortality rate calculations. As a consequence, **the numbers were**

skewed substantially upward. Therefore, the reported "nearly 50 percent" fatality rate – like the smallpox 30 percent fatality rate – was a mathematical absurdity promoted for the sole purpose of frightening the public into accepting massive government regulations and submitting to mandatory vaccination. This was similar to those who were told they may be an "asymptomatic COVID-19 carrier" – a healthy person – who was then coerced into receiving the COVID-19 shots.

Myth #5: The vaccine prevents infection.
Fact #5: No, it will not.

Most people still believe that vaccines prevent them from contracting a disease, a 200-year-old premise that is simply not true. Further, it is assumed that the presence of a vaccine-induced antibody is what prevents an infection, another unproven assumption. The measurement of an amount of antibody in the blood is called a **titer;** titers have not been proven to correlate with protection.[56] Many literature reports and even more clinical observations have definitely demonstrated that fully vaccinated people, who have adequate levels of "protective antibody," can contract the illness for which they have been vaccinated.

Even the CDC admits the smallpox vaccine did not prevent infection. Dr. Harold Margolis, Senior Advisor to the Director of the CDC's Smallpox Planning and Response task force, stated at the St. Louis town meeting that "the vaccine decreased the death rate among those vaccinated by 'modifying the disease,' **not by preventing infection.**" *(emphasis added)* That means, if a person had been vaccinated, they had a milder case of the disease… but they still got the disease.

LEARN MORE

The 1999 JAMA article, "Smallpox as a Biological Weapon Medical and Public Health Management," concluded with this statement:

> "Specific recommendations are made regarding smallpox vaccination, therapy, postexposure isolation and infection control, hospital epidemiology and infection control, home care, decontamination of the environment, and additional research is needed. In the event of an actual release of smallpox and subsequent epidemic, early detection, isolation of infected individuals, surveillance of contacts, and a focused selective vaccination program will be the essential items of an effective control program."

How similar does this sound to the conclusions formed at the Event 201 meeting, a high-level pandemic exercise held on October 18, 2019, in New York? The meeting was hosted by the World Economic Forum, the Bill and Melinda Gates Foundation, and The Johns Hopkins Center for Health Security. At the conclusion of the meeting, experts agreed that it was "only a matter of time" before a pandemic with potentially catastrophic consequences occurred that would require "reliable cooperation among several industries, national governments, and key international institutions." They prophetically predicted "The next severe pandemic will not only cause great illness and loss of life but could also trigger major cascading economic and societal consequences that could contribute greatly to global impact and suffering." Five months later, the world was on fire with COVID-19.[53] From what we have learned about the fallacy of COVID-19 testing, we now know to ask: Did they die from the virus or *with the virus?* Or was the cause of death from something else entirely?

ANOTHER GOVERNMENT-FUNDED VACCINE

Despite the candid comments made by public health officials at the town meetings in 2002 regarding the low degree of harmfulness (low virulence) of smallpox, stories of "what would happen in the event of an outbreak" continued to blare across the airwaves of the mainstream media. At the same time, billions of dollars were poured into emergency planning and vaccine production proceeded.

On May 5, 2003, HHS Secretary Tommy Thompson announced the release of $100 million to "strengthen the public health infrastructure in preparation for a bioterrorism event." The funds, immediately available for use, were in addition to the $1.1 billion set aside in fiscal year 2002 for preparations at the state level and the $1.4 billion already allocated in 2003 for a national smallpox program preparation. This increased the total expenditures in 2003 for bioterrorism preparedness, including research into potential disease agents, treatments, and vaccines, to $3.5 billion – up substantially from funds allocated in 2002. The full details of the CDC and HHS rollout plan can be found in the referenced 370-page report, "The Smallpox Vaccination Program - Public Health in the Age of Terrorism."[57]

The media hype didn't end when the immediate concerns regarding a smallpox terrorist event subsided. In fact, in January 2005, a made-for-television movie aired on the FX Channel was created to show what could happen to a community if smallpox arrived in its town. The show, *"Smallpox,"* was produced in documentary style, creating a fictionalized "look back" to the year 2002 when a smallpox outbreak killed 60 million people. The tag line for the movie was, "It's all true. It just hasn't happened yet."[58] This was one of many predictive programming pieces that have come out over the last 20 years, building up to the global COVID-19 fiasco. After all, the WEF brags that they have been working on their plan for at least 50 years.

When President Carter was sworn into office in 1977, the fallout from the swine flu program was still in full swing. Administration officials asked Dr. Harvey Feinberg, the 1982 president of the Institute of Medicine (IOM), and Dr. Richard Neustadt to review the swine influenza program, focusing specifically on the decision-making processes. Neustadt later compiled their findings into the book, *The Epidemic That Never Was: Policy-Making and the Swine Flu Scare* (1982), which revealed significant flaws in decision-making during the swine flu program.

In a second book, *The Swine Flu Affair: Decision-Making on a Slippery Disease,* written by both Feinberg and Neustadt and published in 2005 further explained and summarized the problems:

- Overconfidence by specialists in theories that came from meager evidence
- Convictions fueled by preexisting personal agendas
- Premature commitment to decisions without enough information
- Zeal by health professionals at the CDC and NIH who pressured their lay superiors in government to "do the right thing" and quickly roll out a vaccine
- Failure to address uncertainties in a way that allowed for reconsideration
- Insufficient questioning of scientific logic vs dogma
- Insufficient questioning of the program's implementation plan
- Insensitivity to media relations and to the long-term credibility of government institutions: CDC, HHS, NIH, and Congress

Does this sound familiar?

Those in charge of Operation Warp Speed and other elements of the COVID-19 pandemic would have been well-served to read the report and the books written about the swine flu fiasco. The occurrences, even the conversations within the swine flu plan (1976), the smallpox plan (2002), and the bird flu plan (2005) are eerily similar to the bigger and better orchestrated COVID 19 plan. Those fanning the flames to create recurrent "pandemic scares" should have listened to Feinberg and Neustadt, who were quick to point out that new influenza strains can occur in clusters, causing small outbreaks without becoming widespread.

Government officials have not learned lessons from the past, demonstrating that each outbreak, past and future, is an opportunity to move forward a much larger agenda. Each event has been a market test to see how far the globalists could push their plans on the citizenry for obedience and total control. Notice how each time, when grass roots and scientific resistance got loud enough and gained the attention of the people, the outbreaks faded away as quickly as they began. Time and resources would then be used to crunch the data and evaluate the outcomes that had been achieved based on these or similar questions:

- What tactics worked?
- What didn't work?
- What should we do more of next time?
- What should we not waste time or resources on?
- What laws had been passed?
- What financial protections for the drug companies had permanently been put in place?
- What recourses had been established to silence opposition?
- By using hyped fear and mainstream media messaging, how much domination were we able to obtain?

The swine flu, smallpox, and bird flu threats and the government's response have been used to craft a template for future power grabs by the pharmaceutical industry, controlling politicians, governments and global institutions.

After the media blitz whips the public into a panic about the threat of a pandemic, Americans tend to fall back into their generally apathetic state. Look at what has happened since the COVID-19 restrictions have been lifted. Most people do not want to participate in forming a plan to keep this from happening again; most just want to go back to their baseline status quo of business as usual, travel, and playing video games. Authorities need to create another scare tactic, something to keep everyone psychologically on edge about the possibility of a "death angel" sweeping round the globe before a vaccine can be developed and released, and the government's next-level control plan can be put in place.

When the swine flu pandemic and the smallpox plan failed to get everyone on board with fear-based mass vaccination campaigns, the government needed a new plan. Let's examine the development of the 2003-5 bird flu pandemic, an event which has permanently secured the legal and financial framework for what became COVID-19 and the playbook for future pandemic charades.

*"We cannot banish dangers, but we can banish fears.
We must not demean life by standing in awe of death."*

~David Sarnoff, radio and television pioneer

CHAPTER 7
A New Playbook Focused on Fear

Many people's indifference toward the overly hyped pandemics reflects a broader disinterest in vaccination programs. This same apathy is increasingly evident toward the annual flu shot campaigns – where alarmist messaging has lost its impact, and public engagement has waned. Unsurprisingly, public health officials are far from pleased.

Every winter it is reported that millions of people around the world get the flu. Coworkers and classmates are home for about a week, sick and miserable. A few – mostly the elderly and infirm – die. We have been told the annual death toll from influenza is 30,000 to 70,000 in the US and a few hundred thousand more around the globe. However, this computer-generated number leaves gaping holes in the government's credibility because medical authorities don't separate and verify those who died of influenza from those who died of an "influenza-like illness" or from complications of the flu, most commonly, bacterial pneumonia.

The number of deaths from the flu has long been overstated. In fact, the American Lung Association kept meticulous records through 2015 that distinguished the total number of deaths from influenza from the number of deaths from pneumonia. For example, in 2010, there were 49,597 deaths due to pneumonia and only 274 deaths reported from influenza. In 2013, there were 53,282 deaths due to pneumonia but only 3,550 deaths from influenza. In those two years, and others, the number of deaths from influenza was a far cry from the 36,000 reported.[59]

More recently, the CDC has changed its rhetoric, proposing the impact from influenza ranged from 3,000 to 49,000 yearly deaths. When actual death certificates are tallied, influenza deaths are, on average, around 1,000 per year, mostly in the elderly. So, while the actual threat is unknown (but likely to be exaggerated), the estimated impact of influenza vaccination is small at best.[60]

Near the end of the COVID era (2023), the data was clear: death from influenza is enormously overstated. The data reported by *Statista* showed that the number of deaths from pneumonia (1,147,399) far exceeded the number of deaths from influenza (22,256), still well under the 36,000 parroted across the airwaves by the mainstream media.[61]

Most people have a casual attitude about the flu vaccine. After an initial response in the fall to advertisements on the radio and the evening news, few pay much attention. The government was finding it increasingly difficult to whip up fear about the flu, no matter how many articles or news reports of "catastrophic concern" were published. So, a new scary disease needed to be put forth. SARS fit the bill.

SARS: THE WARM-UP DANCE

The first case of "mysterious new flu" was reported in South China in November 2002. Named SARS (Severe Acute Respiratory Syndrome), the WHO issued the first global alert in early March 2003. Teams of experts were sent to investigate the outbreak. The ominous concern ramped up quickly and within just a few weeks, the Hong Kong Department of Health issued a quite unprecedented quarantine order to keep residents inside their homes. Mainland China followed suit shortly thereafter, with authorities closing cinemas, libraries and even public schools with the goal of stopping the spread of the virus.

At the same time, scientists began feverishly working to try to determine the cause of SARS. On April 16, 2003, the WHO announced that the pathogen had been identified. It was a member of the coronavirus family "not previously seen in humans."

In Canada, more and more cases began to be reported in Toronto, and Canadian health officials also implemented similar measures to China, telling residents to quarantine and wear masks.

Does this sound familiar?

Over a period of six months, 8,422 people tested positive for the virus in 2003. Asia (China, Taiwan and Hong Kong) had the vast majority of cases at 7,248 reported, including 774 deaths, approximately 10 percent of all **known cases.** But since the total number of cases only represented those ill enough to seek medical help, the actual death rate is unknown and was no doubt far less.

The 2003 SARS experience taught officials a critically important lesson. The economic impact of the six-month SARS period was huge. Although only about 250 Canadians were affected, and only about 40 died, the Canadian Tourism Board estimated the cost of the "outbreak" to be $419 million. Ontario's health minister reported the province's healthcare system cost impact to be $763 million. This estimate included money spent to develop special clinics and stock the facilities with supplies.

SARS also had a significant effect on global travel, in particular the airline industry. Flights to Asia and the Pacific Rim dropped by 45 percent; for example, flights between the US and Hong Kong dropped nearly 70 percent. Singapore Airlines, the world's second-largest airline by market value at the time (US budget carrier

Southwest Airlines is the first), lost $6 million *per day* during April and May during the travel reduction.

Other industries also suffered, including the hotel industry as well as restaurants and retail sales.

Workplace absenteeism affected every industry. The WHO estimated the economic consequences of the worldwide SARS "epidemic" to be more than $30 billion. Undeniably, there is a genuine downside to issuing warnings that turn out to be more hype than substance.

As concerns about SARS quickly faded in late 2003, the promotional efforts for the ramp up of the 2004 influenza vaccine season were hitting bumps. Vaccination rates were low and falling, and manufacturers were moaning about the surplus of flu shots sitting on the shelves. Leaning on their government partners to "do something" to encourage people to get a flu shot, David Morens, an NIH scientist and historian of influenza, went public and emphasized the need to strengthen vaccination efforts, saying, **"Annual influenza vaccination is and _must remain_ among the most important public health priorities."** (*emphasis added*) To condition everyone to get a flu shot that fall, including the "worried well," a plan was presented called the *"Seven Step Recipe for Generating Interest in, and Demand for, Flu (or any other) Vaccination,"* engineered to guarantee the economic success of the 2004-5 season's flu vaccine production line. This "recipe" was developed by Glen Nowak, PhD, the Associate Director for Communications for the National Immunization Program at the CDC.[18]

This is a summary of Novak's Seven Step "recipe". Released for the 2004-5 influenza season, there should be little doubt how intensively the media is used to drive demand for the pharmaceutical product.

Step 1: Start discussing the flu at the beginnng of the "immunization season."

Step 2: Media outlets are to make pronouncements that the "new" strain is anticipated as a "severe illness and/or serious outcomes."

Step 3: Media is to invite local and national medical experts and public health authorities on as guests to "state concern and alarm (and predicting dire outcomes) and urge influenza vaccination."

Step 4: Reports by experts will be used to "frame the flu season in terms [that will] motivate behavior." Recommended language to be used includes, "very severe," "more severe than last or past years," and, "deadly." Phrases should include, "this could be the worst flu season ever," "the flu kills 36,000 people per year," and, "the flu shot is the best way to prevent the flu."

Step 5: The media is urged to report that influenza is causing "severe illness" and is "affecting lots of people." The intent is to "foster the perception" that the flu is serious without the vaccine.

Step 6: The media is given explicit instructions: Use pictures of people getting shots and find families who are willign to tell their story about the flu. The intent is "first to motivate, the latter is to reinforce" the necessity of getting the vaccine.

Step 7: To drive the message home, television anchors are to make references to pandemic influenza and continually reinforce the importance of vaccination.

The meticulously scheduled, mostly fear-based messages were used to convince the uninterested public that not only was the flu shot necessary, *Americans should be demanding it.* By announcing the locations of flu shot clinics throughout a community via local radio stations and evening news, the air waves and their broadcasters became accomplices to the injection of toxic products into humans. The "community service" announcements are actually millions of dollars of free advertising to vaccine manufacturers.

For most Americans, the flu season is usually little more than an inconvenience. Even controversies such as vaccine shortages and contaminated vaccine batches barely made a blip on the proverbial radar screen for most people. For example, a few weeks in the fall of 2003, the media hyped vaccine shortages and showed images of people standing in line for hours to be vaccinated. But by January 2004, so few had gotten flu shots, a vaccine glut resulted, leading to the abandonment of rationing, and the authorities began to urge everyone to once again get in line to eliminate the "vaccine excess."

The CDC admits that the flu shot will not prevent influenza-like illnesses; therefore, many people who get the flu shot will still get "the flu."[62]

Similarly, a person can get the flu shot and still get the flu; adults can get one to three episodes and children can get three to six episodes of an influenza-like illness *each year* even after they have been vaccinated. An "influenza-like illness" (ILI) is a respiratory infection characterized by fever, fatigue, cough, and other symptoms that are identical to what we call "the flu" but the illness is caused by another viral family, such as rhinoviruses, adenoviruses, parainfluenza viruses, metapneumoviruses, the respiratory syncytial virus (RSV), and normally circulating coronaviruses. More than 200 viruses can cause ILI.

Without laboratory tests, doctors cannot distinguish between ILI and influenza because both last for days and rarely cause serious illness or death.

Approximately 20 percent of common colds each year are caused by one of the coronaviruses.[63]

First identified in the 1960s, there are seven human coronaviruses, and four are considered endemic, meaning they are present throughout the year. Here is a list of the seven coronaviruses that can infect people:[64]

1. **Human coronavirus 229E (HCoV-229E)** - Alphacoronavirus
2. **Human coronavirus NL63 (HCoV-NL63)** - Alphacoronavirus
3. **Human coronavirus OC43 (HCoV-OC43)** - Betacoronavirus
4. **Human coronavirus HKU1 (HCoV-HKU1)** - Betacoronavirus
5. **Severe Acute Respiratory Syndrome coronavirus (SARS CoV)** - Betacoronavirus (responsible for SARS pandemic in 2002-4)
6. **Middle East Respiratory Syndrome coronavirus (MERS-CoV)** - Betacoronavirus
7. **Severe Acute Respiratory Syndrome coronavirus 2 (SARS CoV-2)** - most likely a laboratory manipulated Betacoronavirus (responsible for COVID-19)

Coronaviruses circulate widely in animals and in birds, particularly chickens. Of the avian coronaviruses, the one that has been studied most extensively is the Avian Infectious Bronchitis Virus (IBV), which, not surprisingly, causes infectious bronchitis. A highly contagious respiratory illness, an infection can lead to reduced egg production, and, in some cases, damage to the kidneys and reproductive systems. Although avian coronaviruses differ from the human-infecting coronaviruses, they belong to the same *Coronavirus* family and share some of the same structural and replication similarities.

That coronaviruses are found in chickens is more than just a point of passing interest. If a hen is infected with IBV, the virus can be present in its eggs, in the egg white or the yoke, or found externally on the eggshell. Called vertical transmission, the virus can be passed from mother to offspring. Eggs used for vaccine production are called Specific Pathogen-free Eggs (discussed in Chapter 11); it is disturbing to note that even these highly specialized eggs are not routinely tested for the presence of coronaviruses. This means that coronaviruses could be in routine flu shots, and flu shot recipients may have had antibodies against coronaviruses in their bodies from a flu shot or from a previous coronavirus infection. Was anyone tested for corona antibodies prior to receiving the COVID-19 jab? Assuredly not. This could have been a contributing factor to many of the serious side effects that were seen associated with the COVID-19 jabs.

MOVING ON TO BIRD FLU 2004

As the concerns about SARS faded into the spring of 2004, the usual "recipe" started all over again in the fall of 2004 in an attempt to push sales for the annual flu vaccine. "Make a plan, then work the plan," comes to mind. But the same old plan had worn thin. The general public shrugged at the public service announcements, knowing the flu was an inconvenience, not a catastrophic illness. The messages seen everywhere, "It's flu season" (really, flu SHOT season) begins at about the same time every year, with the same regularity as the swallows returning to Capistrano.

We learned retrospectively that the bird flu scare caused similar economic consequences to those experienced in 2024. In 2004, more than 200 million domestic birds were killed in at least ten countries, even if they were not sick and were not infected by the virus. The cost to various local economies was estimated to be in the tens of millions. And based on information that was pumped out daily through every possible media outlet, the bird flu pandemic was predicted to cause the "Next Great Depression" and "the end of life as we know it." But if the apocalypse was coming, few in the US seemed overly concerned. People mostly ignored the gloomy scenarios portrayed by the CDC and the WHO. Officials needed to somehow get the attention of the public and motivate participation in preparedness planning without losing credibility.

Enter risk communication.

The field of risk communication was new to public health discussions in 2005, but it really wasn't new. Dating from the early 1980s, it evolved from several different fields of study: health education, public relations, psychology, risk perception, and risk assessment. The CDC commissioned another "recipe," this time from Princeton risk communication experts, Peter M. Sandman, PhD, and Jody Lanard, MD. Their risk communication plan, published in the journal *Perspectives in Health* was based on the three guiding principles:[65]

- **Precaution advocacy** (*"Watch out!"*): How to alert people to serious hazards when they are unduly apathetic.
- **Outrage management** (*"Calm down!"*): How to reassure people about minor hazards when they are unduly upset.
- **Crisis communication** (*"We'll get through it together!"*): How to guide people through serious hazards when they are appropriately upset (or even in denial).

An updated guidebook, called "The Ten-Step Playbook" soon evolved by blending Nowak's 7-step recipe with the plan set forth by the risk communicators. It was updated to get the nation ready for the coming pandemic. Here are the steps proposed by Sandman and Lanard:

Step 1: Start where your audience is

Officials were advised to use empathy instead of scolding people. The idea was to make "common cause with the public", talk about how horrible the pandemic is likely to be, and get people concerned. In other words, officials didn't tell people the answer, but led them to the conclusion.

Step 2: Don't be afraid to frighten people

Sandman and Lanard advised that fear is fair game: "fear appeals have gotten bad press, but ***the evidence that proves they work is*** *overwhelming."* That said, they advised, *"we can't scare people enough about H5N1.*

Step 3: Acknowledge uncertainty

Sandman used an example of a senior veterinary official from Thailand's public health department. This person stated, "We know it is H5, but we're hoping it won't be H5N1." This highlights two additional risk communication principles: 1) acknowledge uncertainty; and 2) don't overly reassure. Since the 1980s, the CDC has been chanting the mantra that we are "way overdue" for another pandemic. Apparently, the mass media was given a green light to magnify this health concern. Their primary weapon was the creation of ominous warnings and headlines far out of proportion to the actual risks.

Step 4: Share dilemmas

In crisis communication, the tactic of dilemma sharing is designed to humanize the organization making the public health decisions. The whole idea is to give the general population the impression that they have a say, e.g. "we the people" are participating in the planning process. Successful use of this strategy will "reduce the outrage if you turn out to be wrong."

Step 5: Give people things to do

In January 2005, Canadian infectious disease expert Richard Schabas told *The Wall Street Journal,* "Only scaring people about avian influenza accomplishes nothing, because we're not asking people to do anything about it." Schabas suggested also giving people something to do, such as creating plans for catastrophic, global business disruptions. He even suggested having "cognitive and emotional rehearsals – learning about H5N1, thinking about what a pandemic might be like, and planning how to cope."

See how long they've been planning and market testing these tactics?

Practicing for disaster is meant to give a "sense of empowerment," but in real life, may have little practical value. Images of school children hiding under tiny wooden desks during nuclear drills in the 1950s come to mind. In addition, nearly every religious tradition, including Drs. Deepak Chopra, Larry Dossey, and Wayne Dyer, as well as pastors from a number of mega-churches, and inspirational speakers such as Napoleon Hill, Earl Nightingale, and Brian Tracy have defined a consistent, clear message:

"You get what you spend your time thinking about."

Could collective, global "cognitive and emotional rehearsals" that anticipate the worst-case scenario for the disaster, actually make the situation happen? Perhaps visualizing a safe, clean, healthy world, free of all illnesses for humans, birds, and other animals is a better form of "cognitive rehearsal."

Steps 6, 7, and 8 are specific suggestions on how warnings should stress the magnitude of the coming calamity, focusing on "how bad things could get."

Step 9: Guide the adjustment reaction

This boils down to using information to maneuver *(manipulate)* people into a place called a "new normal." This is what is called the Hegelian dialectic: problem-reaction-solution. The solution is what the problem-designers were aiming for from the beginning.

Steps six through nine serve to accentuate Step 2: Don't be afraid to frighten people. Get people fired up. Make them really worried and afraid. Get them to wring their hands and fear present and future pandemics. Get them to stockpile drugs, buy extra food, and store excessive amounts of water. We didn't see a disaster materialize at the Y2K Millennium or with smallpox after 9/11 or with swine flu – but no doubt, a global disaster is just around the next corner that will wipe out everyone and everything. Hurry; pass laws to protect the public. Call up the military. It's coming any minute. Soon. We're due. We're doomed.

Step 10: The last step is to **"inform the public early and aim for total candor and transparency."** Sandman argued that it's almost impossible for governments to be too candid. He warned against declining to answer questions from the press or from the public by using the excuse, "We can't tell you because it's national security."

Admittedly, the last suggestion was, and remains, the most difficult for governments to adopt, especially in the US. The government has collaborated with its many hundreds of agencies to hide so many things from its citizens – from vaccine injury cover-ups that included thimerosal to the known deadly problems with the anti-inflammatory Vioxx. Do government officials have the ability to be "transparent"?

COMPARISONS

It is rather apparent that Sandman's playbook was used to help orchestrate the entire COVID-19 power grab. Let's take a look at the fear factors used in 2004 with the rhetoric that was used during the COVID-19 pandemic.

Step 1: Start where your audience is

Step 2: Don't be afraid to frighten people

Where was nearly every person in America when COVID-19 started in March 2020? They were glued to the daily reports on television as officials hammered home their fear-based messages, the primary psychological weapon. How many times did we see that Chinese gentleman collapse and presumably die from COVID-19 while walking through a mall near a people-mover? How many times did we see terrified people in full-body HAZMAT suits hugging each other without touching each other?

How many hundreds of times were fear-based pictures blasted across the TV screen and social media pages?

Step 3: Acknowledge uncertainty

Step 4: Share dilemmas

Phrases such as, "We don't know when the second wave will come," and "the situation is evolving" were used endlessly to hold us hostage, keep us shut in, and to shut down our businesses. Every day, Drs. Fauci and Birx appeared for their situation update and told the American people, "We're doing the best we can" to get the situation under control, so we can "flatten the curve." As stated by Sandman in 2005:

> "Dilemma-sharing does raise some anxiety at first, but… this leads to better buy-in and better coping down the road. And it reduces the outrage *if you turn out to be wrong*." *(emphasis added)*

Step 5: Give people things to do (or not do)

COVID-19 officials gave us plenty to do. Here are a few:

- Wear face masks, even when in your car alone, and even though more than 150 studies have been published that prove masks don't protect from infection. More recently, it has been published that components in the mask, including high micro- and nanoplastics, volatile organic compounds, acrolein, phthalates, lead, cadmium, and more, can make the wearer sick.[66]
- Stand six feet apart, a completely fabricated number lacking any scientific basis.[67]
- Get tested, frequently and randomly, with a fraudulent PCR nasal swab, even when driving by a testing station.
- Don't sing. Don't play a wind instrument.

- Don't shake hands. Don't touch anyone.
- Don't gather more than 10 people together at a time.
- Don't stay out after 10pm at night.
- Don't visit dying loved ones or those alone in a nursing home.

There are many more. Add to the list all the "duties" you can remember.

Step 6: Speculate responsibly

Step 7: Avoid the "numbers game"

Step 8: Stress magnitude (dramatic warnings)

For months, we heard about the millions who had died from the SARS CoV-2 infection. But the real dramatic warnings should have been about the shots, not an infection which had a negligible mortality rate. As time goes on, we hear more and more about the many millions who have suffered and/or died as a result of being coerced into getting three or more COVID-19 jabs that were not safe, were not protective, and definitely caused harm. An estimate from October 2022 pegged the deaths from the injections to be at about 20 million in the US alone, with more than 2.2 billion people injured globally. That was in 2022; the numbers are no doubt higher now.[68]

In another example, international researchers published a paper in May 2024 that analyzed data from the Italian National Healthcare System. The results showed that COVID-19 specific deaths were not reduced with vaccination and that COVID-19 vaccination did not "save lives" as so many in Washington have proclaimed without evidence. At the time of this writing, hundreds of studies have confirmed this statement and more are forthcoming.[69]

A peer-reviewed study, published in *Public Health Policy and the Law* in November 2024, took the investigation to a deeper level.[70] Researchers reviewed 325 autopsies and one necropsy case. The results were as follows:

1. The mean age of death was 70.4 years. The most implicated organ system among cases was the **cardiovascular system (49%)**, followed by hematological (17%), respiratory (11%), and multiple organ systems (7%).

2. Three or more organ systems were affected in 21 cases. The mean time from vaccination to death was 14.3 days. **Most deaths occurred within a week from the last vaccine administration.**

3. A total of 240 deaths (73.9%) were independently judged as **directly due to or significantly contributed to by COVID-19 jab,** of which the primary causes of death include sudden cardiac death (35%), pulmonary embolism *[a blood clot, usually from the leg, that passes to the lungs]* (12.5%), **myocardial infarction** (12%), VITT - *[which stands for Vaccine-Induced Immune Thrombotic Thrombocytopenia]* (7.9%), **myocarditis** (7.1%), multisystem inflammatory syndrome (4.6%), and cerebral hemorrhage (3.8%).

Conclusion: The consistency seen among these cases with known COVID-19 vaccine mechanisms of injury and death, coupled with autopsy confirmation, **suggests a high likelihood of a causal link between COVID-19 vaccines and death.** *(emphasis added throughout)*

Step 9: Guide the adjustment reaction

The COVID-19 pandemic designers are continuing to "guide" us into *their* New Normal. They are moving us to accept vaccine mandates, vaccine passports, border IDs, iris scans, implantable biometrics, surveillance cameras, travel restrictions, 15-minute cities, and more.

In April 2012, a report was quietly released by the North American Plan for Animal and Pandemic Influenza (NAPAPI) detailing the cooperative agreement developed by the Obama Administration between Canada, Mexico, and the US.[71] The agreement is being pushed forward now.

The NAPAPI Preparedness Plan contained a significant part of the language from the WHO Treaty that was not ratified in the summer of 2024. While the treaty has yet to pass, even with ongoing meetings and international arm-twisting, what *was* passed by the full Security Counsel in September 2024 was the UN's "Pact for the Future." Section 65 of the approved document, labeled "Transforming Global Governance" states, "A transformation in global governance is essential to ensure that the positive progress we have seen across all three pillars of the work of the United Nations (UN) in recent decades does not unravel. **We will not allow this to happen.**" (*emphasis added*)

We are being guided to accept One World governance, which will include mandatory vaccination and more.[72]

Step 10: Be transparent with the public

The last step went completely off the rails during the recent pandemic. There have been continual lies about the massive devastation caused by the COVID-19 jabs orchestrated by the globalists. They are desperately trying to whip up the fear machine again over ebola, monkeypox (mpox), and another round of H5N1 bird flu, threatening that it is more deadly than the 2005 version. If that's true, then it has been weaponized by illegal gain of function research.

As their methodology continues to be exposed, challenged and dismantled, it is time for the citizens of the world to take back control. Now that the new-old plan is out in the open, be mindful of the rhetoric.

Pay attention to the language that has been used – there's more to come.

"The more things change, the more they stay the same."

Jean-Baptiste Alphonse Karr, 1849

CHAPTER 8

Bird Flu Hype and Preparation: 2024

A historical review of what happened during the first bird flu pandemic makes it clear that an algorithm or a check-the-box template was designed and then perfected to be used over and over for each pandemic the WHO and the WEF want to declare and have the countries of the world enforce. Plans are being put into place to protect the next round of pandemic countermeasures. However, the WHO is much more quiet about this upcoming bird flu pandemic than they have been in the past.

Here is a brief timeline of what has happened from 2022 to the time of this writing:

- Beginning in July 2022, H5N1 cases began to be reported sporadically in animals in diverse places around the globe. In the US, government officials began to mention a "bird flu pandemic" vaguely on TV news shows.
- November 2022 and early 2023: a few human cases appeared in diverse locations (China, Ecuador, and Cambodia)

- March 2024: one dairy farmer in Texas tested positive for H5N1. He reported conjunctivitis with no other symptoms.
- March 2024 to present: 4,100 people were tested after being exposed to an infected animal; only 13 were positive.
- March 2024: first reports of H5N1 detected in dairy cows in several states
- April 1, 2024: first reported transmission of H5N1 from cows to humans
- May 9, 2024: FDA Commissioner, Robert Califf, MD warned lawmakers that the US needed to institute countermeasure coverage
- December 18, 2024: ONE person hospitalized with a severe H5N1 infection in Louisiana, the first instance of severe illness linked to this virus in the US

From the CDC website "situation summary" for bird flu reported as of 12/12/2024:

- Dairy cattle: ongoing multi-state outbreak in 16 states
- Wild Birds: widespread, detected in more than 10,000 birds
- Poultry Flocks: sporadic outbreaks affecting 121 million birds in 49 states
- Mammals: sporadic infections from tested dead animals
- Person-to-person spread: **None**
- Current public health risk: **Low** - Globally since 2003, only 23 countries have reported rare, sporadic human infections with H5N1 bird flu viruses to the WHO

Between April 2024 and December 13, 2024, the CDC admits that only 61 cases of H5N1 have been confirmed among dairy and poultry workers. They all described mild symptoms, many with eye redness or discharge (conjunctivitis). The person who was hospitalized was exposed to sick birds in a backyard flock. Otherwise, no other workers have been hospitalized.

Even though the pandemic potential is low, the illness is mild, and no one has contracted the virus or viral illness from eating eggs, milk, dairy products, beef or chicken, more than 500 million chickens, ducks, and turkeys have already been culled, even if completely healthy.

Recall that there are many versions of the HxNy viruses in circulation, including H5N6, H3N8, H7N4, H10N3, H9N2, and others that have infected a small number of humans around the globe for decades. Because the pandemic can be caused by any one of these, and others, on July 18, 2024, the Secretary of HHS, Xavier Becerra, broadened the April 19, 2013, pandemic EUA to include, "pandemic influenza A viruses and influenza A viruses with *pandemic potential,*" with a special focus on H7N9. He determined that by adding nearly every influenza A virus to the list of potential problems, he was covering all his bases. What was the justification for specifically naming H7N9?

> "H7N9 has demonstrated the ability to transmit from poultry to humans, causing two separate human case clusters involving over 400 people and resulting in over 100 fatalities from 2013 to 2014. *While sustained human-to-human transmission was not seen, familial clusters could not be ruled out.*"

Effective as of the date of the signed document, the authorization of emergency use of nasal swab testing for detection of the avian H7N9 virus, as a countermeasure, could begin, without liability.[73]

To accelerate this process, the WHO announced on July 29, 2024 an agreement with the Argentinian manufacturer Sinergium Biotech to accelerate the development and accessibility of a human influenza (H5N1) vaccine using the messenger RNA (mRNA) platform. As of this writing, Sinergium Biotech has not yet started clinical trials for its H5N1 avian influenza mRNA vaccine. The company is still in the preclinical phase, focusing on establishing proof-of-concept using preclinical models.[74]

Elsewhere internationally, Finland began administering a bird flu vaccine for H5N8 in June 2024 even though the vaccine had never been tested on humans. The campaign primarily focused on individuals at higher risk due to occupational exposure, such as poultry workers, veterinarians, and those handling infected animals or samples. Even though Finland only had one case of bird flu in 2024, the Nordic country bought 20,000 doses of vaccine for 10,000 people, each consisting of two injections, as part of a joint European Union (EU) to procure from manufacturer CSL Seqirus up to 40 million doses for 15 nations.[75]

US APPROVED H5N1 VACCINES

As of June 2024, the FDA already licensed at least three bird flu (H5N1) vaccines:

- **Sanofi (for the National Stockpile).**(package insert)[76] *Approved in 2007,* this vaccine, simply called **Influenza Virus Vaccine, H5N1,** is an inactivated, monovalent vaccine indicated for people 18 through 64 years of age. In one of the clinical trials, 151 enrollees were included. Of the 103 adults who were vaccinated, 48 received a placebo. Four serious adverse events occurred in the vaccinated group, including one death and three other serious adverse events (one each: menorrhagia (heavy menstrual bleeding), a cerebrovascular event, and breast cancer). The virus is replicated in **eggs** and inactivated by **formaldehyde.** The final product contains **Triton X100, porcine gelatin** (500 mcg), **thimerosal (mercury)** (50 mcg), **polyethylene glycol (PEG),** and **sucrose** but no antibiotics and no latex. Similar to all other vaccines, this H5N1 vaccine **was not** evaluated for its carcinogenic or mutagenic potential, or for its ability to impair fertility.

- **ID Biomedical Corporation of Quebec (a subsidiary of GlaxoSmithKline).** (package insert)[77] The Influenza A (H5N1) Virus Monovalent Vaccine Adjuvanted, trade named **Q-Pan,** was *approved in 2013* for use in children 6 months to 17 years. Two doses of 0.25 ml are to be given to babies three weeks apart; people 18 years and older are to get one 0.50 ml shot.

  In the original vaccine trials, multiple severe adverse events were reported: a cerebral vascular accident occurred in one subject on day 1 and again on day 9 following the second vaccine dose; on day 21, one subject suffered a pulmonary embolism, and one subject experienced a corneal transplant rejection after the second dose even though the transplant had been 18 years previously. The virus is grown in **eggs,** inactivated with **formaldehyde,** and disrupted with **sodium deoxycholate** (disrupts DNA). The shot is supplied in two vials, one contains the H5N1 antigen in suspension; the other is a vial of **AS03 adjuvant,** a proprietary adjuvant containing **squalene, polysorbate 80,** and highly inflammatory **DL-alpha-tocopherol**. *(details on this and other adjuvants in Chapter 13)*

- **Seqirus.** (package insert)[78] Manufactured in Holly Springs, NC, the third bird flu vaccine was *approved in 2020* under the trade name **Audenz** but uses **H5N8.** Distributed in a multi-dose vial, it has been approved for all people 6 months of age and older. The virus is replicated in **MDCK cells (dog kidney),** inactivated with **B-propriolactone,** and disrupted by the detergent cetyltrimethylammonium bromide **(CTAB).** The vaccine contains **MF59,** a squalene-based oil-in-water adjuvant that also contains the chemicals **polysorbate**

80, sorbitan trioleate, sodium citrate dihydrate, and citric acid monohydrate. Each 0.5ml vaccine dose contains 25 mcg of **mercury.** The American Medical Association and the Centers for Medicare and Medicaid Services (CMS) announced in mid-July that CPT codes have been assigned for bird flu vaccines, specifically the cell-line vaccines, so that doctors could be reimbursed when they do a test for bird flu infection or when they give the shot.

Other H5N1 vaccines (trade names listed below) have been approved by the European Medicines Agency (EMA).[79] They are:

1. Foclivia - Seqiris, eggs, MF59 - approved 2009
2. Aflovov - Seqiris, eggs, MF59 - approved 2010
3. Zoonotic - Seqiris, eggs, MF59 - approved 2023
4. Celldemic - Seqiris, MDCK cells, MF59 - approved 2024
5. Incellipan - Seqiris, MDCK cells, MF59 - approved 2024
6. Adjupanrix - GSK, eggs, AS03 - approved 2009
7. (unnamed) - AstraZeneca, eggs, no adjuvant - approved 2016

MORE ON THE WAY

Moderna: The US government, with the assistance of Biomedical Advanced Research and Development Authority (BARDA) paid the vaccine maker Moderna $176 million to accelerate the development of a pandemic influenza vaccine for bird flu.[80] Moderna's early-stage bird flu vaccine uses the same mRNA technology that allowed the rapid rollout of the COVID-19 vaccines. But given how the mRNA technology works, the project can be quickly *redirected to target a different form of influenza* if a threat other than H5N1 emerges.

They haven't wasted any time to plow ahead into the next plandemic.

But just in case you didn't get your flu shot and you're starting to get the sniffles that may lead to full-blown flu symptoms, doctors can give you a pill to nip it in the bud. They can prescribe Tamiflu designed to stop the flu in its tracks.

Or will it?

*"The young physician starts life with 20 drugs for each disease,
and the old physician ends life with one drug for 20 diseases."*

~Sir William Osler, Canadian Physician, 1849–1919

CHAPTER 9
The Scam of Tamiflu

In addition to the pandemic vaccines, two drugs were introduced in 2005 for the treatment and prevention of influenza. Both gained a great deal of attention. The ideal antiviral drug is effective against all types of influenza viruses, regardless of strain and irrespective of antigenic drifts and shifts. The drug companies thought they had found the answer and GlaxoWelcome capitalized on the concept with its drug, Relenza.

Recall that two protein antigens project from the surface of all influenza viruses. One is called hemagglutinin (H), which plays a role in binding the cell receptors of the host, and the other is the enzyme neuraminidase (N), which plays an important role in allowing the spread of viruses to other people. When a virus enters the host's cells, the (H) protein binds to a molecule sitting on the surface of mucous cells. This lock-and-key configuration opens the door to the cell, allowing the virus to enter and start the process of self-replication.

When new virus particles are formed inside a cell, they are released to infect other cells. However, as they exit, they get coated with a molecule called sialic acid. This coating prevents the virus's key (H) proteins from binding to new cells, effectively trapping the virus. The virus solves this problem with the other protein on its surface, an enzyme called neuraminidase (N). Neuraminidase removes the sialic acid, "cleaning" the (H) proteins so they can attach to and infect new cells. Without neuraminidase, the virus wouldn't spread because its (H) proteins would remain blocked. This understanding led to the creation of drugs called neuraminidase inhibitors, which stop the enzyme from working, blocking the virus's ability to spread.

RELENZA

On February 24, 1999, a special meeting of the Antiviral Drug Products Advisory Committee convened to discuss Relenza (zanamivir), a new product that was set to be accelerated into the market by GlaxoWelcome. Relenza, a powdered medication delivered through a device called a diskhaler, was developed for the treatment of uncomplicated flu caused by influenza type A and type B. GlaxoWelcome's drug application sought approval for use in adults and in adolescents at least 12 years of age. In 2006, the approval age was extended for use in children as young as five years old. Unusual in its scope, Relenza's application was quite different from those typically presented for consideration to the Advisory Committee.

Debra Birnkrant, MD, an FDA official, opened the 1999 meeting by admitting that the committee usually only discussed drugs that were under consideration for treating "serious life-threatening diseases." Regarding Relenza, she went on to say:

> "This is a [drug] application for a disease which is acute and self-limited in the majority of patients, but could potentially infect the entire population and account for a substantial morbidity. This application was granted for a 'priority review' because influenza has the propensity to affect such a large portion of the population."

She closed her introduction by saying that reviewing the application was a way to keep HHS in the loop to prepare for an influenza pandemic.[81]

LEARN MORE

In January 2000, it was announced that GlaxoWelcome intended to merge with SmithKline Beecham. The merger was completed in December of that year to form GlaxoSmithKline (GSK). As of November, 2024, Relenza continues to be manufactured and distributed by GSK.

In 2015, The Antiviral Drugs Advisory Committee at the FDA was officially terminated. Following its dissolution, responsibilities previously managed by this committee were transferred to the Antimicrobial Drugs Advisory Committee. The updated committee provides recommendations to the FDA Commissioner and evaluates safety and efficacy data for drugs aimed at treating infectious diseases, including antivirals.

Given that it was a novel drug utilizing a unique delivery system, Relenza had encountered special difficulties during its clinical trials. A full day of testimonies and questions following the routine opening remarks brought several concerns to light.

The Committee immediately raised questions about the conflicting data GlaxoWelcome presented from its three clinical trials: one conducted in the United States and Canada, one in Europe, and one in the Southern Hemisphere. Of the 1,588 total subjects enrolled in the three studies, only 73 percent had culture-confirmed influenza. The rest – more than 25 percent of the study's participants (428) – were included because they had "influenza-like" symptoms. That created a glaring but unaddressed problem with sample selection: Relenza is only effective against influenza viruses and not other viruses that cause influenza-like illnesses. The Committee agreed that participants who were not confirmed to be infected by an influenza A or B virus should not have been included in the trial.

The primary endpoint of the study involved measuring the "time-to-alleviation of symptoms," an arbitrary determination ranked on a scorecard by study participants. Patients judged their symptoms as "none, mild, moderate, or severe" on a scale of zero to three with regard to fever, cough, headache, myalgia, and sore throat. To be considered "over the flu," all symptoms had to be ranked as none or mild, and the patient's temperature had to be less than 100°F (37.8°C) for at least 24 hours.

The effectiveness of Relenza was dismal. The three trials showed inconsistent findings, with the largest of the three, the North American trial, demonstrating *no effect at all.* In addition, in both of the foreign trials, Relenza showed only modest effectiveness. Nonetheless, GlaxoWelcome attempted to spin the results, calling it a "smashing success," touting that symptoms had decreased by two and a half days in the European trial and one and a half days in the Southern Hemisphere trial. When the numbers were reworked by an FDA statistician, the results equated to a symptom-relief score of a meager 1.8 days in the first trial and a barely noticeable 1.1 days for the second, meaning symptoms were shortened by about 1 day. The bottom line? Relenza was no more effective than doing nothing at all to treat common flu symptoms.

The endpoint determination – the "diary cards" – troubled one of the conference attendees, Janet Wittes, PhD, a statistician and resident in the Statistics Collaborative, Inc. in Washington D.C. She raised concerns about the subjective nature of the cards and questioned the validity of comparing the studies because the cards were distributed in different languages and in different countries. She asked, "I have a question about the diary cards in terms of the translations and the back translations. Given the subjective nature of those responses, how did you calibrate one language against another? How do we know what one observes in one country is the same as in another? How do you know that the translation was perceived the same way across languages?"

Not missing a beat, the answer quickly came from GlaxoWelcome's representative, Dr. Michael Elliot who stated, "We don't have a poll that measures perception. I think we just have to rest on our experience and assume that the translation is true to the meaning." Given that the totals on the self-scored cards were the crucial determining factors for assessing the effectiveness of the medication, his answer was far from reassuring.

Further, the Advisory Committee was very apprehensive about the lack of data regarding the drug's use in high-risk patients, particularly those with preexisting lung conditions, such as asthma. In the studies, "high risk" groups were patients with asthma who averaged 37 years of age. James Stoller, PhD, head of the Respiratory Therapy Department in association with the Department of Pulmonary and Critical Care at the Cleveland Clinic, asked very specific questions about the use of "objective measurements" such as pulmonary function tests or peak flow values to determine the severity of the patient's underlying lung disease.

Once again, Dr. Elliot fielded the question, admitting that objective measures were not used and that the severity of the participant's disease was based solely on the "opinion of the clinical investigator," a determination made by the number of medications the patient was using. In other words, the more medications a person was on, the more severe the asthma was judged to be – another completely subjective criteria. Beyond that, the number of patients in the trials with severe lung disease (such as chronic obstructive pulmonary disease, or COPD), severe cardiac disease, and in the geriatric age group was "very small." The committee had reason for serious concern over the paucity of data involving high-risk patients as they are the group targeted with drugs at the first sign of the flu.

In the end, the Committee voted 14 to 3 *against approval* of the drug. One committee member, Dr. John Hamilton, professor of medicine from Duke University, remarked, "While I appreciate that every attempt was made to identify the endpoints, my impression of the data, especially from the North American study, is that there isn't sufficient efficacy to warrant me recommending this drug for my family or myself."

Incredibly, despite concerns and lack of support by her own committee, Heidi M. Jolson, MD, MPH, Director of the Division of Antiviral Drug Products at the FDA, proceeded to approve Relenza for use five months later, on July 26, 1999. She defended her decision by saying:

> "Relenza had not been shown effective for patients over 65 or those 'with a variety of respiratory, cardiovascular and other medical conditions…' Special precautions are warranted if Relenza is prescribed for patients with respiratory disease. These groups would encompass patients most vulnerable to death from the flu."[82]

Jolson went on to say:

> "I do not believe that the lack of a conclusive finding in the North American study negates the **_robust_ demonstrations of efficacy** *(emphasis added)* in the European and Southern Hemisphere studies, particularly given the inherent difficulties in conducting trials for this indication. Overall, the totality of the data provides evidence that treatment with [Relenza] confers a modest reduction in time to alleviation of influenza symptoms."[83]

The European trial decreased symptoms by two and a half days and the Southern Hemisphere trial decreased symptoms by one and a half days over the placebo. By any measure this is hardly "robust efficacy." Hence, Relenza became the first neuraminidase inhibitor to be marketed in the United States, approved for adults and adolescents to be taken by intranasal spray twice daily for five days beginning *within two days* after the onset of symptoms. The big win for patients, at least from GlaxoWelcome's view, was that the drug could shorten symptoms by about one day when compared with doing nothing at all.[82]

That's right. One day. Again, hardly "robust efficacy."

NO RECALL, JUST "EXERCISE CAUTION"

The Committee had justifiably raised concerns about the safety of Relenza in high-risk patients. Soon after the drug was approved, reports of serious complications started to roll in as the first flu season was getting into full swing.

A mere six months after approval, the FDA was forced to issue a Public Health Advisory highlighting problems with Relenza. Caution was advised concerning its use in patients with underlying asthma or chronic obstructive pulmonary disease (COPD) such as emphysema. The FDA received several reports of deteriorating lung function, ranging from bronchospasm (wheezing) to respiratory arrest (cessation of breathing) following the inhalation of Relenza in patients with chronic lung and heart conditions, including seven deaths that were reported in early usage. By June 2000, Relenza was cited as a suspect in 22 deaths, two which had bacterial infections and should have been treated with antibiotics. During that same flu season, (November 2, 1999 to June 30, 2000), the Canadian Adverse Drug Reaction Monitoring Program received 16 reports of suspected adverse reactions. Six were classified as "serious and unexpected," and one death. But instead of issuing a product recall, the FDA instead issued a warning with a recommendation to use "careful monitoring, proper observation, and appropriate supportive care, including the availability of short-acting bronchodilators" when prescribing this drug.

COMMENTARY

Since 2000, reports of serious side effects related to Relenza have continued, including bronchospasm, anaphylaxis, and psychiatric symptoms such as delirium, abnormal behavior, and hallucinations. Some fatalities have been associated with these adverse events, especially in pediatric patients.

This begs the question: Why would the FDA recommend "careful monitoring" of a potentially life threatening drug that only relieves symptoms of the flu by one day? In addition, why would any doctor be willing to prescribe it?

NEXT TO MARKET: TAMIFLU

Three months after the approval of Relenza in 1999, Tamiflu (oseltamivir) became the first oral neuraminidase inhibitor to be approved. Approval of the pill was based on the results of two double-blind trials conducted in 1997 and 1998 involving less than 2,000 patients. One trial was in the United States; the other involved patients from Canada, Europe, and Hong Kong. Only 62 percent in the study had laboratory testing done to confirm influenza viruses as the cause of their symptoms. Like Relenza, Tamiflu was designed to inhibit the neuraminidase enzyme of influenza A and B viruses; it has no effect against other microbes.

Similar to the Relenza trials, the effectiveness of the drug was judged by having participants complete self-assessment "symptom scores." The "time to improvement of symptoms" was calculated from the time of ingesting the first dose of medication to the time when all symptoms (nasal congestion, sore throat, cough, aches, fatigue, headaches, chills and sweats) decreased to none or mild. Despite the fact that symptom relief was *only 1.3 days sooner* with Tamiflu than with the placebo (doing nothing), the FDA approved the drug for use.

It bears repeating that neuraminidase inhibitors work by "cleaning" the (H) antigen of influenza viruses, allowing them to move to the next cell. They have no effect on other pathogens that cause influenza-like illnesses. Amazingly enough, the drug gained approval after being tested on only 849 people who had culture-confirmed influenza. In an FDA memorandum dated October 25, 1999, the Director of the Division of Antiviral Drug Products, Heidi M. Jolson, MD, MPH, once again defended her approval of the drug by saying:

> "The clinical relevance of the modest treatment benefit is a highly subjective question. It is my opinion that a **one-day reduction** in the duration of moderate-to-severe symptoms, including fever, is likely to be clinically important to many patients. Because influenza symptoms are self-limited in the majority of individuals, it is anticipated that many people with influenza will **neither require, nor desire, treatment** with antiviral medications." *(emphasis added)*

In addition to using Tamiflu for the treatments of influenza, two studies were submitted to the FDA to gain approval for its use as a flu preventative. The first was a small study published in JAMA. Twenty-six subjects were given either 100 milligrams or 200 milligrams of Tamiflu for 26 hours before being inoculated with influenza virus; there were twelve people in the control group. The results showed that eight of twelve given the placebo contracted the flu while eight of the twenty-six who were given Tamiflu did not. In addition, six of the twelve people in the placebo group shed the virus to others after being exposed while viral shedding occurred in none of the Tamiflu-treated group. This difference, six out of twelve, was lauded as a *50% reduction* in viral shedding by the drug companies.[84]

At about the same time, the results of a larger trial were published in a separate JAMA article. This study involved 1,559 healthy, unvaccinated adults who were randomized to receive 75 milligrams of Tamiflu or a placebo, once or twice daily for six weeks during the peak of the influenza season. The incidence of the flu was only slightly less in the group that received Tamiflu (1.2 percent) vs. the group who had received a placebo (4.8 percent), meaning that again, doing nothing was just about as effective as taking a ten-day course of Tamiflu costing up to $100.[85] Based on the marginal results of these two studies, the FDA approved Tamiflu for the prevention of influenza in November 2000.

COMMENTARY

Beyond the lackluster results for both the treatment and prevention of influenza, nearly 10 percent of people who are prescribed Tamiflu can't tolerate the most common side effect – persistent nausea. With the course of treatment costing $100 to $200 (depending on the dose) perhaps the best course of action is to use nasal spray (saline, colloidal silver, and povidone-iodine have all been shown to be effective), be sure your vitamin D level is between 80-100 ng/mL, and have powdered vitamin C ascorbate in your medicine cabinet. These will be at least as effective and are minimal cost. And don't forget to wash your hands frequently, but not obsessively.

STOCKPILING BEGINS

On August 26, 2004, the HHS and the CDC released the first draft of the "Pandemic Influenza Preparedness and Response Plan." In it, Tamiflu was highlighted as the antiviral drug to be stockpiled by the US government and the military as part of its preparation for an influenza pandemic. Government models developed by two international research teams suggested a pandemic could be stopped if a "ring of contacts" around the first human cases were given Tamiflu to prevent the virus from "infecting others." All the hype about the use of Tamiflu during the pandemic overlooked one egregious problem – there was no data regarding the effectiveness of Tamiflu for preventing or treating H5N1.

Even though Tamiflu is designed to inhibit the neuraminidase (N) enzyme of influenza viruses so cleaning the (H) receptor doesn't occur, the process was found to be more effective against some influenza subtypes than others. To test the use of Tamiflu for preventing the flu, the drug was tested against nine (N) subtypes, even though it was generally accepted among scientists that the next pandemic strain – whatever it turned out to be – would have the surface protein N1. In laboratory tests, **Tamiflu's ability to inhibit the N1 neuraminidase failed dismally**. Eight to twelve times the recommended dose of the drug was needed to achieve the same level of neuraminidase inhibition found in other (N) subtypes.

When Tamiflu was tested specifically against H5N1 isolates from Vietnam and Thailand, the hot zone of the 2005 outbreak, an additional three-fold increase in the dose was required to stop its activities, meaning *almost 30 times* **more Tamiflu** would be needed to stop the spread of the H5N1 over the other influenza viruses. Even though the recommended adult dose of Tamiflu for prevention was two 75 milligram pills per day for ten days, it appeared the recommended dose would not deliver enough drug to provide even marginal protection.

But a lack of efficacy has never deterred the pharmaceutical companies from promoting a drug or a vaccine. Therefore, it became widely accepted that higher doses were needed to be prescribed during a pandemic. This constituted an even bigger bonanza for Roche Pharmaceuticals, the Swiss company that, at the time, was the sole manufacturer of Tamiflu. The numbers were overwhelming: 6.2 billion people worldwide taking two pills per day for just ten days would require 124 billion pills. The average cost of a ten-day course of medicine is around $100. Now if 30 times that amount is needed to make a difference … the dollars spent by countries and siphoned into Roche would be staggering.

SIGNIFICANT ADVERSE EVENTS REPORTED

Reports of resistance to Tamiflu soon began to surface. On February 27, 2005, a 14-year-old Vietnamese girl had reportedly received a 75-milligram, once-a-day dose of Tamiflu for three days and then 75 milligrams twice daily for an additional seven days while hospitalized. In laboratory testing, it was determined that her isolated strain had shown resistance to the medication. (Incidentally, she recovered uneventfully and was discharged from hospital on March 14, 2005.)

News of a possibly resistant strain of H5N1 caused articles to be published at lightning speed, reassuring people – and countries – that the resistant bug was merely an "isolated case" and that the billions of dollars that were being spent to stockpile the medication were not being spent in vain. Researchers noted that everyone, including Roche, expected some resistance to Tamiflu once it was in wide use. However, in spite of the pronouncements, as more resistance occurred it was kept under tight wraps.

HIGHLIGHT

Tamiflu (oseltamivir) became available in generic form after its patent expired in 2016 allowing other companies to produce and sell cheaper versions. Generic versions of Tamiflu are now made by companies for other parts of the world, including Hetero Drugs, Cipla, and Mylan (now part of Viatris).

Resistance to Tamiflu (oseltamivir) had been observed more frequently in children than adults, as shown in a 2000 study in Japan involving 50 children. Researchers collected influenza virus samples before and during treatment. Within four days of starting Tamiflu, 18% of the viruses showed resistance. Some types of influenza viruses appear to develop resistance more readily than others, highlighting that there was even more variability in the drug's effectiveness. Sensitivity testing revealed that treated viruses could be ***300-fold to 1,000,000-fold more resistant*** than untreated viruses.[86]

Another Japanese study, the only market that fully embraced Tamiflu, found that 16 percent of viruses developed resistance to the drug each season. "That's one in six. So I would anticipate that in H5N1-infected people that the frequency would certainly be no less," says Dr. Frederick Hayden of the University of Virginia (also co-chair of an international network of scientists who monitor for resistance to neuraminidase inhibitors).[87] The big concern regarding Tamiflu-induced drug resistance, and why it was so heavily monitored, was the potential for the emergence of "mutant" viruses that would be thousands of times more virulent. Could Tamiflu use actually *cause* the pandemic that governments and health officials are trying to avoid?

Roche resolutely denied the FDA's assertion, and pushed to smooth over the FDA's concerns by pushing the position that mutant viruses are "less pathogenic (less disease-causing) than wild type influenza viruses." The FDA wasn't buying it and responded, "It appears that mutant viruses may be shed at high titers [in large amounts] by some subjects before being cleared. Therefore, this reviewer has **not been reassured** that the [mutant] viruses are harmless to the general population (package insert)."[88] *(emphasis added)*

Information about Tamiflu continued to become increasingly more unsettling. Evidence indicated Tamiflu could increase the seriousness of the illness in people with suppressed immune systems. Tamiflu was first prescribed for the elderly and for those with chronic lung diseases based on *an assumption* that those people are more likely to be seriously compromised by the flu. However, many patients with emphysema, COPD, and severe asthma may also be taking Prednisone, a drug that suppresses the immune system. There was essentially no data to support the safety of taking these two drugs together, especially in the geriatric population.

CONCERNS ABOUT TAMIFLU IN KIDS

Beyond the risk of the elderly and the risk of unleashing potentially overly aggressive mutant strains, concerns surfaced regarding the drug's safety in children. On November 19, 2005, the FDA's Pediatric Advisory Committee met to discuss new reports of serious skin reactions, neuropsychiatric events, and deaths associated with taking Tamiflu. According to IMS Health, approximately 24.4 million prescriptions for Tamiflu had been dispensed in Japan between 2001 and 2005; approximately one fifth that number – 5.5 million – were filled in the US during the same period. Pediatric prescriptions accounted for 11.6 million in Japan versus 872,386 in the US.[89]

LEARN MORE

Pediatric Tamiflu Timeline:

- October 1999: FDA approved oral capsules for the treatment of uncomplicated acute influenza in patients one-year of age

- November 2000: Prophylaxis for adults and children 13 years and older

- December 2000: Oral suspension approved

- September 2009: approved for use in infants as young as 2 weeks old

As part of its post-marketing surveillance efforts, reports submitted to FDA Adverse Event Reporting System (FAERS) database were scrutinized, searching for serious and non-serious adverse events in children. FAERS is woefully underutilized by physicians; therefore, the actual number of adverse events was likely to have been much higher than reported. It is estimated that less than 10 percent of adverse events are reported to FAERS or its vaccine equivalent, VAERS, the Vaccine Adverse Event Reporting System.

Query dates from March 22, 2004 through April 22, 2005 encompassed the 13 months post-release; 1,184 case reports for adverse reactions were posted from sources both domestic and abroad. Nearly 16 percent of the events occurred in children (n=190). Among the 75 pediatric case report submitted as "serious side effects," there were eight fatalities (four sudden deaths, three cardio-respiratory arrests, and one case of acute pancreatitis with cardiopulmonary arrest); 32 neuropsychiatric events; and 12 skin/hypersensitivity events and many other miscellaneous adverse events were found in the review. No further action regarding the use of Tamiflu in children was taken by the FDA after they issued their review.

Since Tamiflu's 1999 approval, a number of serious adverse events including anaphylaxis and deaths have continued to be reported. There have been several reports of children who developed influenza, started taking Tamiflu, then died suddenly in their sleep. The skin reactions reported were quite severe and included erythema multiforme and Stevens-Johnson syndrome, which is a severe, potentially life-threatening immune reaction.

Beyond skin reactions, the reports of neuropsychiatric events associated with Tamiflu were highly disturbing and included cases of delirium, convulsions, and encephalitis. The FDA issued a warning after a review of 103 reports of neuropsychiatric adverse events associated with Tamiflu. About two-thirds of the adverse events were reported in children under 17. Early concerns came after the report of three children who experienced very troubling neurological and behavioral symptoms:

> "Two children, a twelve- and a thirteen-year-old male, jumped out of the second floor window of their homes after receiving two doses of Tamiflu. Head CT scans showed no abnormalities in either patient. A third case was an eight-year-old boy who experienced frightening hallucinations and rushed out of his house onto the street three hours after receiving his first dose of oseltamivir. He was rescued by his family from potential traffic injury."[90]

In spite of these serious reports, but true to form, the FDA voted unanimously that Tamiflu had "no links to the deaths in children," that the agency would "continue to monitor adverse events," and Roche was required to provide the Committee "a one-year surveillance update" after this year's flu season, which was not completed or cannot be found.[91]

This type of so-called "surveillance" was, and remains, woefully inadequate. Part of the FDA's mission statement is to protect public health by assuring the safety of biological products, medical devices, etc. This was not ensuring safety; this was ensuring the continued purchase of Tamiflu. In May 2022, Data Bridge Market Research analyses set Tamiflu's market value at $542.88 billion and expects it to reach $862.85 billion by 2029.[92] Everyone, especially parents, should be wary of this drug since it is still in use. Reports of psychiatric events have continued. For example, in 2018 and 2020 reports of children having hallucinations and threatening suicide made headline news across the country.

Tamiflu remains the most used anti-influenza drug 20 years after its approval.

MORE BACKSTORY ABOUT TAMIFLU

Tamiflu was discovered by Gilead Sciences in 1995, patented in 1996, co-developed with Hoffmann-LaRoche Ltd, then commercially launched by Roche in November 1999. The studies that reported its favorable safety profile were funded by Roche. Over time, Tamiflu became one of the highest ever revenue earners for Roche.

During the 1990s, Roche sponsored 40 clinical trials on Tamiflu. In 2003, Kaiser et al. published a meta-analysis of the studies and concluded that Tamiflu "reduces lower respiratory tract complications, antibiotics uses, and hospitalization in healthy and 'at risk' adults."[93] This oft-cited article was also supported by Roche and apparently was what pushed the robust scientific argument for stockpiling the drug in later years.

In March 2009, Roche retained Genentech's research operation, one of the strongest in the pharmaceutical industry, to become a member of the Roche Group. In the first half of 2009, sales of Tamiflu had tripled to 1 billion Swiss francs ($931 million), spurred by retail sales and stockpiling of the drug by governments and corporations.

In 2010 and 2012, two more large meta-analyses were published, one funded by the WHO and the other by Roche, to further support the drug's safety and efficacy. However, a Japanese pediatrician sounded the alarm regarding the inaccuracy of data in the reviews. He called on the Cochrane Collaboration to help investigate the findings.

Cochrane is an international, independent network of researchers and health professionals that do systematic reviews of the literature and, over the preceding 30 years, had published many highly respected summaries on a variety of subjects. In research, the Randomized Controlled Trial (RCT) is considered the gold standard. Cochrane found that the RCTs evaluating Tamiflu, among other scientific errors, "lacked precision, provided low-quality evidence and had poor study design." After a painstakingly thorough evaluation of all the data, Cochrane published its findings in 2014: Tamiflu's benefits had been overplayed and its harms had been underplayed in many of the trials. And there was no evidence that Tamiflu reduced transmission or decreased respiratory complications.[94]

In November 2014, a whistleblower lawsuit was filed by Dr. Thomas Jefferson of the Cochrane Collaboration under the False Claims Act, suing Roche for "falsified scientific conclusions and mounting a high-powered marketing and lobbying campaign to deceive the government about the effectiveness of Tamiflu (oseltamivir) for fighting a flu pandemic." In the case, plaintiffs sought to recover more than $1.4 billion of taxpayer dollars, wrongly spent by the federal government to add Tamiflu to the Strategic National Stockpile. After many years of legal banter, the case was finally unsealed September 10, 2019; Roche was found vulnerable to a judgment in excess of $4.5 billion. The high dollar amount accrued because the False Claims Act mandates not only civil penalties, but payment of triple damages. However, in 2023, for unknown reasons, Dr. Jefferson voluntarily moved to dismiss the case. The dismissal was agreed upon by both Dr. Jefferson and Hoffmann-La Roche, as indicated in a recent court filing with the US District Court for the District of Maryland after a protracted legal battle. No further details are publicly available.

More than two billion dollars were spent to stockpile Tamiflu in the US alone in 2005. The marginally effective, potentially toxic, even potentially dangerous drug is still available to the general public. In 2019, Sanofi acquired exclusive rights to market Tamiflu, with a plan to release it as an over-the-counter (OTC) medication in the US. However, at the time of this writing, the FDA has not yet made the switch and a prescription is still required for the drug.

Let the buyer beware: Tamiflu and Relenza, which provide at best one and a half days of relief from flu-like symptoms, can have lethal consequences.

*"No one should approach the temple of science
with the soul of a money changer."*

~Thomas Browne, English physician and writer

CHAPTER 10

The Vaccine Industry:
A Short Summary of a Big Topic

To fully understand the vaccine business, a brief review of vaccine history is in order.

The industry evolved from surprisingly modest origins. In the 18th century, when smallpox outbreaks were spreading across much of Europe, Englishman Edward Jenner noticed that most milkmaids seemed to escape contracting smallpox. Jenner, a country apothecary, had purchased his medical degree from St. Andrews University in Scotland for the sum of 15 pounds, approximately USD$2,500 today. He made a simple observation: milkmaids boasted blemish-free complexions while smallpox survivors were conspicuous with their facial pockmarks. This led to Jenner's deduction that the milkmaids were somehow protected from the disease, perhaps because they had contracted a milder version of the illness, known as cowpox, from milking the cows.

In 1796, Jenner tested his theory by collecting the pus from a cowpox blister on the hand of milkmaid Sarah Nelmes and injecting it into

James Phipps, a healthy eight-year-old boy. Jenner then repeatedly injected Phipps with cowpox pus over several days, gradually increasing the dosage. He then injected Phipps with smallpox and the boy became ill. However, after a few days, the boy made a full recovery with no apparent effects from the smallpox nor side effects from the vaccine. The experiment was considered to be a success. Although much controversy has surrounded the smallpox vaccine, even in its early stages, the seeds of an industry were sown. Throughout history, Jenner has been given credit as the "Father of Vaccination."[95]

The 19th and 20th centuries saw the introduction of many vaccinations designed to combat various infectious diseases. The rewards, both financial gain and historical acclaim, were noteworthy. Names like Pasteur, creator of the rabies vaccine, and Salk, developer of the first polio vaccine, are routinely mentioned with the same lofty adoration as Newton and Edison. Since Jenner's introduction over 200 years ago, more than 17 childhood and adult vaccines have been put into broad international use. And many more – as many as 200 more – are under development, illustrating how vaccination has become part of the accepted standard of medicine around the world.

During the historic period of production and use, vaccines were largely confined to industrialized countries. For instance, the original smallpox vaccine was offered to all age groups, but children, healthcare workers, and travelers were the primary target. As a result, coverage within a community was patchy. For example, despite the accolades given to its role in eradicating smallpox, it has been estimated that only about 10 percent of the world's population ever received the vaccine. As stated previously, Dr. Tom Mack's opinion was that "even without mass vaccination, smallpox would have died out anyway. It was already on its way out; it just would have taken longer."[96]

After World War II, the development of vaccines rapidly increased in scope but the focus remained primarily on childhood diseases. The research continued with the blessing and full endorsement of the US federal government. The implementation of the National Immunization Program in 1986 was met with near universal approval. With the world's population booming and the standards of living increasing in many former third-world countries, increased purchasing power for vaccines was thought to drive sales and increase profits. The future seemed bright for vaccine makers. However, consolidation was underway. In 1967, there were 26 companies supplying the US market with various vaccines. By late 2004, the number of major vaccine producers had shrunk to six. In 2024, there were 15.

THE VACCINE INDUSTRY

The global pharmaceutical market has experienced sensational growth over the years, and especially in the last few years. In 2023, the total global Big Pharma market had an estimated value of around $1.6 trillion US dollars, comparable to the gross domestic products (GDPs) of countries such as Spain, Mexico, or Australia. This is an increase of more than $100 billion dollars over 2022. By contrast, the global vaccine market (excluding COVID-19 vaccines) was valued at about $53.0 billion in 2024 and, according to FiercePharma, is poised to reach $80.3 billion by 2029, a growth of 8.7%. Comparatively, in 2004, the vaccine sector of the pharma market was valued at only $8 billion.[97]

By any objective measure, $53 billion for the manufacture and distribution of vaccines is a pretty hefty number, especially since it is divided among only a handful of manufacturers. But it is small compared to other companies and sectors within the medical industry. There are at least 100 companies that produce a wide variety of medical products, from MRI machines to surgical instruments, each with a market cap of more than $100 billion. Because vaccines have a short shelf life with relatively slim profit margins per dose, manufacturers have been known to consider the vaccine sector the "charity work" of the industry.

However, drug companies are driven by profits, not by helping others as a "charity." A better way to describe vaccines is that they are a business "loss leader." It's akin to going to the mall and seeing a sign in a window advertising a FREE T-SHIRT JUST FOR COMING IN THE STORE. Once inside, after receiving the free gift, the salesperson works to sell you a $5000 Prada suit. The t-shirt actually costs pennies in comparison to the "win" of selling the expensive suit.

The same can be said about vaccines. They can be given away for free during campaigns at pharmacies, even at business events. The shots can be provided by the manufacturers at low or no cost because giving them away can result in the sale of a lifetime of profitable drugs to address the side effects that may result from the injection of foreign matter into otherwise healthy individuals. The results may be asthma, allergies, ADD/ADHD, eczema, seizure disorders, and other conditions, even cancer. Remember that the money is in the medicine; the expansive profits that come from repeat sale of expensive drugs.

A partial explanation for the comparatively small market share is that prescription drugs are taken day after day, whereas many vaccines are given only once or twice in a lifetime. What keeps sales going is the continuous supply of new customers, primarily children. Over a three-year period (2000-2002), the US Bureau of Statistics posted that there were just over 4 million live births per year. That has dropped to around 3.67 million live births per year (2019-2022.) Nonetheless, that's an average of 77,500 babies, government-guaranteed customers for vaccines, *each week*. Adding influenza and other vaccines to the recommended list for babies has certainly expanded the vaccine sector's market share.

LEARN MORE

The flu shot was added to the pediatric schedule in 2004, with the first shot beginning at six months of age and given annually thereafter for the rest of the child's life. The Gardasil vaccine, to protect against a virus thought to cause cervical cancer, was approved in 2006 for little girls, expanded in 2009 to little boys, and expanded again in 2018 for individuals up to age 45. The new RSV vaccine, Beyfortus (nirsevimab), was conceived to give protective antibodies to preemies and ultra-preemies, but has been expanded to be given to all children up to 24 months of age. These are three of many shots added to the schedule in the last 20 years that have served to balloon the revenues for vaccine manufacturers.

THE PHARMA-CONGRESS DANCE: FOLLOW THE MONEY

Business schools devote entire courses to consumer psychology. Creating the perfect formula for tapping into the psyche of a potential buyer is more art – and sometimes more luck – than science. But whatever the clever angle an institution's marketing division may choose, a few simple truths apply to any business. Chief among them is that while customers pay for products or services in the literal sense, they actually buy something to get a benefit, satisfy a need, or fulfill a demand. When a carpenter buys a drill bit, he is really buying holes. When travelers pay for airplane tickets, they are really buying transportation. Women buy cosmetics, but they are actually satisfying a need for a healthy glow, to cover a blemish, or more abstractly, to recover lost youth.

Vaccine manufacturers do the same thing: provide a benefit, fill a need, or meet a demand by the creation of a new product for a particular market niche. But when customers dig in and ferret out "true" versus "perceived" benefits of a vaccine, the misinterpretation of market demand can send a company into full retreat. The vaccine maker MedImmune experienced the full force of what misjudging a "perceived need" can do to sales and profits.

Information presented at the May 2003 National Influenza Summit showed that approximately 85 percent of Americans between the ages of 20 and 50 go unvaccinated, and nearly 66 percent between the ages of 50 and 64 do not receive the flu vaccine. Assuming that the low flu shot rates were due to resistance to getting a shot, MedImmune anticipated its pain-free, intranasal vaccine, FluMist, would be a smashing success. MedImmune expected its vaccine to become the next blockbuster drug with sales that would push revenues over the $1 billion per year mark. Every Pharma industry watcher agreed. Even with a cost of $46 per dose, compared to $15 per dose for a regular flu shot, FluMist was awarded a prize by *Popular Science* for being one of the best new healthcare products of 2003.[98]

Hundreds of television, radio, and print ads were designed to persuade everyone to take "The FluMist plunge," squirting a drop of influenza vaccine up the nose instead of getting a needle in the arm. In the "most intense, direct-to- consumer marketing campaign ever waged to date for a vaccine," the 9-week campaign was estimated to cost around $25 million. Wyeth, MedImmune's then partner, planned a three-year $100 million campaign to encourage physicians to use the nasal flu vaccine. Airplane advertisements, magazine articles, and rebate coupons from the FluMist website were all part of the blitz. Even scare tactics were employed similar to those used to promote the smallpox vaccine, warning of the high possibility of a bioterror attack using the flu virus.

It was all for naught. The first season for FluMist was a resounding flop. Anticipating sales of four to six million doses, MedImmune executives disappointedly reported a few weeks into the campaign that only about 400,000 doses had been sold in pharmacies and in doctors' offices.

They reluctantly admitted that as many as 80% of the doses that had been produced might be returned unused from distributors. Even when the initial price of $46 per dose was cut by more than 50 percent, no one wanted the vaccine. MedImmune stock plummeted from $24.50 per share to $1.08 almost overnight.[99]

What caused the marketing disaster? Many things went wrong. For starters, the vaccine needed to remain frozen until used, discouraging doctors and pharmacies from handling it. Another problem was timing: since the FDA didn't approve it for use until June, most pharmacies and offices had already ordered their supply of flu shots for the season. From the consumer's perspective, there was a long list of reasons to refuse FluMist. Some said it was the price. Some said there were too many safety concerns since FluMist contained live, attenuated viruses that could theoretically give people the flu (the illness they were trying to prevent), especially those with a weakened immune system. Some doctor's offices refused it because the FDA only approved FluMist for healthy people aged 5 to 49, the group that rarely gets flu shots. Some said it was the side effect profile. For example, it was not approved for kids under the age of 5 because this group had a higher rate of asthma attacks and wheezing within 42 days of the vaccination, compared to children who received a placebo. Perhaps the biggest reason consumers and physicians rejected the product was because there was no proof of efficacy in people over 50 years of age.

Obviously, misinterpreting market demand can be both costly and embarrassing.

Since that time, FluMist has been on and off the market several times because of lack of efficacy in various age groups. Most recently, in the 2022-2023 flu season, it was only 54% effective in preventing the flu in people less than 65 years of age and it was supposedly 71% effective in children. For the 2023-2024 flu season, FluMist was again only approved for people ages 2 to 49.

ENTER THE PANDEMIC VACCINES

The vaccine manufacturers were grumbling that the profit margins were so small they had minimal interest in developing new vaccines – until COVID-19, of course. Given the potential to inject billions of people with multiple doses of their products at a premium price backed by government money, manufacturers all over the world perked up their collective ears and began to change their minds. Every government began meetings with the producers, working on plans for how to quickly ramp up the ability to produce mRNA vaccines. All players were driven by the thoughts of an avalanche of money to follow.

An analysis done in 2021 by the accessibsa project identified a list of at least 120 manufacturers across Asia, Africa, and Latin America with the technical know-how and quality standards to make mRNA vaccines, with 55 plants located in India and 33 in China.[100] Companies identified had both the capacity to manufacture sterile injectables and had been certified by reputable agencies or organizations for good manufacturing practices (GMP). This was the only guarantee consumers had that any of the companies might adhere to international quality standards.[101] To track the research, *The New York Times* set up a manufacturing tracker to follow the clinical trials of the 10 top developers of COVID-19 jabs from early 2020 through August 31, 2022. They tracked many elements of the products' development, including the type of vaccine (e.g., DNA vs. genetic vs. inactivated, etc.). The tracker fully explained, with diagrams, how each type worked, how it was to be administered, how many doses were to be given, challenges for obtaining FDA approval, the number of subjects in each clinical trial, and more. When *The Times* stopped updating the tracker, 42 vaccines were in large-scale efficacy testing, 21 were in early but limited use, 12 had been approved for full use, and 17 trials had been abandoned. Throughout the time period, more than 120 clinical trials were underway.[102] In the end, about 19 companies went into full production, with Pfizer, Moderna, AstraZeneca, and Johnson and Johnson being the obvious big winners.

Having experienced the largest financial boom in the industry's history, Pfizer and Moderna were chomping at the bit to get going with the next blockbuster pandemic vaccine post-COVID. For a short period of time, this appeared to be a bird flu (H5N1) vaccine. The government was quick to play along.

Even though as of June 30, 2024, only three documented cases of humans with bird flu had been identified anywhere in the US, the government, with the help of BARDA, awarded Moderna $176 million in federal funding to develop an mRNA-based human pandemic influenza vaccine against bird flu for people 18 years and older.[103] More on this later.

Another company that scored an early big win for developing an H5N1 vaccine was CSL Seqirus, a seasonal flu shot manufacturer. In early 2022, CSL Seqirus gained a "ready to respond" designation, meaning that if a pandemic was declared, the factory would immediately shift from its seasonal flu shot production and begin manufacturing those required for the emergency. In October of that year, CSL Seqirus received a $30.1 million grant to begin testing H5N1 vaccine candidates.[104]

The following year, in August 2023, the government paid CSL Seqirus $46.3 million for 4.8 million doses of a bulk lot of H5N8 influenza A antigen for the US government. A study enrolled 480 adult participants to evaluate the safety and immunogenicity of a cell culture-derived influenza vaccine using H5N8 or H5N6. The experimental solutions also contained the adjuvant MF59 (more on that chemical later).[105] Then in May 2024, just a few weeks before the Moderna grant was announced, the government selected CSL Seqirus to deliver additional 4.8 million doses of a pre-pandemic, cell-based vaccine that matched the 2024 circulating H5N1 strain. The doses were to become part of the National Pre-Pandemic Influenza Vaccine Stockpile.[106]

HIGHLIGHT

CSL Seqirus' manufacturing facility in Holly Springs, NC, was built with a $2.1 billion public-private partnership contract navigated by HHS and BARDA.

As the largest cell-based influenza vaccine producer in the world, the facility can deliver up to 150 million doses of influenza vaccine within six months of a declared pandemic flu emergency.

THE GOVERNMENT MONEY POTS

What are the agencies within the government that so easily obtain our tax dollars to develop dangerous vaccines to be used against us? Here is a list of a few. There are actually many more, such as USDA, EPA, DoD, etc.

DHHS: The Department of Health and Human Services is the umbrella agency for more than 100 programs. DHHS, usually referred to as simply HHS, has 13 operating divisions, or agencies, with more than 80,000 employees.

> *NOTE:* During a national public health emergency, the Secretary of HHS is the most powerful person in the country.

ASPR: The Administration for Strategic Preparedness and Response (ASPR) has been in operation under various names since the 1950s. After Hurricane Katrina, the division took on more formal duties in 2006 under the Pandemic and All Hazards Preparedness Act. These roles have continued to expand since that time and in July 2022, the ASPR was elevated to an Operating Division within the Department of HHS. ASPR serves as the advisory staff on all public health emergencies.

The agency has doubled in size since 2019 and now has more than 2,000 employees.[107]

BARDA: The Biomedical Advanced Research and Development Authority resides within HHS and, according to its website, BARDA is responsible for the procurement and development of medical countermeasures "that address the public health and medical consequences of chemical, biological, radiological, and nuclear (CBRN) accidents, incidents and attacks, pandemic influenza, and emerging infectious diseases." A countermeasure is "a vaccine, medication, device, or other item used to prevent, diagnose, or treat a public health emergency or a security threat." Remember that word: **countermeasure.**

Two of BARDA's primary projects, Project NextGen and MedicalCountermeasures.gov, have allocated many billions of dollars for the development of the next round of bioterrorism vaccines and medical interventions. BARDA is the official interface between the federal government and the biomedical industry, which essentially means BARDA establishes public-private partnerships and determines if something is worthy of investing in to accomplish its missions then negotiates the contracts. The government allocates the funds, usually as grants. Under US Code Title 42, BARDA was appropriated $611,700,000 for *each* of the fiscal years 2019 through 2023. The funds are to remain available for use "until expended."[108]

The head of BARDA reports to the Secretary of ASPR. Several different sources cite that the number of employees working for BARDA at a given time can vary. However, the most recent and consistent information indicates that BARDA has around 150 employees. That's a lot of power in the hands of a relative few.

RRPV: The Rapid Response Partnership Vehicle is a fund managed by BARDA to accelerate production of Medical Countermeasures. At the time of this writing, the fund has more than 400 members, including 31 non-profits and 12 institutions of higher education. With no initiation fee and no annual membership fees, more members are joining the RRPV all the time. At the time of this writing, the RRPV had 483 members.[109]

BARDA uses Other Transactional Agreements (OTAs) to accelerate collaboration between industry and the federal government.[110] Governed by specific statutory authorities rather than the Federal Acquisition Regulation (FAR), OTAs lack standard oversight mechanisms like mandatory reporting, cost-accounting standards and performance audits. This makes it harder for Congress, watchdog agencies, and the public to track BARDA spending, evaluate performance, and ensure the efficient use of taxpayer funds. OTAs often allow sole-source or limited competition agreements, reducing competition and potentially increasing costs or fostering favoritism. They are also exempt from socioeconomic requirements, such as small business set-asides, which can disadvantage smaller contractors. Additionally, "project creep" – where projects expand beyond their original scope – can lead to significant cost overruns and make it harder to hold contractors accountable for project delays, cost overruns, or failures.

CDC: The Centers for Disease Control and Prevention, headquartered in Atlanta, Georgia, has 10 divisions. The mission of the CDC is to protect public health by "preventing and controlling disease, injury, and disability." This includes promoting vaccines, conducting research, responding to emergencies, collecting and analyzing health data, and collaborating with hundreds of health organizations. The agency currently employs around 15,000 people.

CMS: The Centers for Medicare & Medicaid Services (CMS), headquartered in Baltimore, Maryland, is the largest purchaser of healthcare in the US. CMS is in charge of Medicare, Medicaid, the Children's Health Insurance Program (CHIP), and the Health Insurance Marketplace, providing health coverage for more than 100 million individuals.

Medicare provides health insurance for individuals aged 65 and older, as well as some younger people with disabilities or specific conditions. **Medicaid** provides health coverage for low-income individuals and families, including children, pregnant women, elderly individuals, and people with disabilities. It is a form of medical insurance that covers hospital care, doctor visits, and mental health support, often at little or no cost. It aims to improve access to care for vulnerable populations while allowing states flexibility in program design. The **Children's Health Insurance Program (CHIP)** provides health coverage for children in families with incomes too high to qualify for Medicaid but too low to afford private insurance. The **Health Insurance Marketplace,** created by the Obama administration and the Affordable Care Act, is an internet platform designed to help people find insurance coverage that meets their health needs and budget. CMS has approximately 6,400 employees.

NIH: The National Institutes of Health is a sprawling campus headquartered in Bethesda, MD. The mission of the NIH is to conduct and support medical research to "improve human health, advance the understanding of diseases, and develop effective treatments and prevention strategies." This includes funding research projects, training the next generation of researchers, and promoting the translation of scientific discoveries. The NIH consists of 27 different divisions called Institutes and Centers, each with its own specific research area. As the nation's medical research agency, most areas focus on infectious diseases or diseased organs. The NIH employs 18,500 people.

Altogether, there are more than 122,000 people working for these agencies. Do the math and take a guess on the annual collective payroll for all these folks. The government's money tree is actually your tax dollars, paying for, among other things, the aggressive development of medical countermeasures and biomedical vaccines with you and your children as a target. And all of these products are fully liability-protected, even if they kill you. More on that later.

SHORING UP THE LIABILITY

In 2005, when manufacturers were confronted with a short timeline for the production of millions of doses of a new, untested, pandemic bird flu vaccine, they knew from the swine flu experience 30 years earlier that appropriate funding and insurance safeguards needed to be put in place before proceeding. To get that done, Congress needed to be persuaded: the drug companies had the tools – and the money – to get the job done. They had proof that the payments to Congress worked; it had just been done to get the Medicare Modernization Act passed two years earlier.

LEARN MORE

As reported in *Contingencies*, a bi-monthly trade journal for the actuarial profession, the pharmaceutical industry spent $24.58 million on government lobbying between January 1, 1998 and June 20, 2004. The lobbyists lavished funds and more on each person in Congress in 2002-3 to ensure the passage of the Medicare Modernization Act (MMA), one of the most significant changes ever to the 40-year-old Medicare program. Since its passage, the MMA has been a financial windfall for Big Pharma's profits, but it has been devastating for seniors.[111]

The amount of money spent by lobbyists has steadily increased every year since 2004. According to OpenSecrets.org (*the organization that tracks money in politics*), during COVID-19 in 2020, 2021, and 2022, the amount of money skyrocketed. Almost $1.126 billion was spent on lobbying efforts for pharmaceutical and health products by 1,854 lobbyists, of whom nearly 63% were former government employees. In fact, since 2008,143 members of Congress left to become lobbyists in the health sector.[112]

The lobbyists went to work. Billions of dollars were instantly available to ensure every part of the vaccine development process was in place to ramp up and roll out the new bird flu vaccine. These funding mechanisms included research grants, tax credits, advanced purchase commitments, and most importantly, laws that would absolve the companies and their products from ALL liability if issues arose from a marginally tested, unsafe product.

As the vaccine solution was put in the vial and headed toward the arms of all Americans, a few questions started to be raised. What made this pandemic influenza vaccine any different than the annual flu shot? As an egg-based product, would it also have contaminants and stray viruses? What about adjuvants and other chemicals? What was coming through that needle?

"May we assume, therefore, that chicken cell substrate vaccines are safe? With biological products, as with crossing the street, there is no such thing as absolute safety."

~Robin A. Weiss, University College London, UK

CHAPTER 11

Influenza Vaccines: What's Coming Through That Needle?

In terms of process, the method for manufacturing pandemic vaccines was only marginally different from the steps used to make the influenza vaccine that is produced each year. Even though cell-based vaccines are becoming more popular and mRNA flu shots are on the horizon, egg-based influenza vaccines represent the majority of flu vaccines currently offered. With more than thirty years of experience with the commercial scale application, egg-based manufacturing is a well-defined process. Some background of the manufacturing process will provide an understanding of both the annual flu shot and the pandemic vaccine first created in 2005. The new mRNA H5N1 vaccines will also be discussed.

THE ANNUAL FLU SHOT

Each year between January and March an FDA advisory panel selects the three influenza strains that are expected to be the most widespread strains during the upcoming flu season. Influenza virus detection assays are used in public health laboratories in all 50 US states. There are currently 152 national influenza centers (NICs) in over 129 countries that conduct year-round surveillance for flu viruses as part of the WHO Global Surveillance System. Five viruses are selected then sent to the seven WHO Collaborating Centers for Influenza. The process is an "educated guess", which the CDC admits. They send the selected "seed virus" to the FDA for approval prior to distributing it to the manufacturers for production. In 2004, there were two primary manufacturers of influenza vaccines for the US market, Chiron and Sanofi-Aventis. Today there are seven: AstraZeneca, GlaxoSmithKline (GSK), Novartis, Sanofi-Pasteur, Sanofi-Aventis, Mylan/Viatris, and Seqirus.

The annual flu shot contains three or four strains: two strains of influenza A and one or two of influenza B. Most commonly, two of the strains are the same as the preceding year's shot; one new strain is selected each year and then modified in the lab. The new viral strain and a second influenza virus, known to grow well in eggs, are injected into fertilized chicken eggs. The genes from the two viruses "mix together" through the reassortment process, forming as many as 256 possible newly created genetic combinations. From there, one virus is selected. Is this an "exact match" the CDC talks about so often?

Researchers select ONE virus for the season's vaccine that has both the (H) antigen from the upcoming year's virus and the internal genes from the virus that grows well in eggs. The new virus, along with the two other strains from the previous year, make up vaccines for the current season.[113]

The next few manufacturing steps are tricky. The original flu shot production is a slow, cumbersome process utilizing 500,000 fertilized chicken eggs *per day* for up to eight months. Hundreds of millions of eggs are purchased to become mini- incubators for the cultured viruses. Workers use a labor-intensive process known as candling, the examination of every egg by hand with a specialized light. This process allows for the handler to discard any eggs that have not been fertilized, do not have a growing embryo, or have cracks in the shell.

When the embryos are approximately 11-days old, the eggs are labeled with specific identification numbers and placed in a tray with the blunt end up. The tops are cleaned using a 70 percent ethanol wipe and a tuberculin needle is used to punch a small hole into the shell over the air sac. The amniotic membrane of the chicken embryo (the egg white) is then injected with a drop of viral-containing solution. Enough solution is contained within each syringe to inoculate three eggs. The puncture hole in the shell is sealed with a drop of glue and the eggs are maintained for two to three days in a temperature-controlled environment between 91.4°F and 93.2°F (33°C and 34°C, respectively). During that time, the viruses infect the lungs of the developing embryo and begin to rapidly replicate.

Several days later, the eggs are placed into a cooler and chilled to 39°F (3.8°C) overnight. The next day sterile forceps are used to chip open the shell and the fluid from the three similarly inoculated eggs is collected into a test tube. The gooey viral suspension is then centrifuged – sometimes more than once – to remove as much chicken blood and tissue from the solution as possible. Some residual egg protein remains within the final product. Even though the recommendations have changed over time, people with an egg allergy are still advised against receiving an egg-based flu shot.

LEARN MORE

Over the years, many studies have been published that say the same thing that the American Academy of Family Practice (AAFP) says on its website: *(paraphrased)*

> The vaccines that may contain egg protein are measles, mumps, rabies, yellow fever, and influenza. Even though someone may be intolerant to eating egg-containing foods, he or she may still have an egg allergy to injected proteins. However, in a review of 27 published studies, a total of 4,172 patients with egg allergy received 4,729 doses of egg-based inactivated influenza vaccine with no cases of anaphylaxis. Therefore, ACIP recommends that egg-allergic people receive inactivated influenza vaccine as a single dose, without prior vaccine skin testing, and be observed for 30 minutes afterwards for any possible allergic reaction. If the person reacted to the ingestion of eggs with *hives only,* the vaccine could be administered in a primary care setting. If the person's reaction to the ingested eggs was more severe, it was instructed for the vaccine to be administered in an allergist's or immunologist's office.[114]

I've often wondered how the presence of a doctor or giving the vaccination in a medical office somehow mitigates the risk of anaphylaxis after a flu shot, which has been estimated to be approximately 1.35 people per million doses. It has also been estimated that 70 million flu shots are administered on average each year. That means approximately 100 people per year have an anaphylaxis reaction to a flu shot. The risk of paralysis from Guillain-Barré Syndrome (GBS) is approximately 1-2 per million doses administered. Is the risk worth it?

After this "purification" step, a test is performed to detect the presence of the H antigen; if none is detected, the specimen is discarded. If H antigen is present, the solution is submitted for further chemical processing before it is placed into ampoules for sale. The entire process, from egg selection to viral harvest, takes at least six months.[115]

FROM EGG TO NEEDLE: THE ADDED CHEMICALS

After the viral particles are separated from the egg yolk, they are inactivated with formaldehyde, a known carcinogen.[116] Some brands of influenza vaccines also add 500 micrograms of **gentamicin**, a broad-spectrum antibiotic, to inhibit the growth of bacteria that may be in the suspension. The surface antigens, (H) and (N) are separated using **Triton X-100,** a detergent commonly used in laboratories and is added to viral vaccines at different stages of the manufacturing process. The chemical separates the surface antigens, increasing the probability that a B-cell can identify the (H) antigen to form an antibody.

Triton X-100, made by Dow Chemical, is formed by a reaction between polyethylene glycol (PEG) and ethylene oxide. Given the large number of reported allergic reactions to PEG, scrutinizing a vaccine's package insert to see if the manufacturing process used Triton X-100 is important because traces of Triton X-100 remain in the vaccine solution. This chemical may be an under-recognized and ignored contributor to allergic reactions after vaccination. Triton X-100 may be a "hidden" ingredient that leads to the anaphylactic reactions seen with the COVID-19 jabs, which is known to contain PEG.[117] Additional product information on this compound states the following:

> Triton X-100 is a 100% active ingredient, and is often used to solubilize (break down) proteins. Triton X-100 has no antimicrobial properties. It is considered a comparatively

mild detergent. Other uses (besides vaccine manufacture) include household & industrial cleaners, paints & coatings, pulp & paper, textile, agrochemicals, metal working fluids, oilfield chemicals.[118]

More chemicals go into the influenza vaccine solution including: **tributyl phosphate,** another detergent, **polysorbate 80,** an emulsifier, **sucrose** (table sugar), sodium phosphate-buffered isotonic salt solution, and **gelatin,** a stabilizer. **Resin** is mixed in to eliminate "substantial portions" of these chemicals even though residual amounts remain in the final product. **Thimerosal,** the mercury-based preservative, is added to the multidose vials of the flu vaccine.

COMMENTARY

There can be cross-reactivity between polysorbate 80 and polyethylene glycol (PEG). While polysorbate 80 and polyethylene glycol are chemically distinct molecules, they both belong to the group of chemicals called non-ionic surfactants and share similar properties. Cross-reactivity can occur in individuals who have had hypersensitivity reactions to one of these substances. This was an ignored concern regarding the cause of anaphylaxis seen early on in the distribution of COVID-19 jabs which contained PEG. Many may have been previously sensitized by the ubiquitous nature of polysorbate 80 that is found in food products, cosmetics, and childhood vaccines.

After detailing this vivid description of the toxic chemical soup used to manufacture influenza vaccines, the thought of injecting it into your body – or the body of your baby – should be repugnant. For those not repulsed by the idea and are still on the fence about the necessity of a flu shot, perhaps knowing that the vaccine won't prevent you from getting the flu will help sort out the decision.

First published in 1999 and periodically thereafter, the Cochrane Reviews on the effect of vaccinating healthy adults with influenza vaccines have been telling. The most recent review done in 2016, assessed 52 clinical trials that included more than 80,000 adults. The final analysis included 15% of the studies thought to be well designed and correctly conducted. It was concluded that flu shots give only a small protective effect against influenza, as 71 people would need to be vaccinated (NNV) to avoid one case of influenza. Vaccination may have little or no appreciable effect on hospitalizations (low-certainty evidence) or number of working days lost.[119]

There are more than 200 viruses that cause influenza-like illnesses (ILIs), which produce the same symptoms as influenza viruses: aches and pains, headache, cough, and runny nose. Without laboratory tests, doctors cannot distinguish between influenza and ILI because both conditions last for 7 to 10 days and rarely cause serious illness or death. The Cochrane Review found that the number needed to be vaccinated (NNV) to avoid one case of an ILI is 29.

In 2014, a meta review of 90 studies, also published by the Cochrane, concluded that influenza vaccination had very limited effect on reducing symptoms, on reducing hospitalizations, or on the number of missed days from work in pregnant women. In fact, flu shots had an average NNV to protect against ILI in pregnant women of 92 and an NNV of 27 against laboratory-confirmed influenza in newborns from vaccinated women.[122]

If this is true for garden variety influenza, wouldn't the same be true for a new pandemic bird flu strain? There is little doubt that a new H5N1 vaccine will come with the same criteria: It will be experimental, it will have no proof of safety, it will lack efficacy, it will have no long term studies, it may be released under an EUA, Emergency Use Authorization, and it may be given countermeasure protection, all similar to the COVID-19 shot. And instead of being made with eggs, it will be made using the mRNA technology. mRNA-based influenza vaccines are in various stages of research and development by pharmaceutical companies and collaborations including Moderna, Pfizer, GSK, Sanofi, Arcturus, and Seqirus (CSL).

Keep these studies in mind as the hype for mass vaccination begins once again.

LEARN MORE

The concept of "number needed to treat" (NNT) was introduced in the medical literature in 1988 by Laupacis et al.[120] Although the NNT was originally conceived for use in research studies, the NNT has become valuable for helping physicians select therapeutic interventions. The term NNV, or number needed to vaccinate, is essentially the same. NNV measures the preventive benefit of vaccination for a population while NNT measures the direct therapeutic benefit of a treatment to an individual. The ideal NNT is 1, where everyone improves with treatment and no one improves with control. **The higher the NNT or the NNV, the less effective a treatment is.**

For the COVID 19 shots, the NNV had different values for different populations, ranging from approximately 40 for older individuals to 600 for younger individuals, to prevent one hospitalization or one emergency department visit, showing how the jabs were not at all helpful.[121]

SPECIALIZED EGGS?

The eggs used in the production of the influenza vaccines are purchased by the tens of millions each season. An entire industry has evolved for the purpose of providing eggs for vaccine research and production.

Produced by specific pathogen-free (SPF) flocks, the birds have been certified to be free of contamination from *certain* microorganisms. Keep that word in mind.

The chickens are raised vaccine-free in isolated, air-filtered buildings that are expensive to build and to maintain, making the SPF eggs much more expensive than eggs available at the supermarket. The designation SPF is used to refer to these high maintenance birds, which are tested frequently to ensure the "microbiological integrity" of the flock is maintained.

In addition to testing the birds, their eggs are also closely inspected to guarantee the specific pathogen free status. The eggs are tested for 25 to 38 viruses and bacteria to confirm the absence of the specific pathogens on the list. If none of the listed agents are detected the egg is reported as "pathogen free."

The number of viruses and bacteria that eggs are screened for is finite, even though there are nearly an *infinite* number of potential agents from which to choose. To screen for every microbe would be completely time and cost prohibitive. So in theory, *if* human vaccines are made from SPF eggs, and *if* the standards of Good Manufacturing Practice (GMP) are maintained, vaccines *should* be free from specific pathogens and safe for human use with little concern about cross-species contamination.

The truth is, each egg is a new experiment.

Disturbingly, there is a wide difference between "specific pathogen-free" and "pathogen free." The distinction has long been important. First written about in 1997 in the January/February edition of the CDC's *Public Health Reports Journal,* it was acknowledged that "although it is not possible to produce a completely uncontaminated animal, it is possible to produce an animal [or egg] certified to be free of *specific pathogens.*"[123]

More recently, the Division of Technical Resources at the NIH released a bulletin on SPF animal research facilities in 2021 as a reminder of how the facilities must be designed and operated to receive the certification. The news report states the following:

> SPF animals are distinct from gnotobiotic animals, which are completely germ free and require sterile facilities. SPF facilities must be designed and operated to provide pathogen-free environments (though not sterile) to protect the health of the animals and the veracity of the research conducted within. An SPF facility can be as small as a microisolator housing a few animals, but a more typical facility is a dedicated suite consisting of one or more procedure rooms and holding rooms located within a larger general-purpose vivarium. Animals are either bred within the SPF facilities or introduced after quarantine and rigorous testing to confirm they are [specific] pathogen-free.[124]

Could unidentified pathogens present in eggs be passed into the finished product of the current, and future, pandemic influenza vaccines? Could viruses that are harmless to their animal host be dangerous to humans? This grave concern is more than theoretical because harmful "extra" viruses have been passed on through vaccines before.

EXTRANEOUS VIRAL CONTAMINATION

Over the last 15 to 20 years, researchers have recorded a litany of serious disease-causing transmissions from vaccines. In the 1940s, hepatitis B was transmitted via the albumen used to stabilize the yellow fever vaccine.[125] Between 1955 and 1962, at least a third of all polio vaccines were thought to be contaminated with the cancer-causing monkey virus SV40.[126] (For a full discussion on the contamination of the polio vaccines with SV40, see the book by Debbie Bookchin and

Jim Schumacher, *The Virus and the Vaccine: The True Story of a Cancer-Causing Monkey Virus, Contaminated Polio Vaccine, and the Millions of Americans Exposed*, St. Martin's Press, 2004.) Similarly, human blood products, blood-derived materials, and clotting factors have transmitted infectious viruses. Multitransfused hemophiliacs have acquired long term hepatitis from contaminated Factor VII and Factor XI products. Fortunately, these infections occur much less frequently now than before 1985. However, other transfusion-transmitted infections that have occurred include hepatitis A (HAV), hepatitis B (HBV), hepatitis C (HCV), hepatitis G (HGV), and HIV.[127]

Eggs are currently used to manufacture several vaccines other than flu shots: measles, mumps, and yellow fever. If only a portion of the bird flu H5N1 vaccines are made from eggs, they will have a risk of contamination too. The chart (provided with the permission from AVSBio Laboratories), is an example of infectious agents that eggs are commonly tested for. If these pathogens are absent from the eggs, they are labeled SPF eggs. Given the hundreds of known viruses and bacteria with which they could be contaminated, this list is dangerously short.

EXTRA VIRUSES IN EGGS

One virus that has garnered a great deal of attention because of its confirmed presence in vaccines is called endogenous avian leukosis virus, or ALV. Nearly 45 years ago it was found that seemingly healthy hens could transmit ALV to their eggs and then it could be passed into vaccines. Found in all chicken cell lines, ALV is known to affect large segments of the modern poultry industry. Because it is found in all commercial chickens and their eggs, humans are exposed on a consistent basis. ALV is considered a "parent" virus because it can transform into other potentially cancer-causing viruses through recombination or mutation. Viruses that derive from ALV include several members of the Rous sarcoma virus (RSV) family.

These viruses can be oncogenic and are known to cause tumors in chickens:

- avian myeloblastosis virus
- avian myelocytoma virus
- avian erythroblastosis virus
- Fujinami sarcoma virus
- and others that are less common

Egg Quality Comparison Guide (Table 1)

Agent	Antigen	Test	Premium	Premium Plus	Research
Avian Adenovirus Group I	CELO-Phelps	AGP	X	X	X
Avian Adenovirus Group II (HEV)	Domermuth	MFIA	X	X	X
Avian Adenovirus Group III (EDS)	CLKKT5D	HI	X	X	X
Avian Encephalomyelitis	van Roekel	MFIA	X	X	X
Avian Influenza (Type A)	T/W/G8	ELISA, AGP	X	X	X
Avian Nephritis Virus	G4260	MFIA	X	X	X
Avian Paramyxovirus Type 2	Yucaipa	MFIA	X	X	X
Avian Reovirus (Av. Orthoreoviruses)	S1133	AGP, MFIA, IFA	X	X	X
Avian Rhinotracheitis Virus (Turkey Rhinotracheitis or Avian Pneumovirus)	UK	ELISA	X	X	X
Avian Rotavirus	Ch-2	AGP	X	X	X
Avian Tuberculosis (Mycobacterium Avium)	M. avium	CO, PM	X	X	X
Chicken Anemia Virus	DelRose	IFA		X	X
Endogenous GS Antigen	p27	ELISA			X
Fowl Pox	Conn	MFIA, CO	X	X	X
Hemophilus paragallinarum (Avibacterium Paragallinarum)	Serovars A,B,C	CO	X	X	X
Infectious Bronchitis - Ark.	Ark 99	MFIA	X	X	X
Infectious Bronchitis - Conn.	Conn A5968	MFIA	X	X	X
Infectious Bronchitis - JMK	JMK	MFIA	X	X	X
Infectious Bronchitis - Mass	Mass 66579	MFIA	X	X	X
Infectious Bursal Disease Type 1	M4040(2512)	MFIA, AGP	X	X	X
Infectious Bursal Disease Type 2	M4040(2512)	AGP	X	X	X
Infectious Laryngotracheitis	UC A92430	ELISA, AGP	X	X	X
Lymphoid Leukosis A, B	RSV-RAV A,B	MFIA	X	X	X
Avian Lymphoid Leukosis Virus J (ALV J)	Hc-1	MFIA	X	X	X
Lymphoid Leukosis Viruses (Antigen)	A,B,C,D,E,J	ELISA	X	X	X
Marek's Disease (Serotypes 1,2, 3)	SB-1	AGP	X	X	X
Mycoplasma gallisepticum	A5969	SPA	X	X	X
Mycoplasma synoviae	WVU 1853	SPA	X	X	X
Newcastle Disease	LaScta	MFIA	X	X	X
Reticuloendotheliosis Virus	ATCC 770 T	IFA, AGP	X	X	X
Salmonella pullorum-gallinarum	K Polyvalent	SPA	X	X	X
Salmonella species		IA	X	X	X

Test abbreviation key:
AGP = Agar Gel Precipitin
CO = Clinical Observation
ELISA = Enzyme-Linked Immunosorbent Assay
HI = Hemagglutination Inhibition
IA = Isolation of Agent
IFA = Indirect Fluorescent Antibody
MFIA = Multiplexed Fluorometric Immunoassay
PM = Postmortem
SPA = Serum Plate Agglutination

2025 AVSBio Technical Guidelines for SPF Eggs chart. Used with permission.

Like other avian retroviruses, ALV can be transmitted through direct contact, contaminated environments, or vertical transmission from infected hens to their eggs. One group of researchers who studied the actions of ALV writes, "Serial passage of a retrovirus that does not carry an oncogene, with high frequency, will lead to the emergence of new viruses that can transduce oncogenes..." [128] That is professional double-speak for the following: Given the right growth conditions, ALV can transform into closely related viruses that are known to be cancer-related.

Another virus discovered in 1985, called endogenous avian retrovirus (EAV), is also a known contaminant of influenza vaccines. This virus is present in all breeds of chicken and, because of its endogenous nature, cannot be eliminated from most flocks even with stringent biosecurity measures.[129] EAV has an associated enzyme called reverse transcriptase. The job of this enzyme is to copy the genetic material of the RNA of the virus into DNA, reversing the normal flow of genetic information, which is normally copied from DNA to RNA. Since 1982, researchers have identified the presence of EAV and reverse transcriptase in influenza vaccines. In 1997, reverse transcriptase activity was also found in chicken embryo fibroblast cultures.[130]

Soon thereafter, in 1999, Tsang, et al. detected the presence of EAV, ALV and reverse transcriptase in the measles and mumps vaccines. They tracked the enzyme's origin back to the cell cultures in which the viruses had been grown. Considering the numerous regulations requiring cell cultures to be free of known chicken bacterium and viral pathogens, this was an alarming discovery. Knowing how the reverse transcriptase works in living cells, could it be possible that vaccines containing reverse transcriptase were weaving viral genes from chickens (EAV and/or ALV) into the human genome and could they become oncogenes in humans?

That was a sobering thought.

In a follow up study later that same year, a PCR analysis looked for ALV and EAV sequences in peripheral blood mononuclear cells (a special type of white blood cell) in 33 children who had received the measles and mumps vaccination. The results were negative. Tsang, et.al. were quick to point out that this ONE small study was enough to eliminate the concerns that ALV, EAV, and/or reverse transcriptase found in the vaccine were not found in the blood of the vaccine recipients. They quickly retracted their previous concerns, saying this single study should "provide reassurance for current immunization policies."[131]   It is noteworthy that other researchers disagreed with the conclusion of Tsang and her group. Even though the risk for humans appeared to be low, it wasn't zero.

COMMENTARY

A test group of 33 kids put the concern to bed. *Really?* Note the research done by Dr. Tsang's group was funded, at least in part, by the National Vaccine Program Office, a division of HHS. I wonder how much pressure was applied by the vaccine manufacturers to ensure that the "belief in vaccines" would remain unquestioned? No one will ever know.

Given the behavior of viruses in mammalian cellular cultures, a blood serum test cannot always provide the evidence of the presence of a virus in mammals. What if the virus has been incorporated into tissues at the time of the blood draw? It would not be found in the bloodstream or even inside of circulating white blood cells.[132] But like so many disturbing questions about the safety of vaccines that should cause the industry to pause production and evaluate the concerns, researchers were focused on proving the absence of the adventitious (extra) viruses and disproving the activity of reverse transcriptase, rather than documenting the presence of the extra viruses and searching for harm they may be causing.

AVIAN VIRUS CONTAMINATION AND CANCER

The issue of avian virus contamination has long been discussed by government agencies that regulate the production of egg-based vaccines. The CDC, FDA, Center for Biologics, Evaluation, and Research (CBER), and other branches of the public health service have convened on many occasions to discuss the implications of vaccine contaminants.

Co-sponsored by the FDA and CBER (one of its divisions), a workshop named *"Evolving Scientific and Regulatory Perspectives on Cell Substrates for Vaccine Development"* was held on September 10, 1999. Experts convened from government and industry to once again discuss the problems of vaccine contaminants. Dr. Phil Minor from the National Institute of Biological Standards and Control (NIBSC) – the CBER equivalent in the United Kingdom (UK) – was the first speaker of the morning of the meeting's sixth session. Minor gave a straightforward introduction, voicing concerns over the problem of animal viruses contaminating human vaccines. Of note, Dr. Minor was paid by GlaxoSmithKline, manufacturers of MMR, to act as an expert witness in the impending UK High Court MMR/autism cases. GSK is one of three UK companies that were the subject of the litigation at the time, the other two being Aventis Pasteur MSD and Merck.

There was little argument among researchers that avian retroviruses (ALV and EAV) and reverse transcriptase had been detected in influenza vaccines and other vaccines made from eggs for a very long time. What they did not agree upon, however, were the effects the viruses may be having on humans, including the possibility that they may be causing cancer. Also, even though the studies had concluded, there was no evidence that avian oncogenic viruses could replicate in humans or that they were involved in human cancer or multiple sclerosis (MS), the lack of evidence is not the same as lack of proof.

"Lack of evidence" means that there is yet to be sufficient information or data to support a claim, while "lack of proof" suggests that something has been definitively shown to be false or untrue. In other words, just because there isn't evidence to support an assertion doesn't necessarily mean the assertion is false; it may simply mean that the "smoking gun" has not yet been found.

Extra viruses in the vaccines are considered to be completely benign by some researchers. These contaminants, called "free riders," have not been found to interact in any way with the immune system or other cells of the vaccine recipient. However, considering all contaminants to be completely benign has a glaring flaw – even though many inactive viruses have been tested and are indeed harmless, not all viruses have been tested. If some – *even one* – is found to have the ability to replicate, it could very well cause harm.

Attempting to determine the effect a viral contaminant may have on human cells and on the human genome has an added complexity. Part of the normal life cycle of a retrovirus involves integrating, for a variable period of time, into the host's DNA. The virus can insert itself and "become invisible" to the immune system and beyond the reach of antibodies used to identify and remove it. This also means the virus is beyond the scope of the researcher's testing tools, such as PCR testing. Researchers are unable to find a retrovirus if it has already been embedded into human DNA.

Chicken cell cultures are not the only concern for the source of viral contaminants found in vaccines. Bovine (cow) sera are used for the production of the following vaccines: rubella, chickenpox, shingles, hepatitis A, rabies, polio, and some flu shots. Nearly 100 percent of the commercially available bovine serum is contaminated with bovine viruses, particularly bovine diarrheal virus (BVDV). This begs the questions: Are we incorporating chicken and cow genetic material into the human genome? By administering vaccines, are we altering the genes of future generations in unknown ways?

A well-researched, highly documented paper published online in 2003 by an obvious industry insider under the pseudonym Benjamin McReardon has been widely read and quoted. The paper described in detail the problem of not knowing whether a viral particle is active, inactive, or dormant. If it is active, viruses such as ALV have the capacity to activate cancer-causing genes within the host's cells:

> "Considering that ALV can, for example, easily capture the human oncogenes [called] 'erb' and 'myc,' and these two oncogenes are strongly associated with common forms of human breast cancer, it seems the issue of ALV vaccine contamination risk should deserve a high level of attention. A well-known microbiology text reinforces these concepts by teaching, "Proto-oncogenes become incorporated into retroviral genomes with surprising ease."[133]

It has been said that the seeds of cancer lie within us. The human genome contains at least 50 genes called proto-oncogenes, which under normal conditions, keep a watchful eye over excessive cell division and keep it under control. However, when a proto-oncogene is converted into an active oncogene, uncontrolled cell growth can occur. When cells undergo rapid, unchecked cell division the possibility for abnormal cells to arise and replicate is more than a theoretical concern. This is the start of cancer.

EFFECTS ON THE GLOBAL POPULATION

As discussed, published research has documented the presence of viral contaminants in egg-based vaccines. If the flu shot were given only once in a lifetime, the load of stray viruses delivered in a single shot would have minimal consequences on the human genome. But the influenza vaccine is recommended for infants starting at six months of age, and is intended to be given annually for the rest of that child's life. Could potentially cancer-causing retroviruses and other viruses be incorporated into a child's genome from infancy and thereafter be done so without detection, leading to health problems later in life?

It's not an unreasonable question.

LEARN MORE

A proto-oncogene can be activated by a variety of mechanisms including the insertion of viral DNA into the host's genome. In October 2023, Dr. David J. Speicher and his research team published a paper reporting that they had independently tested 27 modRNA vials, the greatest number of unopened vials of COVID-19 vaccine to date. High levels of residual plasmid DNA were found in both the Pfizer and Moderna COVID-19 modified mRNA jabs. When the vaccine vials were tested by fluorometry, the total DNA levels greatly exceeded the regulatory limit by 7 to 145-fold.[134] The Pfizer COVID-19 modRNA vaccines also contained an SV40 promoter-enhancer-ori, **which may play a role in facilitating transport of DNA into the nucleus.**[135] *(emphasis added)* The study confirmed the earlier work of Kevin McKernan and Dr. Philip Buckhaults.[136] Was the massive international increase in turbo cancers caused by the ingredients in the COVID-19 jabs?

Samuel S. Epstein, MD, (1926-2018) was, at the time of his death, the chairman of the Cancer Prevention Coalition and professor emeritus of Environmental and Occupational Medicine at the University of Illinois School of Public Health, Chicago. In a report released on May 9, 2002, he stated that the incidence of cancer has steadily increased since passage of the 1971 National Cancer Act, which launched the "War Against Cancer." In the US, for example, the age-adjusted cancer incidence rate in 1975 was 335 per 100,000 people (earliest data available), compared to around 439 per 100,000 in 2022. This represents a notable increase over the decades despite fluctuations in specific cancer types. Globally, cancer incidence rates have also risen, reflecting broader trends in industrialization, urbanization, and lifestyle changes affecting risk factors for cancer.

Certainly, a laundry list of environmental causes have been implicated in the exponential rise in cancer: paternal and maternal exposures to alcohol, drugs, and cigarettes; exposure to occupational carcinogens such as dioxin and thousands of environmental chemicals; pesticides in the home, lawn, and garden including glyphosate; pet flea collars; and consumption of sodium nitrites in meat. Our food now contains more than 10,000 different food additives that have not been studied for cumulative or combined toxicity.

But what about the elephant in the living room?

A child receives approximately 73 vaccine doses of 16 different vaccines from birth to 18 years of age, depending on the specific brand of vaccine. With the addition of the new RSV vaccines and the COVID-19 jabs, many will receive even more. The regimen includes 100s of doses of chemicals, some with carcinogenic properties. Does early exposure to this chemical soup, contaminating viruses, and reverse transcriptase lay the groundwork for increased susceptibility to cancer as children grow into adulthood?

WHAT'S AT STAKE?

The risks of the incorporation of retroviruses into human DNA have gone up substantially since the influenza vaccine was added to the pediatric vaccine schedule in 2004, targeting six to twenty-three-month-old babies. With the specter of another pandemic influenza on the horizon, more alarms need to be raised. With each egg-based vaccine, the risk that abnormal viruses will be introduced into the human genome goes up exponentially. With manufacturers moving toward cell-based cultures (dogs, monkeys, etc.) and mRNA platforms used to make faster and cheaper vaccines, what else will be coming through that needle to poison us?

The logarithmic increase of exposure to viral contaminants caught the attention of a few concerned researchers at the previously mentioned September 1999 CBER workshop. Dr. Martin Myers from the National Vaccine Program posed a thoughtful question regarding the long-term safety of egg-based vaccines. Dr. Myers asked:

> "As I sit and count the number of immunizations that various populations receive [that contain] these retroviral particles, I wonder if there is any data on sero-responsiveness in longitudinal [studies]?" *(meaning, have we followed these children over an extended period of time to see if they have developed antibodies to viral contaminants?)*

An even more appropriate question would have been, "Have we looked for health problems in these children to see if they have been caused by the vaccine viral contaminants?" And note this was 25 years ago; many vaccines have been added since that time.

A response came quickly from James S. Robertson, PhD, from NIBSC. He interrupted Myers stating, "There is no evidence for any increase in the incidence of childhood cancers since the introduction of the measles and mumps vaccination program" [in 1963].

This comment was as incomplete as it was inaccurate. A more accurate answer would have been, "We have not identified any increase in childhood cancer caused by retroviruses," which begs the question: Are researchers actually *looking for* an association between vaccine retroviruses and cancer? In research, you can't find what you're not looking for. Finding an association between retroviruses in vaccines and cancer would be disastrous for both the vaccine and the cancer programs. Because no one wants to find this association, funding for this type of research was, and is in short supply.

At the end of his presentation, Dr. Phil Minor again addressed the group, summarizing his concerns this way:

> "...the issues that I have been dealing with really have to do with primary cells that come directly from animals. I think there is no doubt in my mind that this is the main source of concern in terms of human health."

His conclusions were echoed by a CDC virologist, Dr. Walid Heneine, also in attendance at the workshop. Dr. Heneine publicly cautioned the importance of not generalizing about the hypothesis that "no harm" is being caused by the accidental avian viruses in vaccines. She mentioned the research conducted in 1997 by Weissmahr, et al. at the EPA which demonstrated that, because viral contaminants *were capable of replicating,* they may be capable of causing harm.[137] In addition, Dr. Heneine suggested that "prudence be followed" because even though the presence of some viruses are known, other disease-causing viruses may be present although they have not yet been detected.

What's coming through that needle could, indeed, be deadly. And we haven't explored all that is being injected into the human body via vaccination.

The worst is yet to come.

"Today, the NIH is working with vaccine makers to develop new cell-culture techniques that will help us bring a pandemic flu vaccine to the American people faster in the event of an outbreak... and it would allow us to produce enough vaccine for every American in time."

~Pres. G. W. Bush, November 1, 2005

CHAPTER 12
Human and Animal Cell Lines

S anofi-Pasteur, the vaccine division of the Sanofi-Aventis Group, was the first to partner with HHS when the roll out of the first bird flu vaccines began in 2005. Over the preceding year, *(did they know what was coming?)* the company had negotiated five production agreements with the US government using the pandemic H5N1 virus.

The first contract, signed in May 2004, was an agreement between Sanofi-Pasteur and Fauci's NIAID to produce 8,000 investigational doses of H5N1 vaccine for a phase I human clinical trial. The doses were manufactured at the Swiftwater, Pennsylvania facility and the human trials took place at three university-based centers throughout the US: The University of Rochester in New York, the University of Maryland at Baltimore, and the University of California, Los Angeles. The first trial, which included 452 healthy adults, was designed to assess the immune response and safety profile of the experimental vaccine. The results of the three-month trial came in at the end of August 2004 and were mixed at best.

As reported in *The New York Times*, a positive antibody response only occurred in 115 of the participants (25.4 percent) with two doses of vaccine (an initial dose and a second dose given four weeks later.) NIAID Director Anthony Fauci was quoted in *The Times* story as saying, "It's good news. We have a vaccine." However, it wasn't all good news, especially for the manufacturers. The vaccine required 90 micrograms of viral (H5) antigen – remember that number – to elicit an antibody response and it had to be given twice (a total of 180 micrograms.) This immediately created a monumental challenge to production capacity. In comparison, the annual flu shot requires only 15 micrograms of (H) antigen per shot. The solution to "stretching" the effect of the antigen? The addition of a toxic adjuvant. More on that below.

In a subsequent *Wall Street Journal* report dated October 14, 2005, Fauci reported that based on the preliminary results, the two million H5N1 doses ordered by the US government would only cover about 450,000 people. Infectious disease expert Michael Osterholm, MD, expressed concern about the supply issue, stating that 12 times the amount of antigen would be needed to get the same response as a typical flu shot AND to cover the entire population.

The industry's explanation for this lack-luster response to the H5N1 antigen was that this "new virus" had never been "seen" before by the immune system and the system needed to be "primed" to generate an adequate response. However, this created a serious contradiction. If H5N1 was as dangerous to humanity as portrayed in the media, then a small amount of the antigen should generate a huge immunological response. This didn't appear to be the case. Not then. Not now.

A more feasible explanation – then AND now – was that the H5N1 virus doesn't present a threat. This assumption was confirmed by the New England Journal of Medicine article, published in September 2005, that said:

> "The relatively low frequencies of influenza A (H5N1) illness in humans despite widespread exposure to infected poultry indicate that the species barrier to acquisition of this avian virus is substantial."[138]

In simple terms, that means that the idea of a bird flu virus "jumping species" to infect a human was, and remains, highly improbable. It also explained why the thousands of people who had been exposed to their chickens that were infected with H5N1 in 2003 only had mild sniffles or no symptoms at all. The same happened with bird flu in 2024. The most prevalent symptom in a farm worker who tests positive is conjunctivitis.

The news that much more H5N1 antigen was needed to meet vaccine demand meant that standard production methods would be inadequate. Each flu shot factory has a limited production capacity, partially due to the space constraints needed to house millions of eggs. In addition, the process requires up to six months to produce a single lot of vaccine with no margin for error and no capacity to ramp up production if the effectiveness was found to be dismal. A new type of vaccine production was needed, including new factories. Anticipating this need, the attention of manufacturers was drawn on a new technology – cell-based influenza vaccines.

CELL-BASED TECHNOLOGY

First described in the mid-1990s, all major players in the vaccine industry have been working for decades to develop cell culture technology for flu shots. They were searching for a methodology that could be rapidly scaled any time the government thought there was an emergent need for more vaccines.

Although new for making pandemic vaccines, cell-culture technology for making standard vaccines was hardly new. This process has been used since the 1950s for the production of polio, measles, mumps, and tetanus vaccines. Different from the tedious egg-based technique, cell-culture methods grow viruses in large steel vats filled with living cells. The viruses, which need living tissue to replicate, enter the cells and rapidly start to divide, allowing for large-scale harvest within a matter of days. While the egg-based method requires at least six months and a large amount of human-power to produce viruses for millions of vaccines, the cell-based method, from start to a finished product, creates a large batch in approximately 60 days. That is the potential of five to six viral harvests every three weeks.

Cell-line technology has not been used on a large scale, primarily for logistical reasons – it would require a complete retooling of existing production facilities to create the new manufacturing process. None of the manufacturers were willing to invest the millions of dollars and the five to seven years required to build new vaccine production plants, unless, of course, the government puts up the money. Their perspective was rather like, "if it ain't broke, don't fix it." But with the specter of repeated pandemics looming on the horizon, the need for hundreds of millions of doses of vaccine, with the windfall of profits, and tens of millions in federal dollars available to pay for the capital improvements, the reasons and the means were in place to proceed.

Sanofi-Pasteur was the first to sign the agreement to build a new cell line-based manufacturing facility and the first to secure government funding for preliminary vaccine trials. On April 1, 2005, HHS awarded Sanofi-Pasteur a $97 million contract to expedite the construction of the new plant. This five-year grant facilitated a rapid overhaul of their existing manufacturing facility in Swiftwater, Pennsylvania, which had been producing influenza vaccines for more than 50 years and was responsible for several flu shot brands, including Fluzone – the only influenza vaccine at the time (2003) approved in the US for children aged six to thirty-five months. The renovated facility, spanning 145,000 square feet (13,470 square meters) and costing $150 million, was completed in July 2007. In May 2009, the FDA approved its production of vaccines in time for the 2009-2010 flu season. This initiative created more than 100 new production jobs and had the capacity to produce at least 300 million doses of influenza vaccine annually – enough for every person in America.

As of 2024, there are between 10 and 15 major production facilities in the US that utilize cell line technology for vaccine manufacturing, and the specific number can vary over time. This includes companies like Seqirus, Sanofi, Pfizer, Moderna, Johnson & Johnson, and others that produce a variety of vaccines.

LEARN MORE

As of 2024, this list of vaccines utilizes human and animal cell line technology in their production:*

COVID-19 Vaccines
1. **Pfizer-BioNTech (Comirnaty)**: HEK293T cell line.
2. **Moderna (Spikevax)**: HEK293T cell line.
3. **Johnson & Johnson (Janssen)**: PER.C6 cell line.

Influenza Vaccines
1. FluBlok: *Sf9* insect cell line.
2. FluLaval: MDCK cell line.
3. Afluria: MDCK cells.

Hepatitis A Vaccines
1. Havrix: MRC-5 cell line.
2. Vaqta: MRC-5 cell line.

Rabies Vaccines
1. RabAvert: VERO cell line.
2. Imovax Rabies: VERO cell line.

Varicella (Chickenpox) Vaccines
1. Varivax: MRC-5 cell line.
2. ProQuad: MRC-5 cell line. (MMR + Chickenpox vaccine)

Zoster (Shingles) Vaccine
1. Shingrix: MRC-5 cell line.
2. Zostavax: MRC-5 cell line.

Measles, Mumps, and Rubella Vaccines
1. MMR II: WI-38 cell line (rubella) and MRC-5 cell line. (measles & mumps)

Other Vaccines
1. **Dengvaxia**: (Dengue Vaccine): VERO cell line.
2. **Rotavirus Vaccines**:
   - RotaTeq: VERO cells.
   - Rotarix: MDCK cells.

3. **Human Papillomavirus (HPV) Vaccines**:
   - Gardasil: HEK293 cell line used in development; not in the final product.
4. **Japanese Encephalitis Vaccine**:
   - IXIARO: VERO cell line.
5. **ACAMBUS 1000:** (vaccinia) MRC-5
6. **RSV Vaccines**:
   - Arexvy: HEK293
   - Abryvso: HEK293
7. **Polio Vaccines:**
   - IPV: (Inactivated Poliovirus Vaccine): VERO cell line. Some formulations may also have used the WI-38 cell line.
   - OPV: (Oral Poliovirus Vaccine): Historically, MRC-5 cell line, then grown in VERO cell line.

*cell lines are:

HEK293T: human kidney of an 8-week-old aborted fetus. 1973.

PER.C6: human retinal cells 18-week-old aborted fetus. 1990s.

Sf9 cells: derived from the fall armyworm. 1990s.

MDCK: kidney of an adult female Cocker Spaniel. 1950s.

MRC-5: lung tissue of a 14-week-old male fetus. 1966.

WI-38: lung tissue of a 12 week-old female fetus. 1962.

VERO: kidney of an African green monkey. 1962

FETAL CELL LINES

Although the idea of growing viruses in eggs to create a vaccine may sound repulsive to some, the choices for cell line vaccines are no less offensive. Two cell lines from aborted fetal tissue, WI-38 and MRC-5, have been used to make MMR vaccines since the 1960s.

The use of human cell lines for vaccine production started in 1962 with the **WI-38 cell line,** established by Dr. Leonard Hayflick and his team at the Wistar Institute (WI) in Philadelphia. WI-38 was derived from the lung tissue of a 12-week-old female fetus that had been legally aborted in the UK for therapeutic reasons. While looking for a cell line that would replicate and be stable for many generations, multiple other WI cell lines were developed using the fetus. For example, cell lines were established from tissue extracted from the kidneys, liver, heart, skin, and brain.

As it turned out, lung cells were the easiest to culture and had the most desirable growth characteristics, including long-term stability. WI-38 cells are diploid, meaning they contain two sets of chromosomes and exhibit typical human cell characteristics. Because the cells have a finite lifespan, they typically undergo about 50 doublings before entering senescence, a state where they no longer divide. The finite life span of the WI-38 cells sets them apart from precancerous or cancerous cell lines that divide in perpetuity.

The rubella vaccine, developed in 1963, was the first to use WI-38 cells. Later, the use of WI-38 cells expanded to other vaccines, including hepatitis A, varicella (chickenpox), and an older version of the shingles vaccine (Zostavax; no longer on the market.) That the cells originated from an aborted fetus has long raised ethical debates surrounding the use of fetal tissue in medical research. In addition, the presence of residual human DNA from the diploid cell lines raises concerns that the foreign DNA could integrate into a developing infant's genome, potentially causing genetic mutations, trigger autoimmune disorders such as type 1 diabetes or rheumatoid arthritis, or worse, promote cancer as previously discussed.

Vaccine safety testing has not adequately addressed the theoretical risks posed by residual DNA, even small amounts of 5 to 10 nanograms per dose, from different genders into infants. For example, WI-38 cells originate from a female fetus and the MRC-5 cells originated from a male fetus. There are gaps in understanding the potential long- term effects of injecting a full set of opposite gender chromosomes into a rapidly developing baby before two years of age. The FDA and CBER say the fragments are "unlikely to cause harm." But the full effects are not known.

About the same time that WI-38 cells were commercialized the **MRC-5 cell line** was developed by researchers at the Medical Research Council (MRC) in the UK, specifically by a team led by Dr. Paul J. van der Eb and Dr. Michael J. O'Neill. MRC-5 cells were derived from lung tissue of a 14-week-old male fetus and have since become widely used in various applications in medical research and vaccine production.

PER.C6 cells are human cells that originated from the retina of an 18-week-old fetus by researchers at Crucell (now part of Johnson & Johnson). The original retinal cells were extracted, and frozen in liquid nitrogen in 1985. They were thawed in 1995 for the complex creation of the PER.C6 cells. The fetal retina cells were first exposed to Adenovirus 5, which transformed them into perpetually dividing cells. The biological culture used to grow the cells is called a **designer substrate.** That this biological material can be harmful to humans is more than a theoretical consideration.

When test animals were injected with Adenovirus 5 alone, no tumors were formed. However, when mice were injected with liquid from the designer substrate, tumors appeared. There are many reasons the growth medium could cause tumor formation. Among these are the use of genetically modified ingredients, the presence of foreign DNA, oncogenes from stray contaminating viruses, growth factors from the modified proteins in the platform, and more. The FDA has long been aware of this concern because it was reported in a meeting in 2001, but research using designer substrates has continued.[139, 140]

LEARN MORE

Fetal cell lines are also widely used in scientific research, especially in areas like virology, oncology, and genetics. Some cosmetic companies, such as Clinique, LaMer, Olay, and Pantene have used fetal cell lines, at least in the past, in research for anti-aging products. However, the use is controversial and not widely publicized. Many brands are moving away from the technology due to public backlash.

Senomyx was a biotechnology company focused on creating flavorings for the food and beverage industry that would reduce the amount of sugar, salt, MSG, and fat in foods while preserving flavor. However, Senomyx used HEK293 cells from human fetal kidneys in flavor research which raised ethical concerns, particularly from pro-life groups. When it became known that Senomyx had partnered with major food and beverage companies, including PepsiCo, Nestlé, and Campbell Soup, the idea was repulsive to consumers. Even though no cells were in the final products, calls rang out to boycott these companies and others that used Senomyx's technology.

In 2018, Firmenich, a Swiss flavor and fragrance company, acquired Senomyx. Since the acquisition, it's unclear to what extent HEK293 cells continue to be used in the development of new flavorings under Firmenich's leadership. However, Firmenich hasn't made any announcements regarding either a continuation or a halt of this specific practice, although they have issued a statement saying no cells are found in the final products.

The PER.C6 cells are primarily used in research, but they were used to develop Johnson & Johnson's COVID-19 vaccine (also known as the Janssen or the J&J vaccine). Even though the CDC website insists that all fetal cells are removed from the final vaccine product, as we will see, a restricted number of cells are allowed in the solutions that are injected into a person's arm.

HEK293 cells were derived from a <u>h</u>uman <u>e</u>mbryonic <u>k</u>idney in the early 1970s, hence are referred to as HEK. Canadian scientist, Frank Graham, originally developed the perpetually dividing cell line from kidney cells obtained from Dutch researcher Alexander Van der Eb, who attested that the cells were derived from human fetal tissue, although he was uncertain if the cells came from an aborted fetus or from a miscarriage. The cell line is officially named HEK293, referring to the 293rd experiment conducted to finalize the creation of the immortalized human cell line. The immortalized HEK293 cells could potentially acquire mutations or become genetically unstable over time, which could increase their potential to become truly oncogenic (cancerous), particularly if they are exposed to other factors that promote tumorigenesis. Researchers have many tools available to determine if the cells have become unstable and should be discarded. The key is to be sure all cells are eliminated, a difficult process.

The 293 cells come in many different subtypes. One of the most common versions is HEK293T, which has been transformed by the oncogene antigen SV40, allowing for easier and faster replication of SV40-based plasmids. This was the cell line used in the COVID-19 jabs made by Johnson and Johnson (Janssen) and AstraZeneca (Vaxzevria). HEK cells have been extensively used in research. In fact, a 2020 paper from the Witherspoon Institute reported 58,094 scientific papers had been published using the HEK293 cells; certainly many more have been published since that time.[141]

VERO CELLS

Beginning in the mid-1990s, manufacturers began discussing the development of the cell line for pandemic influenza vaccines. Preliminary studies indicated that VERO cells should be a good choice for growing influenza A and B viruses.[142] First used by Salk in the 1950s to produce polio vaccines, VERO cells were derived from the kidneys of African green monkeys.

The cells have been under fire for many years due to the reported contamination by a cancer-causing adventitious virus, Simian Virus 40 (SV40).

LEARN MORE

While many well-known cell lines are derived from aborted fetal tissue, other cell lines may originate from embryonic tissues such as the placenta, tumors, or cancerous tissues that are not directly linked to abortions. The exact origins of some cell lines can vary, and it's important to refer to specific literature for precise details. This is a partial list of cell lines from fetal tissue:

1. **WI-38**: Derived from lung tissue.
2. **MRC-5**: Derived from lung tissue.
3. **HEK293** and **HEK293T**: Derived from kidney tissue.
4. **PER.C6**: Derived from retinal tissue.
5. **IMR-90**: Derived from lung tissue.
6. **Lambda.hE1**: Derived from liver tissue.
7. **Fetal Human Dermal Fibroblasts (FHF)**: Generally derived from fetal skin, but can vary.
8. **FRhL-2:** Derived from human kidney tissue.
9. **FL**: Derived from fetal lung tissue.
10. **JEG-3**: Derived from a choriocarcinoma (tumor) of placental tissue.
11. **NTERA-2**: Derived from a testicular tumor, not directly from fetal tissue.

Researcher and Assistant Professor of Pathology at Loyola University Chicago, Dr. Michele Carbone, was in a head-to-head battle with the FDA and the NIH for years over his research that linked SV40 to specific types of slow growing human tumors. The biologic criteria for a causal association between viruses with tumors include:

1. the presence of virus before the onset of the disease,
2. the presence of virus in the tumor's tissues,
3. viral persistence – the ability of a virus to remain in a host organism for an extended period, often without causing noticeable symptoms or disease,
4. the location of virus at the appropriate sites [e.g., within the tumor], and
5. the disease can be avoided by prevention of the viral infection.

Carbone had found all of those criteria were met when he studied the slow-virus, SV40.[143] Carbone's research discovered that when SV40 was injected into hamsters, the same types of tumors developed that occurred in human cells infected with SV40. The tumors were ependymomas and choroid plexus tumors (brain tissue); mesotheliomas (lung tissue); and osteosarcomas and sarcomas (bone tissue).

Even though these findings may seem to have only scientific interest, they hold significant implications for public health and the health of the population. SV40 was a contaminant in the polio vaccines administered widely from 1955 until 1963, most likely inoculating many millions of people with a known tumor-causing virus. Using VERO cells for the production of a pandemic influenza vaccine targeting every person in the world could have had the same disastrous implications.[126] (For the complete, well-written discussion regarding the polio vaccine, SV40, and Dr. Carbone's work, see the book by Debbie Bookchin and Jim Schumacher, *The Virus and the Vaccine: The True Story of a Cancer-Causing Monkey Virus, Contaminated Polio Vaccine, and the Millions of Americans Exposed* (St. Martin's Press, 2004).

Recall that CBER is a division within the FDA. The CBER website states that it works "to protect and enhance the public health through the regulation of biological and related products including blood, vaccines, tissues, and gene therapies." The website goes on to state:

202

*"Although medical products are required to be safe, **safety does not mean zero risk**, since all medical products are associated with some level of risk. A safe biological product is one that has **reasonable risks**, given the patient's condition, the magnitude of the benefit expected, and the alternatives available. The choice to use a biological product involves balancing the benefits to be gained against the potential risks."*[144] *(emphasis added)*

Who determines the definition of "reasonable risk"?

As far back as 2000, CBER was disturbed enough over the carcinogenic potential of VERO cells that it issued a memorandum stating each manufacturer who used VERO cells from the master cell bank must do "tumorigenicity testing," to determine if the VERO cells ensure that residual VERO cells in their formulation did not induce tumors. The memo went on to state that, based on extensive internal discussions, consultation with outside experts, and comments received from the Vaccines and Related Biological Products Advisory Committee (VRBPAC) during a meeting held on May 12, 2000, the Committee had "residual concerns" the manufacturers needed to address. The CBER memo acknowledged that, even though the WHO's "acceptable limit" for the number of residual VERO cells per vaccine was 10 nanograms per dose, CBER wanted **all the cells out**. CBER also wanted the right to assess the cancer-causing risks of each vaccine lot on a "case-by-case basis for all viral vaccines."[145] That is an overwhelming amount of concern. If the CBER was willing to admit that level of apprehension over the cancer-causing potential of VERO cells in vaccines and put forth a zero-tolerance rule regarding residual VERO cells in the final product, the concern was – and is – absolutely real.

Complications from the use of VERO cells in the manufacture of influenza vaccines quickly began to emerge. In 2002, Baxter Healthcare Corporation received regulatory approval in the Netherlands to develop a new influenza vaccine, PrefluCel, using the company's VERO cell technology.

COMMENTARY

Clearly, CBER was aware and disquieted over the carcinogenic potential of VERO cells and wanted manufacturers to take every available precaution to eliminate the cells from vaccines under development in 2000. But VERO cells have long been utilized in smallpox, polio, and rabies vaccines, and more recently in rotavirus, yellow fever, Japanese encephalitis, dengue, Ebola, and even the COVID-19 vaccine, Covaxin (Bharat Biotech, India). The intense concern should have also been extended to the use of other animal cells used to make vaccines, whether the animal is a monkey, a dog, a chicken (fibroblasts), a cow (bovine serum), or a chinese hamster because measurable amounts *of these animal cells are allowed* in the end products.

Baxter was pursuing regulatory approval of PrefluCel in other European countries and had plans to initiate clinical trials in the US. However, on December 9, 2004, Baxter announced that it had voluntarily suspended enrollment of participants in the Phase II/III clinical study for PrefluCel due to a *"higher than expected rate of mild fever and associated symptoms"* being reported among clinical trial participants. Norbert G. Riedel, Baxter's chief scientific officer explained, "Based on the preliminary data we've seen, the rate of fever and *associated symptoms* observed with the current formulation of PrefluCel has been higher compared to other vaccines available on the market." The clinical trials were stopped without further explanation. No definition of the "associated symptoms" was given and no further testing was forthcoming.

With continued experimentation, Baxter was finally able to get PreFluCel approved by the Austrian Agency for Health and Food

Safety (AGES) on September 30, 2010. It was widely distributed across 15 countries in Europe for use only in adults. However, soon after its release, AGES and the European Medicine Agency began receiving reports of allergic reactions (including anaphylaxis), influenza-like symptoms, and ocular reactions following administration of PreFluCel. The lot numbers were tracked and the vials causing the reactions were found to be from the predominant batch distributed across the European market. Four days later, Baxter issued a voluntary recall of all of the nearly 230,000 doses on the market in all nations as a "precautionary measure."[146] No additional seasonal flu shots have been released to the market that were developed using VERO cells and Baxter's application has long expired. VERO cells didn't work in the past for flu shots; they won't work in the future either.

VACCINES FROM INSECTS

Protein Sciences Corporation had been working since the 1990s to develop a patented influenza vaccine using an insect cell designer substrate. The rationale behind this novel approach was to bypass the use of chicken eggs for production. The vaccine strategy was finally refined and it was used to produce the vaccine, FluBlok. The process is complex. It starts with removing the hemagglutinin proteins (H) from the surface of the three viruses chosen by the WHO to be in the current season's flu shot. The (H) proteins are inserted into a second virus, forming a **baculovirus,** a type of virus that infects insects. The baculovirus is then inserted into cells of the fall army worm, *Spodoptera frugiperda.* The baculovirus rapidly replicates, creating large quantities of (H) antigen to be harvested and used to make the vaccine. In several early Phase I and II trials conducted by NIAID with over 600 participants, FluBlok demonstrated a robust antibody response in humans.[147]

The baculovirus expression system was thought to be advantageous over egg-based flu shots for several reasons:[147]

- The production could be rapidly scalable and reproducible. Preparations of FluBlok could be completed in less than two months.
- Since FluBlok does not contain egg antigens, concerns about egg allergies were removed and the production costs are much lower without the need for bio-containment facilities for chickens and eggs.
- Manufacturing does not require use of an extensive number of chemicals to purify the (H) antigen. Therefore, the amount of residual toxic chemicals in the vaccine is minimized.

First approved in 2013 for adults 18 to 49 years old, the application was soon expanded to adults of all ages in 2016 and in 2023, it was approved for use in pregnancy. The success of the product got the attention of Sanofi. In 2017, Protein Sciences was acquired by Sanofi for $750 million to strengthen its position in the flu vaccine market.

MDCK CELLS FROM DOGS

Another cell line used in flu shot production is the MDCK cells, short for Madin-Darby Canine Kidney cells. First isolated in 1958 by researchers S.H. Madin and N.B. Darby from normal kidney cells of a healthy female cocker spaniel dog, the cell line was then transformed into perpetually dividing, immortalized cells. In the 1950s and 1960s, the ability to scale up cell culture systems for large-scale vaccine production was limited because the cells were challenging to work with. In addition, regulatory agencies were cautious about using cell lines from a dog for human vaccines. Advances in bioreactor technology and cell culture media in the 1970s and 1980s made MDCK cells more practical for industrial applications. By the 1990s, researchers better understood how to genetically stabilize and optimize MDCK cells for vaccine production. The use of MDCK cells for **flu vaccines** gained traction in the late 1990s and early 2000s as part of the shift away from using eggs. Flucelvax, approved in the US in 2012, is recommended for adults and children two years and older. Flucelvax and Flucelvax Quadrivalent (approved in 2016) are the only vaccines produced using MDCK cells, and to a smaller degree, Influvac (made by Mylan in Europe).

LEARN MORE

What's the difference between a "designer substrate" and "immortalized cells"?

- A **designer substrate** in vaccine manufacturing is not a solution or a serum but rather a **biologically engineered environment** to produce key components of a vaccine. It is customized to the specific type of vaccine. Designer substrates have the potential to introduce contaminants, impurities, or other unknown risks, especially since these systems often use genetically modified cells or organisms. This can lead to long-term safety and health risks.

- **Immortalized cells** have been manipulated to replicate in perpetuity while retaining their original characteristics. Using modern gene editing tools, such as CRISPR/Cas9, specific genes can be introduced to promote immortality and enable continuous division. Vaccines produced using genetically modified or immortalized cells can lead to unpredictable long-term health effects.

Solvay Pharmaceuticals, a Dutch company, had been working with MDCK cell-cultures to produce influenza vaccines for 15 years when the first bird flu pandemic began to evolve. In fact, Dutch authorities awarded Solvay the first cell-based vaccine license in 2001. In June 2005, the company submitted an FDA application for approval of its cell-derived influenza vaccine. Part of the application included a commitment to build a state-of-the-art cell-based, Level 3 vaccine manufacturing facility in Marietta, Georgia.

In May 2006, HHS granted more than $1 billion to five pharmaceutical firms to develop cell-culture manufacturing facilities within the US. Solvay, one of the five, received $298 million for "the development and testing of new influenza vaccines including pandemic vaccines that are produced using cell-based MCDK technology and the development of a master plan to manufacture, formulate, fill and package annual and pandemic influenza vaccines in a new US-based facility," the company said in a press release at the time.

But the expansion plans never came to fruition. In October 2008, Solvay announced that it was canceling plans to build the second vaccine manufacturing plant, a $386 million project that both Birmingham, Alabama and Athens, Georgia had been competing for. The plant would have made both seasonal and pandemic flu vaccines – but just as the final site selection was about to be completed, the company announced that with the drop in flu shot sales in the post-pandemic environment, the deal no longer made economic sense. Millions of doses of flu vaccine each year had been tossed in the trash. For example, 27 million of the 140 million doses made for the 2007-08 flu season were not administered, representing money wasted for the manufacturers – and for the US taxpayer.[148] Changing the direction of its business, in 2009, Solvay sold its vaccine division to Abbott Labs and later, the division was sold again to AbbVie. The only two flu vaccines currently made using MDCK cells are **Flucelvax** (both the standard and quadrivalent versions).

As it turns out, MDCK cells have not been widely used in vaccine manufacturing for several reasons:

- Viruses do not proliferate well in dog kidney cells.
- Regulatory approvals have not been easy to obtain for safety reasons.

- The cells have specific nutritional and environmental requirements for optimal growth, which can complicate large-scale production.
- Other cell lines worked better for propagating large quantities of viruses needed for vaccines.

MORE ON CELL LINE CONTAMINANT CONCERNS

The FDA's latest recommendations on cell lines and designer substrates are detailed in a 50-page document titled *Guidance for Industry: Characterization and Qualification of Cell Substrates and Other Biological Materials Used in the Production of Viral Vaccines for Infectious Disease Indications.*[149] Released in February 2010, this document outlines procedures for testing cell lines for residual cellular DNA, oncogenicity (cancer-causing potential), tumorigenicity (tumor-forming potential), presence of contaminating adventitious (foreign) viruses, and residual bovine and porcine cells, among other factors. A relevant section on page 37 is excerpted here (lightly edited for clarity):

> "Residual DNA might be a risk to your final product because of oncogenic and/or infectivity potential. There are several potential mechanisms by which **residual DNA could be oncogenic**, including the integration and expression of encoded oncogenes or **insertional mutagenesis** following DNA integration. You should limit **residual DNA**, such as when the virus is passed through VERO cells, to **less than 10 nanograms per dose** as recommended by the WHO.
>
> Because injected DNA is taken up (absorbed) approximately 10,000-fold more readily than orally administered DNA, we recommend limiting residual DNA to **less than 100 micrograms per dose for oral vaccines**. If you are using

cells with **tumorigenic phenotypes** (cells that came from tumor cells) or other characteristics that give rise to special concerns, more stringent limitation of residual DNA quantities **might be needed** to assure product safety." *(emphasis added)*

In the same bulletin (p.14), an additional glance is given to producing vaccines using cells taken from tumors:

"Use of **tumorigenic and tumor-derived cells** for vaccine production is associated with additional issues. This document **does not provide guidance** on a pathway for licensure of live-attenuated or minimally purified vaccines produced in these cells. You should perform additional testing **if your cell lines are tumorigenic or derived from a tumor.**" *(emphasis added)*

Note the caveats of **"should,"** **"we recommend,"** and **"might be needed."** Instead of strict requirements and stringent standards, the bulletin has the words **"contains nonbinding recommendations"** at the top of every page. Why in the world would cancerous (tumorigenic) cells be used to make vaccines, knowing that some of those cells would end up in the final product? *How can they say this is "safe," as in "safe and effective"?*[149]

As previously mentioned, the FDA is fully aware that using cell lines to make vaccines comes with risks that in many ways are no different than the risks associated with using eggs. The cells can become contaminated with adventitious viruses that are potentially deadly. An FDA memo from 2000 acknowledged the risks:

"The experience in the early 1960s with SV40 contamination of poliovirus and adenovirus vaccines and the continuing questions regarding whether SV40 could be responsible for some human neoplasms [cancers] underscores the importance of keeping viral vaccines free of adventitious agents [viral contaminants]. **This is particularly important when there is a theoretical potential for contamination of a vaccine with viruses that might be associated with neoplasia [cancer].** It is unclear whether neoplastic cells have a greater or lower risk [of contamination] than other types of cells. However, if their growth in tissue culture is not well controlled, there may exist additional opportunities for **contamination of cells with a longer lifespan.**" *(emphasis added)*

And it gets worse. The same FDA memo went on to say:

"In addition to the possibility of contamination of cell substrates...the use of immortalized, neoplastic human cells to develop [vaccines] raises theoretical concerns with regard to possible contamination with TSE/BSE agents."

TSE is Transmissible Spongiform Encephalopathy, a condition that includes a group of rare degenerative brain disorders characterized by tiny holes in the brain tissues, giving a "spongy" appearance when viewed under a microscope. When this condition occurs in cows it is called BSE or Bovine Spongiform Encephalopathy, commonly known as "mad cow disease." In a study published in 2004, researchers found:

"The susceptibility of a cell line to TSE infection cannot be predicted on the basis of its country of origin or its level of expression of the cellular prion protein. Thus, testing cells for TSE susceptibility might be necessary for **all cell lines** that are routinely used in vaccine production and in other medical applications."[150]

A similar investigation was done in 2011, and researchers reported that while they did not find any BSE agents in the cell lines that were tested, given the long incubation time (years) that is needed to elicit disease in this primate model, they advised that longer models were needed to fully evaluate the samples and added:

> "We must caution that even cell lines susceptible to TSE infection have shown widely different responses when exposed to various TSE strains. Furthermore, the emergence of atypical forms of BSE raises new concerns, i.e., cell lines resistant to infection with the original classic BSE might not resist infection by newer strains of BSE."[151]

Creutzfeldt-Jakob disease (CJD) is a specific type of transmissible spongiform encephalopathy (TSE) marked by rapidly worsening dementia and other neurological symptoms. CJD results in severe disability and often death within months or a few years after symptoms present. TSEs are a broader group of brain diseases caused by infectious proteins called prions. These diseases, affecting both humans and animals, share the common feature of brain damage due to prions. While each type of TSE can have different symptoms and ways of spreading, they all involve the abnormal buildup of prions in the brain, *leading to progressive neurological decline.*

A number of reports have suggested an association between COVID-19 infection, COVID-19 jabs, and initiation of accelerated neurodegenerative diseases, including Alzheimer's disease (AD) and Creutzfeldt-Jakob disease (CJD). These diseases and several other neurodegenerative diseases have a common association: they are caused by the misfolding and aggregation of human brain proteins.[152]

A recent study (2024) from Seoul, South Korea investigated the association between COVID-19 vaccination and the onset of Alzheimer's disease and its prodromal state, mild cognitive impairment (MCI). The large study analyzed data from a random sample of 50% of the city's residents aged 65 and above, totaling 558,017 individuals. Findings showed that within three months of their last shot, those people in the mRNA-vaccinated group exhibited a significantly higher incidence of AD and MCI when compared to the unvaccinated group. No significant relationship was found with vascular dementia or Parkinson's disease.[153] The pressing question arises: Why is cell line technology allowed to be used to make vaccines, especially given its potential to cause cancer and the risk of contaminants that can have devastating neurodegenerative consequences?

Despite significant evidence and expert concerns, the FDA continues to overlook the potential risks associated with using foreign cells for vaccines.

FDA and CBER could simply say STOP using contaminated cells and cells made from tumors. This situation raises serious alarms about the hasty approval of these products, especially in light of the adverse effects that have been reported in people who have received one or more COVID-19 vaccines.

COMMENTARY

What if people who received the COVID-19 vaccine are experiencing two issues in their brain at the same time? One issue could be neurodegeneration caused by the spike protein and the lipid nanoparticles in the vaccine. The other could be a prion-related disease resulting from the use of cell lines in the vaccine production.

Recall the Johnson & Johnson vaccine (Janssen) was made using the cell lines HEK293 and PER.C6. Similarly, AstraZeneca's vaccine (Vaxzevria) used HEK293 cell lines. Bharat Biotech (Covaxin) and Sinovac (Coronavac) developed their COVID-19 shots using VERO cells. CoronaVac was one of the most widely distributed vaccines globally due to Sinovac's ability to quickly scale production. It was particularly favored by countries in low- and middle-income regions due to ease of storage.

The precedent for human experimentation and the exploration of the human genome was established long ago, and this practice continues to advance at an alarming pace.

ENTER MRNA TECHNOLOGY

The discovery of protein synthesis pathways, where DNA is transcribed into mRNA which is then translated into proteins by ribosomes, resulted from contributions by several key scientists over many years. It began in the early 1940s when George Beadle and Edward Tatum conducted their groundbreaking experiments with *Neurospora crassa* (a fungus), leading to the formulation of the "one gene, one enzyme" hypothesis. At the time of their research, the understanding of genetic material was limited. While it was known that genes played a role in heredity, the chemical and structural nature of genes was still unclear. Beadle and Tatum's experiments demonstrated a direct relationship between genes and specific biochemical pathways, but they had not yet identified DNA as the molecular basis of those genes.

Watson and Crick's discovery of the structure of DNA in 1953 provided the molecular explanation for how genetic information is stored and replicated, ultimately connecting the earlier findings of Beadle, Tatum, and others to the physical structure of genes. These findings were further supported by the 1958 experiments conducted by Matthew Meselson and Franklin Stahl, reinforcing the idea that DNA serves as the template for RNA production.

In the 1960s, Marshall Nirenberg and Heinrich Matthaei provided the first insights into how ribosomes, discovered by George E. Palade in 1955, linked amino acids to form proteins. Around the same time, in 1961, two teams independently discovered that mRNA acts as an intermediary in the transmission of genetic information from DNA to the ribosomes for protein synthesis. The team of François Jacob and Jacques Monod were French biologists celebrated for their groundbreaking work on gene expression, earning them the 1965 Nobel Prize in Physiology or Medicine, which they shared with André Lwoff. The other team, Sydney Brenner and Matthew Meselson, also made significant contributions to molecular biology. Brenner, a South African-born biologist, was recognized for his research on the genetic code and RNA structure, while American biologist Meselson gained acclaim for his work on DNA replication. Together, these two teams advanced the understanding of molecular genetics and received the Nobel Prize in 2002. The processes of translation (mRNA to protein) and transcription (DNA to mRNA) are fundamental to cellular function. All of these researchers and more contributed to the understanding of this complexity.

NORMAL PROTEIN SYNTHESIS

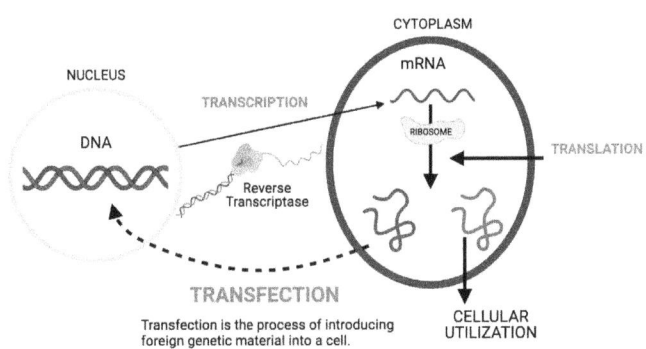

Created by Dr. Sherri Tenpenny
www.DrTenpenny.com

powered by Biorender.com

Scientists had developed methods to synthesize mRNA in the lab in the 1970s, but early efforts to get the strands of RNA into cells were met with significant challenges. Naked RNA in general circulation was degraded swiftly. Lipid nanoparticles (LNPs) were considered early on as a way to encapsulate and protect mRNA from being attacked by circulating enzymes. However, it had been known for more than a decade that injected lipid formulations were toxic, caused severe immune reactions, and actually delivered very little mRNA into the cells.

It took 20 more years of research to advance the use of mRNA in living organisms. In the 1990s, Katalin Karikó and Drew Weissman achieved the breakthrough by modifying the strands of mRNA. While working at the University of Pennsylvania, they were able to replace the terminal nucleic acid uridine with pseudouridine, which enhanced the molecule's stability, drastically reduced its immune-stimulating effects and allowed for indefinite translation. This change essentially gave mRNA an "on" button to indefinitely produce the protein it was programmed to make, and the cell had no ability to turn it off.[154] This innovation laid the foundation for moving forward with mRNA-based therapies.

Throughout the 2000s, biotech companies such as BioNTech (2008) and Moderna (2010) began exploring the use of mRNA for vaccines and other therapies. The US government and the Department of Defense, primarily through BARDA's alliances, have invested at least $31.9B to develop, produce, and purchase mRNA COVID-19 vaccines, including sizable investments that began as a partnership with Moderna in 2010.[155] At the same time, advancements in lipid nanoparticle (LNP) technology facilitated the delivery of mRNA into cells with a reduced inflammatory response. Early clinical trials focused on the use of mRNA vaccines for influenza and cytomegalovirus (CMV). The emergence of COVID-19 in late 2019 accelerated the push to use the new mRNA platform. By January 2020, the genetic sequence of the SARS-CoV-2 virus had been published, prompting both Moderna and BioNTech to design mRNA vaccine candidates. Rather than taking many years to develop and test them as required for existing vaccines, they produced their injectable, Pfizer-BioNTech (BNT162b2) and Moderna (mRNA-1273), within months, which received emergency use authorization (EUA) in December 2020.

At the beginning of the COVID-19 pandemic, the US federal government invested at least $2.3B for more R&D of the mRNA COVID-19 vaccines. An additional $29.2B was spent by BARDA and the Department of Defense to purchase 2 billion doses of vaccine to vaccinate the entire US population.[155]

DISASTROUS RESULTS

The release of mRNA vaccines as covered countermeasures legally shielded them from all liability. The result was disastrous. More than 3,400 peer-reviewed papers have been published since 2020 detailing the extensive list of side effects causally linked to the COVID-19 injections. Even though a plethora of adverse events and death reports were pouring in, Pfizer and the other manufacturers were eerily silent.

Wanting to see the preliminary research study data, a Freedom of Information Act (FOIA) request was submitted to Pfizer in 2022 from the nonprofit Public Health and Medical Professionals for Transparency (PHMPT), a group of about 200 doctors, scientists, professors, public health professionals, and journalists including Aaron Kheriaty, MD, Harvey Risch, MD, PhD, and Peter McCullough, MD. PHMPT appealed to the Federal Court to force Pfizer's hand.

Pfizer wanted to bury data from the early field trials where so many adverse events were reported that Pfizer was forced to hire hundreds of additional employees to record and track the catastrophic details. Not only did Pfizer refuse to answer the FOIA request, Pfizer wanted the FDA to agree to *not release the findings for 75 years*. Attorney Aaron Siri, of Siri & Glimstad, who represented the PHMPT group said that the rate of release was "set so slow" that the documents would not be fully released until "almost all of the scientists, attorneys, and most of the Americans that received Pfizer's product, have died of old age."

Which was clearly Pfizer's intent.

In a stroke of brilliance, US District Court Judge Mark Pittman in Fort Worth, Texas, ruled in favor of the plaintiffs. He saw through Pfizer's bluff and ruled that the FDA must immediately make public 12,000 pages of data it used to make decisions about approvals for Pfizer/BioNTech's COVID-19 vaccine – and then release the next 55,000 pages and continue to release 55,000 pages every 30 days until all 450,000 requested pages were made public.[156] To grasp the magnitude of this project, one package of paper for your printer contains 500 sheets of paper. Imagine having *900 packages* of printer paper piled on a table. That's 450,000 pages.

HIGHLIGHT

On December 6, 2024 Judge Pittman ordered the FDA to release, by June 30, 2025, the entire EUA file that Pfizer used to apply for emergency use, which could amount to *one million additional pages* of documentation and incriminating information against Pfizer, Moderna, and the COVID-19 jabs.[157]

Within the first tranche of the court-ordered document release was a 38-page report called, "Cumulative Analysis of Post- Authorization Adverse Event Reports of PF-07302048 Received through Feb. 28, 2021." Pages 30 to 38 of that document lists **more than 1,200 conditions,** diseases, and syndromes reported during the field trials for the shot, side effects that were known *before* the jab was released to the general public.[158]

In their book, *The Pfizer Papers*, Naomi Wolf, Amy Kelly, and teams of more than 3,000 professionals analyzed the 450,000 pages of clinical trial evidence. Wolf and her volunteer team of analysts took on the massive project, uncovering evidence of seriously flawed research. The documents revealed that Pfizer and the FDA were thoroughly aware, as early as November 2020, before the mRNA shots were rolled out globally, that the jabs were neither safe nor effective but rather dangerous, even deadly. The detailed reports, organized into chapters in the book, highlight severe harm to the neurological system and women's reproductive health. They also found that vaccine-induced myocarditis is not rare, mild, or transient, but instead is significant and long-lasting. The book contains MRI scans, full reports, pathology slides, and a myriad of charts and graphs. It is a full-color analysis of the extensive crimes against humanity caused by these jabs and their creators. Wolf and her co-author, Amy Kelly, should receive the Nobel Prize for investigative reporting.

The mRNA vaccines have inflicted so much extensive damage that a new disease category has emerged, called "CoVax Disease," which defines multi-system, multi-organ conditions. *The Pfizer Papers* expose how the collusion between Big Pharma, the US government, and healthcare entities are shielded by the broad legal immunity granted by the Public Readiness and Emergency Preparedness Act (PREP Act), as discussed in Chapters 16 and 17 of this book.

Over 1.6 million individuals have submitted VAERS reports regarding their injuries; it's important to emphasize that VAERS captures only a small fraction of injuries, less than 1%. Financial analyst Edward Dowd, author of *"Cause Unknown: The Epidemic of Sudden Deaths in 2021 & 2022 & 2023,"* asserts that in the US alone, COVID-19 vaccines have led to 26.6 million injuries and 1.36 million disabilities. Globally, it is estimated that around 5 billion people have received at least one dose of the COVID-19 vaccine. Using the same mathematical estimates he applied to the US data, Dowd suggests that between 7.3 million and 15 million people may have died from the jabs, and between 29 million and 60 million people worldwide may have been disabled. Most countries lack a reporting system comparable to the databases maintained in the US, making accurate estimates more difficult to assess.

COMMENTARY

The FDA and CDC were aware as early as 2022 of the massive number of serious adverse events and took no action. In fact, not only did they allow the rollout to continue, but Fauci, Birx, Walensky, and the mainstream media also urged the public to receive two shots and every subsequent booster. COVID-19 vaccines have been approved for the 2024-2025 fall season for infants six months and older, despite a worldwide outcry from doctors, researchers, and scientists demanding the removal of all mRNA vaccines from the market. The shots are still available from Pfizer and Novavax; additionally, Moderna currently has at least eight mRNA vaccines waiting for approval.[159]

There has been a surge in interest and in research to apply mRNA technology to infectious diseases beyond influenza, including HIV, RSV, and Zika, as well as cancer treatments. Despite a small but growing international group of physicians and other healthcare professionals adamantly calling for a complete, worldwide moratorium on mRNA vaccines, pharma is continuing to expand the use of mRNA vaccines for genetic diseases, and even to inject into plants and animals.

Beyond the mRNA and lipid nanoparticles, there is a long list of toxic chemicals that are spread over the multiple doses of 17 different vaccines injected into children. Some of the most egregious are the vaccine adjuvants. Learning about them, it is disturbing to think about injecting these substances into infants.

"Not all chemicals are bad. Without chemicals such as hydrogen and oxygen, for example, there would be no way to make water, a vital ingredient in beer."

~Dave Barry, American author, columnist, and humorist

CHAPTER 13
Details on the Adjuvants

Vaccine clinical trials are primarily interested in two results: 1) any reactions or side effects, usually only monitored for five to fourteen days of receiving the vaccine; and 2) the development of an "adequate antibody response." If the number of reactions was "acceptably" low and the antibody level was found to be "acceptably" high, the vaccine is considered to be "safe and effective."

But there are problems with this conclusion. For one, it can take much longer than 14 days to develop an autoimmune reaction or other type of side effect; in fact, it can take months, sometimes many months, even years. No long-term studies have been designed to investigate the potential evolution of these problems. These studies are expensive and time-consuming. Manufacturers conclude that the number of future severe reactions are so small that they are not statistically significant, and not worth the time nor the money to study. And of course the FDA, the IOM, and the study investigators themselves, have the liberal prerogative to declare "no causal relationship exists" between the shot and the reported side effect.

The second problem is the definition of "effective" used by clinical investigators. Clinicians and the general public interpret "effective" to be a synonym for "protective." In other words, if a vaccine is determined to be *effective,* the person who receives it assumes they are protected from infection. However, in vaccine research, "effective" is defined as the vaccine's ability to induce an "acceptably high" antibody response called a **titer.** The assumption is that if titers are elevated, protection is assured. And it is also assumed that the higher the titer level, the greater the protection.

This assumption has never been proven. In fact, the mainstream medical journal *Vaccine* published an article in 2001, clearly stating, *"It is known that, in many instances, antigen-specific antibody titers do not correlate with protection."*[160] *(emphasis added)* This means you can get a vaccine, develop an antibody response, and still contract the infection you were trying to avoid. In addition, you assume all the risks that come with being injected with the toxic solution.

In 2003, vaccine manufacturers were scrambling to create pandemic bird flu shots for "every man, woman, and child" in the US, a concept first introduced by former head of Health and Human Services (HHS), Tommy Thompson (2001-2005), while the same manufacturers were scurrying to make a post-9/11 smallpox vaccine. But even with billions of federal tax dollars to grease the wheels, it would be years before the speedy cell-based flu vaccines would be ready for mass marketing. In the meantime, manufacturers contrived a way to stretch the scant amount of available bird flu vaccine antigen to provide injections for millions of recipients in the event the government announced that they are needed. How did they do this? How do they continue to do this even today? With the addition of adjuvants.

FIRST GENERATION ADJUVANT: ALUMINUM AND MF59

Adjuvants are molecules, compounds, or macromolecular formulations designed to enhance both the immediate and long-term immune response to viral antigens. However, they also pose risks of toxicity or long-term immune effects. By definition, adjuvants are classified as "pharmacologically active drugs," yet they are said to be inert and cause minimal harm. This raises a significant question: how can a substance be both "pharmacologically active" and simultaneously be "inert without biological activity"?

The first adjuvants were used in 1925 by French researcher, Gaston Ramon. He found that by adding breadcrumbs, agar, tapioca, starch, or oil lecithin to vaccines, he could increase the antibody response to diphtheria and tetanus antitoxins. Although these substances are no longer used, adjuvants are regularly added to vaccines and are grouped chemically into "classes" based on the adjuvant's mechanisms of action. For example, hypertensive drugs are grouped together based on how they work; one can be classified as a "beta-blocker" and another as an "ACE-inhibitor," based on its effect in the body. Adjuvants are similarly grouped based on the type of immune response they are thought to induce.

The most commonly used adjuvants in human vaccines are the aluminum-based mineral salts – specifically hydroxide, phosphate, sulfate, or mixed forms collectively known as "alum." More than 80% of current vaccines contain aluminum salts. Aluminum adjuvants have been in widespread use for nearly 90 years. Despite this, medical science still has a remarkably poor understanding about their mechanisms of action, and surprisingly little research has been conducted on the long-term effects of these adjuvants.[161]

Aluminum-based mineral salts and the squalene-based adjuvant MF59 (discussed below) are known as first-generation adjuvants. These compounds effectively stimulate a robust antibody response through the TH2 adaptive immune pathway. However, they have limited impact on the TH1 pathways, which are part of the innate immune response – the immune system we are born with.

FDA regulations have long regulated the amount of aluminum allowed in a single vaccine: it cannot exceed 0.85 mg of aluminum per dose. However, to match the global WHO recommendations, this regulation was amended in 1981. Since that time, up to 1.25 mg of aluminum per individual dose has been permitted (21 CFR Title 21. Vol 7. Sec. 610.15).

Concerns have been raised about the total amount of aluminum a vaccine recipient may get on a single day when multiple vaccines are administered. For example, on a typical vaccination day, a 10 pound (4.5 kg) infant typically receives DTaP, HepB, Hib, and Prevnar, all containing aluminum.[162]

HIGHLIGHT

In 1981, only three vaccines were routinely given: MMR, DTP, and polio. There was only a small amount of aluminum in the DTP vaccine. But today, children receive multiple doses of 17 different vaccines, sometimes 6 or 7 shots on the same day. There are concerns that the maximum dose of aluminum may be exceeded when these vaccines are added all together. Is anyone checking?

In healthy people, most aluminum that is ingested or injected is effectively eliminated. Most of the aluminum absorbed is excreted within the first week after exposure, but the process can vary widely, depending on age and many health factors, taking anywhere from a few hours to *several years*. More than 95% of aluminum taken into the body is removed by the kidneys, while about 2% is excreted through the gallbladder.

Infants are particularly vulnerable to aluminum toxicity because their immature kidneys may struggle to eliminate it. At birth, their kidney function (indicated by glomerular filtration rate) is low and does not reach full capacity until nearly two years of age.[163]

As of August 2023, a child who received every vaccine recommended on the pediatric vaccination schedule from birth to 18 years of age, would have received nearly 12,000 micrograms of aluminum. This total would increase by around 110 micrograms if the child received a vitamin K shot that contains aluminum. (Hospira, a company acquired by Pfizer in 2015, produces a brand of vitamin K that includes both aluminum and benzyl alcohol.) As a result, infants may struggle to effectively eliminate aluminum from their bodies.

Another major concern also arises when someone, especially a child, needs intravenous nutrition, known as parenteral nutrition. This feeding method is usually used in situations such as abdominal surgery, prolonged diarrhea, bowel obstructions, or severe malnutrition, where normal digestion isn't possible.

There are two types of parenteral nutrition: Total Parenteral Nutrition (TPN) and Partial Parenteral Nutrition (PPN). TPN provides complete nutrition through an intravenous line for individuals who cannot use their digestive systems at all. In contrast, PPN is designed to supplement specific nutrients or provide additional calories for those who may still be able to eat a limited amount of food and need extra support.

Concerns about aluminum contamination have been widely discussed in relation to TPN and PPN. Aluminum can be present as a contaminant in trace elements, such as calcium gluconate, magnesium sulfate, and various trace element mixtures. Additionally, some phosphate binders used in these nutritional therapies contain aluminum. When aluminum accumulates in various tissues (particularly the brain), it can lead to neurotoxic effects that can impair cognitive function and overall neurological health. In the bones, accumulated aluminum can contribute to conditions like osteoporosis, making bones weaker and more susceptible to fractures. Aluminum binds to the proteins that are supposed to remove it from the body, leading to even more serious health issues over time. High aluminum levels can damage the liver and the kidneys. Since this is true for aluminum administered through TPN and PPN, the total amount of aluminum injected in vaccines should be more closely monitored.

THE QUEST FOR NEW ADJUVANTS

In clinical trials for new vaccines, animals are often injected with live viruses or bacteria to observe their immune responses. Sometimes, the chosen pathogen is so potent that it immediately kills the animal. In these cases, the pathogen needs to be "attenuated," or weakened, before it can be tested in humans. The downside of using the weakened organisms is that they may be "ignored" by the immune system, resulting in little to no response from the adaptive immune system.

SCAN TO SHOP

Learn much more about aluminum adjuvants in Dr. Tenpenny's course. Just scan the QR code to go to the course, and get 10% off on the Aluminum course. Promo code is DRTCOURSE

(https:shoptenpenny.net/products/aluminum)

LEARN MORE

Based on the 2025 Child and Adolescent Immunization Schedule provided by the CDC, the following vaccines are recommended for children from birth through 6 years of age. Almost every dose will contain aluminum:

- **Hepatitis B (HepB):** 3 doses
- **Rotavirus (RV):** 2 or 3 doses, depending on the vaccine used
- **Diphtheria, Tetanus, and Acellular Pertussis (DTaP):** 4 doses
- **Haemophilus influenzae type b (Hib):** 3 or 4 doses, depending on the vaccine used
- **Pneumococcal conjugate (PCV13):** 4 doses
- **Inactivated Poliovirus (IPV):** 3 doses
- **Measles, Mumps, Rubella (MMR):** 1 dose
- **Varicella (Chickenpox):** 1 dose
- **Hepatitis A (HepA):** 2 doses
- **Respiratory Syncytial Virus (RSV):** 1 dose

The CDC recommends children aged 6 months to 4 years receive these vaccines annually:

- **Influenza (Flu):** 2 doses in the first year of vaccination, then 1 dose annually
- **Moderna COVID-19 Vaccine:** 1 dose OR
- **Pfizer-BioNTech COVID-19 Vaccine:** 2 doses

Developing new adjuvants has been challenging because their usability depends on the amount of toxicity observed in animal studies. However, decades of experimentation have shown that "predictions about safety, potency, or efficacy in humans for a particular adjuvant **cannot** be reliably made from [animal] models. In addition, in preclinical studies of vaccine adjuvants, **the same adjuvant can enhance, inhibit, or have no effect at all.**"[164] (emphasis added)

Adjuvants are added to vaccines for two main reasons. First, they are supposed to keep the vaccine antigen at the injection site longer, allowing the immune system more time to recognize the antigen as "foreign" and produce antibodies against it – this is known as the "depot effect." Second, adjuvants trigger inflammation at the injection site, which stimulates the release of cytokines. This inflammatory response boosts antibody production and helps the immune system "remember" the pathogen for future protection. However, these are suppositions as the true effect is not fully understood.

The injection of adjuvants and other chemicals throw the immune system's highly organized, finely-tuned processes into disarray. It's like setting off a small explosion under a pile of dry leaves and then trying to predict where each leaf will land, an impossible task. The reaction that occurs within each vaccine, within each individual, is hardly "inert." Every shot is truly a new experiment with far-reaching consequences.

The research to find an adjuvant to replace aluminum began in the 1970s when UCLA Medical Center scientist, Carl M. Pearson, began experimenting with a variety of edible oils. His assumption was that because the oils were naturally occurring, they could be metabolized by the body safely. The first trials, performed in 1973, used peanut oil-based adjuvant but this choice was soon abandoned.[165] A wide variety of substances were explored in the 1970s and 1980s as adjuvants, with testing of these particles:

- **Liposomes**: biodegradable vesicles that consist of two lipid layers surrounding an aqueous core that contains the antigens. In this structure, the lipid layers allow part of the antigen to protrude through the lipid bilayer, exposing it to the immune system. The liposomal vesicle gradually breaks down over time.

- **Virosomes**: a type of delivery system similar to liposomes, but utilizes a viral shell that lacks genetic material. The viral envelope encapsulates the antigen, allowing a part of the antigen to protrude through the shell, similar in design to a liposome.

- **Chitosan**: a polysaccharide derived from the shells of crabs and shrimp.
- **Saponins:** compounds made from plants and/or marine animals. Saponins form foam and have the ability to cause red blood cell hemolysis (breaking them open and rendering them useless). The most widely used saponins are Quil A and QS-21.

    - **Quil A** is composed of more than 23 different saponins. Used experimentally in animals, **it is too toxic for human use** because it can cause severe local reactions, granulomas, and severe hemolysis.
    - **QS-21** is derived from *Quillaja saponaria,* the bark of a Chilean tree. Widely used as an adjuvant in veterinary vaccines, **QS-21** has been used in a number of human clinical trials, mainly for cancer vaccines and for infections causing HIV, malaria, and hepatitis B. *(Note: It is an enigma to me where the idea to inject **tree bark** into the human body came from, assuming it would not induce side effects or have long-term consequences.)*

- **ISCOMS,** which stands for **immune-stimulating complexes**, are partially purified fractions of Quil A. ISCOMs induce large amounts of inflammatory cytokines. They are costly to make, difficult to manufacture, are highly toxic with many safety concerns, and fortunately, are not used in humans.

From the 1980s and into the 1990s, research continued using oils, hoping to find an adjuvant that didn't induce an antibody response specifically to the oil. Many different oils were tried. Finally, in 1995, Chiron Corporation (which later became Novartis) filed a patent for **MF59,** an adjuvant comprised of squalene and two emulsifying agents, Tween80 (polysorbate 80) and Span85, a biodegradable surfactant made from a fatty acid (oleic acid) and combined with sorbitol (a sugar). Mixed together, these compounds form an oil-in-water emulsion with uniform droplets less than 1 micron in diameter. When co-administered, these antigens elicit a strong antibody response.

MF-59 AND SQUALENE

At first glance, squalene appeared to be an excellent choice as an adjuvant. Naturally produced in the liver, squalene plays a key role in the metabolic pathway that generates human hormones and serves as a direct precursor to cholesterol. It circulates in the bloodstream and is particularly abundant in the skin. Additionally, significant amounts of squalene are stored in fat tissue, muscles, and lymph nodes. Beyond its presence in the body, squalene is also found in various foods such as eggs and olive oil, as well as in over-the-counter medications, health supplements, and cosmetics.

Up to 80% of the oil in a shark's liver is squalene, and shark liver from the spiny dogfish (considered one of the most abundant shark species in the ocean), initially provided the source of squalene for MF59. However, due to concerns of oceanic sustainability, alternative sources were chosen to make MF59: vegetable oils, such as olive oil, rice bran oil, and sugarcane; fermented yeast; and sometimes, it was produced synthetically. The majority of commercially obtained squalene is used in the cosmetics industry, but a portion is used to prepare vaccine adjuvants.

The well-referenced book published in 2004, *Vaccine A: The Government Experiment That's Killing Our Soldiers and Why GIs Are Only The First Victims*, written by award-winning investigative journalist, Gary Matsumoto, gives an excellent visual for the difference between ingesting an edible compound and injecting it into the body:

"Intuitively, this premise seems somewhat dubious: Your body can metabolize the cheeseburger that you ate for lunch, for instance, but you couldn't liquefy it in a blender and inject the resulting slurry [into your arm], and expect to feel well in the morning."

This holds true for squalene from shark oil and other edible oils that are injected in a vaccine. The description on the patent application for MF59 states:

"Any metabolizable oil, particularly from an animal, fish or vegetable source, may be used herein. It is essential that the oil be metabolized by the host to which it is administered, **otherwise the oil component may cause abscesses, granulomas or even carcinomas,** or (when used in veterinary practice) **may make the meat of vaccinated birds and animals unacceptable for human consumption** due to the deleterious effect the unmetabolized oil may have on the consumer."[166] *(emphasis added)*

Scientific data, published in peer reviewed journals, explained that injected squalene is not "metabolized" like food passing through the intestinal tract. In biochemistry, injected squalene droplets are considered to be "metabolized" when immune cells engulf them, transport them through the lymphatic system, then "present" them to the B-cells to form antibodies to neutralize and remove them. In other words, squalene molecules are not broken down and excreted from the body like olive oil on a salad; the lipid molecules deposited in tissues result in toxic reactions.

In 2001, Holm, et al. injected dozens of metabolizable oils including squalene into rats and found that all the oils were toxic, inducing arthritis with varying degrees of severity. Based on their ability to cause arthritis, the oils were assigned "arthritis scores," ranging from (+), considered to be mildly toxic, to (++++) which was "guaranteed to cripple." Squalene was given a score of (+++).[167]

In addition, all squalene-injected rats developed an MS-like disease that left them crippled, dragging their paralyzed hindquarters across their cages. Similarly, when molecules of squalene are injected into humans, even at tiny concentrations of 10 to 20 parts per billion, the oil led to destructive immune responses, such as autoimmune arthritis and lupus.[168]

Several mechanisms have been proposed to explain these reactions. Metabolically, squalene stimulates an immune response excessively and nonspecifically. A study was conducted using electron microscopy to examine neurological tissue of mice after they had been given 20g/kg of squalene for four days. The devastating effects of the squalene were seen in both the central and peripheral nervous system.

Researchers documented swollen astrocytes (brain cells) and disintegration of myelin sheath throughout the brain. Peripherally, the myelin sheaths were destroyed and the nerves were compressed. It was concluded that squalene "produces pathological changes in both the central and peripheral nervous systems."[169]

Granted, this was a very large dose of squalene. However, even trace amounts are not harmless. In immunology, parts-per-billion (ppb) is a substantial dose. A mere 10 ppb concentration of squalene translates into roughly 184 trillion molecules of squalene and an equal number of potentially destructive immune responses. More than two dozen peer-reviewed scientific papers from ten different laboratories throughout the US, Europe, Asia, and Australia have documented autoimmune disease in animals injected with squalene-based adjuvants.[168] The most likely mechanism for this destruction is a process called molecular mimicry. For example, an antibody formed against the squalene in MF59 can then cross react with the body's own squalene (or cholesterol), causing severe inflammation and destruction of the tissue or organ. By definition, this is autoimmune disease. And, depending on which organ is attacked, it can lead to debilitating disease, even death.

MF59 is capable of creating a hyper-immune response within the TH1 (innate) immune system. Once the immune system is activated, or "turned on," there is no "off switch." The long-term reactions are unknown. Following patients long-term, looking for delayed reactions, no matter how serious they may turn out to be, is not what the vaccine industry is interested in studying.

In spite of the identified risks, MF59 was licensed for use in 1997 in the European influenza vaccine, Fluad. The new adjuvant was chosen because the aluminum adjuvant did not substantially increase the antibody level in elderly patients who received a flu shot, but when MF59 was added, the antibody response more than doubled. The vaccine was deemed "safe and effective" by the investigators but the results of the study appeared to have some serious flaws. For example, the clinical trial only involved elderly people in nursing homes; the average age was 71.5 years. If autoimmune problems such as fatigue, joint pain, pain, headache, muscle aches, and malaise developed in this geriatric population, doctors might attribute these complaints to old age and investigators would attribute these complaints to "anything but" the vaccine.

HIGHLIGHT

Fluad was initially approved in 1997 in Italy. Chiron, the original manufacturer, was purchased by Novartis in 2006. By the time Fluad was approved in the US in November 2015, it had already been licensed in 38 countries, including Canada and 15 European countries. Fluad Quadrivalent was approved in the US in 2020; it has been available since the 2020-2021 flu season.

The squalene in MF59 is not the only cause for concern. One of its components, polysorbate 80 (Tween 80), is said to be inert but it is far from it. Studies as far back as 2005 have revealed that Tween 80 can cause severe anaphylactoid reactions, which are potentially fatal conditions characterized by a sharp drop in blood pressure, hives, and breathing difficulties. Researchers concluded that the severe reaction was not a typical allergic response characterized by IgE antibodies and the release of histamines, but a serious disruption within the immune system.[170]

The warning given by Matsumoto in his book regarding the widespread use of MF59 is sobering: "The unethical experiments detailed in [my] book are ongoing, with little prospect of being self-limiting because they have been shielded from scrutiny and public accountability by national security concerns." He was referring to the anthrax vaccine and the military. Squalene-containing adjuvants are a key ingredient in a whole new generation of vaccines intended for global mass immunization. Because of this, are widespread problems just over the horizon?

GSK: THE ADJUVANT SYSTEM

Fifty years after aluminum had been in widespread use, second generation adjuvants were trialed and classified as strong immunostimulants. In the late 1980s, GlaxoSmithKline (GSK) began to develop adjuvants to stimulate an antibody response against difficult pathogens, such as malaria and HIV. Combining the various molecules that had already been tested in humans (MPL, QS-21, CpG) with classical adjuvants (aluminum, liposomes, oil-in-water emulsions), the results became a proprietary adjuvant technology. Over a 5-year period, 10 different Adjuvant System compounds were designed to induce a strong immune response with an acceptable reactogenicity (side effect) profile. Currently there are four in use to potentiate immune responses to vaccines: AS01, AS02, AS03 and AS04.[171]

Let's examine each of these individually:

AS01: consists of monophosphoryl lipid A (MPL) and liposomes containing the saponin QS-21. As mentioned previously, MPL is derived from the cell wall of a *Salmonella* bacteria and QS-21 is an extract from the bark of the *Quillaja saponaria* tree.

AS02: combines monophosphoryl lipid A (MPL) with aluminum hydroxide (alum). It induced high reactogenicity (causing severe adverse reactions) and due to safety concerns, AS02 was phased out in favor of AS01.

AS03: this oil-in-water adjuvant contains 11.86 mg of α-tocopherol (vitamin E), 10.69 mg of squalene, and 4.86 mg of polysorbate 80. The α-tocopherol is a synthetic form of vitamin E; it is not extracted from plants. While the addition of a vitamin may sound like a good idea, it is an injected oil and induces a very strong, very toxic cytokine response.

AS03 was used in the H1N1 pandemic influenza vaccines. In 2009, the vaccine **Pandemerix,** which has been removed from the market, was found to increase the risk of narcolepsy in children in Australia and Finland. Narcolepsy is a chronic neurological disorder where the brain loses its ability to regulate the normal sleep-wake cycle. AS03 has been tested in malaria and HIV vaccines, but is not currently used in either of these experimental shots. However, it was reintroduced in 2024 for one of the approved bird flu vaccines. These were discussed in Chapter 8.

AS04: To overcome the problem of its water-insolubility, 50 μg of MLP was adsorbed onto 500 μg aluminum hydroxide or aluminum phosphate. The adjuvant has been used in human papilloma and hepatitis b vaccines in Europe.

AS04 was used in **Cervarix,** a vaccine against human papillomavirus (HPV) types 16 and 18. This vaccine was taken off the market in 2016 due to the more widely used Gardasil which had captured most of the market share and quite possibly due to more widespread reactions from the AS04 in Ceravarix.

Adjuvants, although they are said to be safe, effective, and inert, can lead to serious health problems. In fact, this was written more than twenty years ago:

> "The absolute safety of adjuvanted vaccines, or any vaccine, **cannot be guaranteed,** so the risks must be minimized. Undesirable reactions can be grouped as either local or systemic, with local reactions ranging from pain and itching to severe systemic reactions ranging from **autoimmune disease to cancer.**"[172] *(emphasis added)*

A partial list of side effects associated with adjuvants includes the following:[172]

- Local or acute inflammation, including the formation of painful abscesses, persistent nodules, ulcers or draining lymph nodes
- Induction of fever, muscle pain, joint pain and headaches – much like the flu
- Anaphylaxis (shock), hives, and vasculitis
- Systemic toxicity to tissues and organs
- Induction of autoimmune disorders
- Cross-reactivity with human cells, causing glomerulonephritis (renal failure) and meningoencephalitis (brain swelling)
- **Immune suppression**
- Genetic events: carcinogenesis (cancer); teratogenesis (birth defects); and abortogenesis (causing abortions)

The goal of injecting these toxic molecules is to generate a high IgG antibody level, no matter the cost to the individual. Over the years they have been given the name "protective antibody." But what if they are not "protective"? And what if we use the IgG test indiscriminately for "diagnosing" a variety of conditions?

DETAILS ABOUT IGG ANTIBODIES: DO THEY PROTECT?

Physicians are taught in medical school that there are five primary types of antibodies (immunoglobulins). They are classified into IgG, IgM, IgA, IgD, and IgE. (I learned them by memorizing the acronym G-A-M-E-D.) They are distributed throughout the body, and each has a different function. The most prevalent and most highly studied are the IgG antibodies. There are four distinct subclasses of IgG termed IgG1, IgG2, IgG3, and IgG4. They differ considerably in their physical and biological properties and the pattern of the four serum IgG subclasses is used to diagnose different autoimmune diseases. In addition, the presence of an elevated IgG level can indicate many diverse conditions.[173]

We "hang a lot of hats" on the IgG antibody test, which doctors order frequently. The results can lead to life-changing diagnoses and treatments. But what does it really mean if you have an elevated (positive) IgG level on a blood test?

- **Does it mean you have an allergy?**

  Food allergy testing uses an IgG assessment to screen your blood for food or environmental allergens. If you are found to have an IgG antibody against, say, chicken or casein, or grass or mold, you are diagnosed with a food or environmental allergy. You are told to avoid those items and perhaps recommended to start getting allergy shots to block the allergic reaction.

- **Does it mean you have a chronic infection?**
  - If you are tested for HIV and found to have an IgG antibody against the human immunodeficiency virus, you are diagnosed with HIV/AIDS.
  - Rapid tests are done, most often in a medical office setting, to quickly assess for an associated infection – such as the flu, mono, strep throat, or SARS CoV-2. If the test is positive, you are "diagnosed" with a viral illness and treated accordingly.

- **Does it mean you have an autoimmune disease?**
  High levels of IgG autoantibodies are associated with many autoimmune diseases. Conditions are often diagnosed when an elevated IgG antibody level is present and targeted against a specific tissue type. Examples include:
  - Thyroid tissue - results in a diagnosis of Hashimoto's thyroiditis, an autoimmune disease of the thyroid.
  - Joints - A specific IgG antibody called rheumatoid factor (RF) – results in a diagnosis of rheumatoid arthritis.
  - Here are a few other autoimmune conditions diagnosed, at least in part, by specific tissue IgG antibodies include:[174]
    - Primary Sjogren syndrome
    - Systemic lupus erythematosus (SLE)
    - Systemic sclerosis (SSc)
    - Primary biliary cirrhosis (PBC)

- **Does it mean you have cancer?**
  Elevated levels of IgG are often found in a long list of cancers including:[174]
  - breast cancer
  - cervical cancer
  - ovarian cancer
  - prostate cancer

- kidney (renal) cancer
- bladder cancer
- nasopharyngeal cancer
- laryngeal, oral, and salivary cancer
- esophageal cancer
- stomach cancer
- thyroid and parathyroid cancer
- lung cancer
- colon cancer
- pancreatic cancer
- liver cancer
- acute myeloid leukemia

- **Does it mean you have had an infection and won't get it again? (you are naturally immune)**

  - Conventional medicine would call this a "protective antibody," but the medical literature is full of case reports where a person had the infection, had an elevated IgG antibody but then had a recurrence of the same infection.

- **Does it mean you've been vaccinated and have generated a "protective antibody"?**

  - People are vaccinated for a long list of conditions. In fact, as of 2023, vaccines are available against 33 human diseases. If you have an IgG antibody after vaccination, the medical establishment says you are "protected." But you can still contract the illness even if you have been fully vaccinated and have what is considered to be an adequate level of "protective antibody." It has happened with:

    - **Mumps**: Outbreak among fully vaccinated school-age children and young adults, Portugal in 2019/2020.[175]

- **Measles:** A fully vaccinated woman contracted and then spread the measles.[176]
- **Pertussis:** Clinical presentation of pertussis in 70 fully immunized children in Lithuania.[177]
- **COVID-19:** Fully vaccinated is defined as two shots and one booster. All COVID-19 infections in vaccinated individuals are termed 'breakthrough' infections. Breakthrough infections have occurred in more than 30% of people. A study of inmates across 33 California state prisons showed that 75% of fully vaccinated individuals contracted COVID throughout the six month period of the study.[178]
- **Tetanus:** An Unusual Case of Evolving Localized Tetanus Despite Prior Immunization and Protective Antibody Titer.[179]

Does it mean you've had the illness in the past OR does it mean you've been vaccinated?

Can you tell the difference?

Example: Chickenpox

Chickenpox is a condition thought to be caused by the varicella-zoster virus. It manifests as a fever and an itchy, blister-like rash that starts on the chest and back and then spreads over the entire body lasting 3 to 10 days. A positive IgG test result indicates that a person has antibodies either from past varicella disease OR from vaccination.

CDC says that laboratories cannot distinguish whether the antibodies were from a past episode of varicella or vaccination.

Example: Measles

Measles is a red, blotchy rash that usually appears first on the face and behind the ears, then spreads downward to the chest and back and finally to the feet. It is generally associated with a cough, runny nose, conjunctivitis, and a fever. The symptoms last 7 to 10 days with nearly everyone experiencing complete resolution and complete, natural immunity. There were 12 cases of measles reported in the US in 2020. A positive IgG test indicates that a person has antibodies either from having measles in the past OR from vaccination.

CDC says laboratories cannot distinguish whether the antibodies were from a past episode of measles or vaccination.

Example: Rubella

Rubella is best known for its distinctive red rash. It is also called German measles or three-day measles. Although most children experience mild or no symptoms, rubella may cause theoretical risk in unborn babies, "theoretical" because there were only 6 cases of rubella and no cases of congenital rubella were reported in 2020.

CDC says laboratories cannot distinguish whether the antibodies were from a past episode of measles or vaccination.

What if you have too little IgG?

People with natural IgG deficiency are more likely to get infections. It's not known what causes IgG deficiency, but it is generally thought to be an immune deficiency disease. A blood test that measures all of the immunoglobulins, but particularly IgG, can diagnose this condition.

So:

1. An elevated IgG *may* indicate you have a food or environmental allergy. However, this test can be inaccurate. For example, what if your test shows an absence of an IgG antibody to dairy, and therefore, you may eat dairy, even if you always vomit, get a rash, or have diarrhea after eating dairy.
2. An elevated IgG level *may* mean you have a chronic infection OR you may have had an infection in the past OR you may have an autoimmune disease OR you may have cancer. Hmm.
3. If you have an IgG elevation *after vaccination*, are you said to be "protected" (immune) even though you can still contract the infection?
4. If you have elevated IgG level after an exposure, but you have never had the illness and are NOT vaccinated, you are still said to be "protected" (immune).

Confusing? Yes. Very confusing.

Why do we place so much importance on antibodies, especially IgG antibodies, which can represent so many things?

WHAT'S MISSING

An IgG antibody is not the signature for "being protected." It is a marker of chronic inflammation and contamination. The formation of an antibody is the RESULT of something abnormal in the body, especially in the bloodstream, that needs to be neutralized and eliminated. Something foreign causes the B-cells to form and release the antibodies. Think of all the ingredients in a vaccine. There are chemicals, metals, animal cells, adjuvants, and more. The IgG antibodies are released as the clean-up crew to get the junk out of the body and removed from the blood.

A blood test measuring the IgG level (coupled with a list of symptoms) identifies a "disease." Why would the body suddenly and without reason attack its own organs? Truth is, the provoking particle needed to be removed.

So the question remains:

Why are these compounds – aluminum, mercury, squalene, polysorbate 80, polyethylene glycol, liposomes, virosomes, crab shells, tree bark, *Salmonella* cells, and more – being injected into the human body? What are the long-term consequences of this misguided attempt to produce antibodies to prevent something as usually benign as the flu?

WHO ARE THE QUACKS?

Dr. Stephen Barrett launched *Quackwatch.org* in 1997, focusing on exposing questionable health practices. As of December 2019, the website had received over 16 million home page visits, and it continued to be actively maintained in 2024. The home page states:

> "This site focuses on health frauds, myths, fads, fallacies, and misconduct. The main goal is to provide quackery-related information that is difficult or impossible to get elsewhere."

Its mission has been "to combat health-related frauds, myths, fads, and fallacies."

Over the years, alternative, holistic, and integrative medicine practitioners have been mercilessly attacked by this "protector of society" for everything from the use of vitamins and supplements to advocating acupuncture and colloidal silver. Done under the guise of "Investigating questionable claims, answering inquiries about products and services, reporting illegal marketing, and attacking misleading advertising on the Internet," the careers of many honest, hard-working doctors and practitioners who were practicing sensible, evidence-based, non-pharmaceutical based medicine – and getting people well – have been seriously damaged both personally and professionally by the accusations of the self-proclaimed caretaker at "Quackwatch."

Now, imagine this scenario:

> An alternative medicine practitioner declares he has created a way to protect a child from an infectious disease. He created an injectable suspension that contains multiple viruses combined with a variety of cells originating from a monkey, a dog, a caterpillar egg, or retina cells from an aborted human fetus. Into the mix he added some cow blood (bovine serum) and chicken parts (fibroblasts). To purify and stabilize the solution, he added formaldehyde, polysorbate 80, PEG, lipid nanoparticles, aluminum, mercury, and a variety of other chemicals. To generate the best response, he added adjuvants made from squalene, tree bark, and bacterial cells. Proclaiming this potion to be a "wonder drug," the new injectable was marketed for use by everyone in the world – from pregnant women, to newborns, to seniors.

What would Quackwatch.org – or State Medical Boards, the FDA, and the US government – do to this "alternative" product and to the practitioner? He would be declared a heretic (maybe a lunatic), dragged into court, prosecuted, have his license to practice medicine revoked, and assigned exorbitant fines for poisoning the population. Depending on what happened to the innocents who believed his rhetoric and received the injected product, he may be convicted of malpractice, or even charged with murder.

Knowing what is in a vaccine, how it is made, and its potential health-devastating ramifications, why aren't the companies that make them, the doctors who prescribe them, and the nurses who administer them held liable for distributing a "quack therapy"?

Recall Dr. Heneine's observations at the 1999 CBER meeting, that "specific pathogen-free" eggs are not the same as "pathogen- free." Knowing what's coming through that needle – is very important to your life, especially since studies have pointed out serious concerns – vaccines have not been proven safe nor have they been shown to be nearly as effective as proponents want us to believe.

How did we get to this place of blindly believing doctors and trusting that pharmaceutical companies create products to eliminate disease and keep us well? How did the government get involved with our personal health and why did doctors stop taking care of our families to become beholden to the medical system? The answers may surprise you.

"When we give government the power to make medical decisions for us, we, in essence, accept that the state owns our bodies."

~ US Representative Ron Paul (R-TX)

CHAPTER 14

How Public Health Became Weaponized

Before the world experienced COVID, the concept of mandatory vaccination was a crazy possibility. Vaccination laws are passed and monitored at the state level, not mandated or enforced at the federal level. In 2002, I decided to purchase the URL www.CoalitionAgainstMandatoryVaccination.com (link not active.) I tried to warn everyone in the Health Freedom and Patriot movements that we were going to be faced with mandatory vaccination in the not-so-distant future. I urgently warned that we needed to organize, formulate a plan, and prepare to fight back. My concerns were not only shut down, the concept was scoffed at…by *everyone*. I was met with many disapproving and condescending comments including, "That's crazy. They'd never go that far," and "How would they enforce it? No one would give up their right to refuse and just comply."

And here we are.

But planning for the nationwide draconian shutdowns, mask mandates, and quarantines started long before 2020. The plan even began before the time when I tried to rally the troops in 2002.

BEGINNINGS OF PUBLIC HEALTH PRACTICES

The Greek philosopher, Hippocrates (460 to 377 BC), frequently referred to as "the Father of Medicine," was also one of the original thinkers on health. His followers believed that eating well, getting adequate sleep, and daily exercise were important to balance the *humours,* which were thought to be responsible for health and disease. His message was that the health of the individual was important to the health of the entire Republic, the Roman Empire.

Likewise, the Romans believed that cleanliness was important for overall health. Through empiric observation they concluded that unclean water, an accumulation of sewage, and a lack of personal cleanliness led to illness. Without even a basic understanding of microbiology, they built public toilets and sewage systems. By AD 100, they had constructed nine aqueducts to carry fresh water into Rome and other population centers. The public baths were places for social congregation and to discuss both commerce and politics. Similarly, in the Far East, Baghdad opened its first hospital in the 800s and twenty years later, had more than 60 facilities across its vast plains. Numerous cities within the Persian empire had also built public baths and complex sewage systems.

After the decline of the Roman Empire, during the next 800 to 1000 years referred to as the Dark and Middle Ages, healthy food, fresh water, and sanitation were nowhere to be found. Hence the widespread epidemics of typhoid, bubonic plague, cholera, and smallpox fill the history books. One of the earliest uses of quarantine was during the "Black" plague epidemics of the Middle Ages. Due to widespread commerce and the risk of importing the illness that at the time had no known cause, Mediterranean seaports instituted thirty days of sanitary isolation before any foreigner could enter the city. In the early 1400s, the isolation period was extended from 30 to 40 days by the Venetians to protect the city from incoming plagues. The 40-day rule remained the standard for centuries.

During the early 1600s, the first US colonies began as a series of seaports peppered along the Eastern seaboard, built to host ships arriving from Northern Europe loaded with immigrants and supplies. Quarantines were instituted to protect the coastal cities from infectious epidemics. Outbreaks of smallpox and cholera, rampant in the 1600s, were often slowed or stopped with the use of quarantine. By the 1700s, the most serious, widespread infection was yellow fever, arriving from Africa and the Caribbean with the growth of the slave trade.

LEARN MORE

Yellow fever is an infection transmitted by the female *Aedes aegypti* mosquito. Today, the infection occurs only in tropical areas, particularly in parts of South America and Sub-Saharan Africa. But in the early 1800s, it was one of the most widely known and feared pestilence of the western hemisphere. It is spread between humans and monkeys through a typical mosquito bite. The infection cannot be spread from person to person. Nearly 85% of people fully recover within a few weeks with only supportive treatment. Once recovered, the person has long term immunity. A few people unpredictably progress to a toxic form of the illness, which can lead to liver and kidney failure, seizures, and coma. An estimated 50% of people who experience the intoxication stage of the infection will die.

Early colonial governors took the spread of infection seriously, especially yellow fever.

The **Massachusetts Quarantine Act of July 1701** held the individual who brought the illness to the shores accountable and fined them heavily, requiring them to pay all associated costs and damages that resulted from the infection. The Act also required all infected individuals to be held in strict quarantine for several weeks after going ashore. Nearly 100 years later (1796), the **Relative Quarantine Act** became the first federal law to control the spread of infection entering through the ports. Repealed in 1799, it was replaced with **The Act Respecting Quarantine and Health Laws** which authorized army and naval officers to assist local and state officials with enforcement of the quarantine as necessary.

In 1798, Congress passed **The Act for Relief of Sick and Disabled Seamen Act.** Within the Act were provisions to establish the **US Marine Hospital Service (MHS)**, operated and funded through the Revenue Marine Division of the Treasury Department. Treasury funds were used to create a loose network of hospitals along coastal and inland waterways to care for sick merchant seamen. The system was paid for by taxing American seamen 20 cents a month; in essence, this was the first national medical insurance program.

HIGHLIGHT

It may seem odd that the Marine Hospital Service (MHS) was placed within the jurisdiction of the Department of the Treasury. According to *Treasury.gov*, many functions of the early federal government, regardless of fiscal significance, were placed under the watchful eye of the Treasury. Examples include the Postal Service, which was part of the Department of the Treasury from its inception in 1775 until 1829. The General Land Office, which later became the Department of the Interior, was part of the Department of the Treasury from 1812 to 1849. The oldest division of the US armed service, the Coast Guard, remained under the arm of the Department of the Treasury until 1967.

In the mid-1800s, a yellow fever outbreak was brought to the US by immigrants fleeing the aggressive epidemic in the Caribbean. In 1858, the outbreak killed over 4,800 people in New Orleans. Twenty years later, another yellow fever outbreak spread across the Mississippi Valley, infecting more than 100,000 people, and leaving 20,000 dead. Congress took action and passed the **National Quarantine Act of 1878** that gave the Surgeon General of the MHS the authority to quarantine ships entering and exiting coastal seaports. This was the first legislation that allowed the federal government to be involved in health regulations.

From 1880 to 1900, this period will long be remembered for the global mass migration to the US from many parts of the world. During those 20 years, more than 9 million immigrants arrived in New York City Harbor and Ellis Island, making it the second busiest global port, after Hamburg, Germany. The travel conditions could only be described as unspeakable squalor. The combination of filth, cramped quarters, and malnutrition in the steerage of the trans-Atlantic steamships became the "perfect storm" for pestilence to arrive on the eastern seaboard. Once landed, several families, often 12 or more people, often lived together in a 625 square feet (58 square meters) tenement where they ate, slept, and expelled excrement. This was long before running water, electricity, refrigeration, adequate ventilation, and standard sewage removal were considered a normal standard of living. As described in Howard Markel's book, *Quarantine!*:

> "Contemporary accounts of life in urban slums during the 1880-90s was that of overcrowding and unsanitary living conditions. Tenements housed people in stifling, windowless, poorly ventilated rooms. The Lower East Side of New York could be summarized by the odor of rotting fish, the putrid meat, the decaying vegetables, the immense amount of animal waste in the streets, and the stench of 82,000 unclean humans living and working in the housing units."[180]

In February 1892, a widespread typhoid outbreak began in the crowded flats on the Lower East Side. With the first report of typhoid disease, the New York City Health Department roared into action and began an intensive sweep of the city. The dragnet inspected everything from boarding homes to slum ghettos. Those who were ill were transferred to the dismal quarantine facilities, commonly described as places to be "avoided at all costs." The city's holding facilities were harsh and inadequate. The laundry, sleeping, and dining room facilities were almost always situated near improperly maintained, overflowing toilets. The quarters had cots that were stacked closely together and were so filthy that those who arrived were "not likely to return home alive." Forcing those without symptoms to be confined into the detention centers alongside those with active typhoid infection increased the probability they would also become ill and possibly die.[180]

But as horrible as the conditions were in quarantine, separating the majority of those who were ill from those who showed no signs of infection eventually quelled the spread of the infection. By May 1892, the typhoid outbreak was burning itself out and by winter, the outbreak was over.

FROM TYPHOID TO CHOLERA

As typhoid fever was waning over the fall months of 1892, American newspapers were reporting huge loss of life and westward spread of a cholera epidemic in Russia. Estimates were imprecise, but reports suggested a nearly 50% death rate among nearly 650,000 cases of cholera. Americans were rightfully concerned about cholera arriving with the immigrants along with the other infections that were well documented. In August, officials in the busiest port in the world, Hamburg, Germany, were forced to admit they were dealing with an uncontrolled cholera epidemic, brought to their city from immigrants fleeing the harsh living conditions of Eastern Europe.

Hamburg's health officials were anxious to rid the city of the human vectors and continued their daily steamship schedules, sending boats around the world loaded with passengers who were ill with cholera. In the six weeks between September 1 and October 14, 1892, 997 vessels, nearly 81,000 passengers, and thousands of tons of baggage were inspected by the small quarantine staff at the NY harbor. The arrival of such large numbers of humans and cargo at the Port of New York the summer of 1892 created unimaginable challenges for the burgeoning public health system with a small cadre of physicians. With little knowledge of pathogen transmission, they had few tools to deal with the epidemic. In the cramped, filthy, turn of the century sailing ships, the microbe infested, watery diarrhea quickly soaked bedding and floors, spreading through all of the onboard supplies. Infected people often died within days due to the rapid dehydration resulting from copious, uncontrollable diarrhea.[180]

LEARN MORE

Since the middle of the 12th century, cholera has been one of mankind's most feared infections. A waterborne disease, cholera is caused by *Vibrio cholerae,* a comma-shaped bacillus which is transmitted between humans via contaminated water or food. The onset of the illness is sudden but subtle, starting with a nonspecific sense of simply not feeling well. Within hours, intense abdominal cramping was followed by violent waves of vomiting and explosive, watery diarrhea. Profound dehydration and shock could quickly ensue, especially in infants and children. Prior to the advent of appropriate hygiene and antibiotics, the death rate from cholera ranged from 30 to 80 percent.

Public health officials in New York handled the 1892 cholera epidemic with fear, prejudice, and scapegoating against immigrants, especially Russian Jews. Hamburg officials later affirmed this group of immigrants was most likely **not** the source of communicable disease, confirmed by their religious rituals and strict adherences to cleanliness.

These examples of yellow fever, typhoid, and cholera from horrific public health conditions form the basis for modern day quarantines during COVID that were called "lockdowns." Reviewing history gives insight into why similar circumstances were entertained during COVID-19.

Fast forward to today: Similar tactics have been used to single out and discriminate against unvaccinated children and adults.

GOVERNMENT EXPANSION INTO HOSPITAL CARE

Political debates and power struggles dragged on for years over which agency within the federal government should be in control of the nation's public health. **In 1893,** the **Rayner-Harris National Quarantine Act** was passed and was quickly signed into law by outgoing President Benjamin Harrison. The Act expanded the role of public health at the federal level and authorized the Marine Hospital Service (MHS) to place every quarantine station across the nation under one federal agency.

Even though the states retained the right to own and operate quarantine stations, Rayner-Harris suggested that in the event of a national emergency, local stations "should consider" turning over control to MHS and the Secretary of the Treasury. With these enactments, Rayner-Harris became an early model for federal control and the early prototype for monitoring Americans in the name of "public health."[180]

Port officials were given discretion to detain newcomers arriving from ports if they felt the detention would prevent the spread of infection. While never exercised, the president was given the **ability to suspend immigration** as he deemed necessary for public health and safety. Chicago was an early adopter to the MHS nationwide plan. Immigrants could only proceed into Chicago from the eastern ports if they had a **certificate of examination and/or a certificate of quarantine** signed by a physician who was part of the US Marine Hospital Service.

COMMENTARY

Can you see the similarities happening today within this federal act that was passed in **1893**?

- Quarantine stations: the forerunner of repeated COVID testing stations.

- The evolving concept for vaccine passports, signed by a physician, to show you are "protected" and "non-contagious."

- Detention of immigrants for testing, while not exercised on our southern border, has been "on the books" for more than a century.

- Executive Order (EO) 13769, signed by President Trump, titled "Protecting the Nation from Foreign Terrorist Entry into the United States." The EO called for a 90-day suspension for people entering the US from seven countries: Iran, Iraq, Libya, Somalia, Sudan, Syria, and Yemen. These countries had previously been identified as a high potential for terrorism with travel to the United States.

A WIN FOR PUBLIC HEALTH

It's difficult to imagine the state of filth that Americans had become accustomed to living with. For example, the average life expectancy in New York City and Brooklyn in 1880 was only 36 years. The 1912 annual report from the New York City Health Department included:

"...the removal of 20,000 dead horses, mules, donkeys and cattle from the streets in addition to nearly half a million smaller animals such as pigs, hogs, calves and sheep, which amounted to disposal of more than 5 million pounds of spoiled poultry, fish, pork and beef which eventually ended up in the municipal water supplies."

It should be no surprise that the report also noted more than 343,000 complaints had been filed over the foul smell due to poor ventilation and unlicensed manure dumps.[181]

An early, big win for public health was the decline of widespread outbreaks of infectious disease. Modern-day public health, including the CDC and the WHO, wants to give the credit to the ever-increasing vaccination program. But that was not the reason.

In 1872, the introduction of water filtration was the most significant step towards improving public health in America. Initially aimed at addressing discoloration and removing bad taste and foul odor, filtration soon proved to be a game-changer. It not only eliminated turbidity, foul color, and nearly 99% of the swarming bacteria but also set a new standard for the "quality" of treated water. However, when outbreaks continued to occur, chemists experimented with several disinfecting methods, including boiling, ultraviolet rays, ozone, copper, and silver. However, cost considerations and ease of use produced the clear winner: **chlorine.**[182]

First used in the paper and textile industries, **calcium hypochlorite**, is a stable, white solid that contains 65% available chlorine and dissolves easily in water. It was cheap, readily available, and easy to use on a large scale. It was already being used in the late 1800s to clean the water in the Chicago Stockyards.

Jersey City, New Jersey, was the first urban area to use chlorine to clean its water. In 1899, the city contracted to build a dam, reservoir, and pipeline to bring water from the Rockaway River, 23 miles away. But when the project was done, city officials were not pleased with the outcome. At certain times of the year, sewage polluted the reservoir and city water supply. A lawsuit followed, arguing that the water was not "pure and wholesome" as the contract required. The construction company was ordered to remove contamination sources and build a new watershed area. When that was done, the city filed another lawsuit, balking at the project's steep cost – equivalent to over $175 million today.

During the time it took to build the new dam, bacteriological techniques had advanced significantly. On September 26, 1908, Jersey City began chlorinating its water. George A. Johnson, of the engineering firm Hering & Fuller, was hired to oversee operations. He developed the chlorine feed system that would deliver millions of gallons of purified water to the city each day. Since then, the system has continually introduced various forms of chlorine into the water supply. As of September 26, 2024, the chlorinating system has been in continuous use for 116 years.

LEARN MORE

When Jersey City began chlorinating its water in 1908, calcium hypochlorite was applied at doses around 0.5 to 1.0 milligrams per liter (mg/L) or possibly higher, depending on water conditions and contamination levels. This was enough to kill pathogens but sometimes resulted in noticeable chlorine taste or odor. Today, the typical residual chlorine in drinking water is 0.2 up to 4.0 mg/L. For consumers who find the taste or smell of chlorine unpleasant, simple solutions included using an activated carbon water filter (removes the chlorine) or letting the water sit uncovered in the refrigerator for several hours (chlorine dissipates into the air). Chlorine in water becomes toxic when the concentrations exceed 50 mg/L.

After chlorination proved successful in Jersey City, many cities quickly adopted it with impressive results.[183] In 1900, waterborne diseases caused nearly a quarter of all reported deaths in major cities. By 1936, widespread adoption of clean water technologies cut overall mortality from infectious diseases by about 43%. By 1941, around 85% of US drinking water was chlorinated. Combined with sand filtration, chlorination reduced typhoid fever deaths by more than 90% by 1956.

The cornerstone of this revelation and review comes from a paper by Cutler and Miller from Harvard University, published in 2004:[184]

> "We show that the introduction of water filtration and chlorination systems led to major reductions in mortality, explaining **nearly half of the overall** reduction in mortality between 1900 and 1936. Our results also suggest that **clean water was responsible for three-quarters of the decline in infant mortality and nearly two-thirds of the decline in child mortality.** The magnitude of these effects is striking. Clean water also appears to have led to the **near eradication of typhoid fever,** a waterborne scourge of the 19th and early 20th centuries."[185] *(emphasis added)*

Therefore, clean water technologies, not vaccination, are likely the most important public health interventions of the 20th century.

The massive number of immigrants who came to the US in the late 1800s brought with them pathogens associated with poor hygiene. Four vaccines – typhoid fever, cholera, rabies, and plague – had been developed late in the 1800s, but none were widely used, nor were they very effective. Few treatments existed for infection. Penicillin, the first antibiotic, was not discovered until 1928 and not put into widespread use until the early 1940s. The only routinely given vaccination was smallpox.

By 1868, more than 95% of Chicago's inhabitants had been inoculated with the smallpox vaccine. After the Great Chicago Fire of 1871, vaccination was required to receive relief supplies. Despite a near-100% vaccination rate, the city was hit with a devastating smallpox epidemic in 1872. More than 2,000 people contracted smallpox, and the death rate was more than 25% among those who became infected. The fatality among children under five was the highest ever recorded.

Vaccinating the entire city did not create herd immunity, and it did not protect the population from contracting smallpox. Despite these – and many other failures – vaccination is continually promoted as one of the "greatest medical achievements of modern civilization." The **real heroes,** the technologies that changed the course of history and public health, are rarely mentioned: *clean water, sewage treatment for municipalities, and electricity to support refrigeration.*

In the 21st century, more than half of the world's population still lives in small cities or rural areas, particularly in regions like Sub-Saharan Africa and South Asia. Many of the poorest communities lack access to clean drinking water and reliable sanitation, with a significant number of people still practicing open defecation. Without adequate nutrition, purified drinking water, or refrigeration to protect food from flies, maggots, and other pathogens, health issues and infections remain a leading cause of illness and death in developing countries. As far back as 2005, the World Bank, in conjunction with the World Sanitation Program (WSP.org), found a 47% reduction in diarrhea and death by dehydration among children in remote villages by improving their sanitation.[186]

Rotary International, the WHO, UNICEF, the Global Alliance for Vaccines and Immunizations (GAVI), WEF, and the Gates Foundation have poured *tens of billions* of dollars into vaccinating malnourished children who lack sanitation, water, refrigeration, safety, and education. Instead of pushing money into polio, measles, and rotavirus vaccines, think of the global problems that would be solved if those same dollars were allocated to the most important health intervention in the world's history: **clean water.**[187]

THE POWER GRAB CONTINUES

The Marine Hospital Service (MHS) had been reorganized and renamed the Public Health and Marine Hospital Service in 1902 and later shortened to the Public Health Service (PHS) in 1912. Government involvement in public health began to accelerate with the passage of the **Social Security Act** in August 1935. Enacted during the depths of the Great Depression (1929 to 1941), it aimed to support the elderly, the infirm, the poor, and the children who were suffering most. Social Security changed people's minds about the government; they began seeing the government as a protective force rather than as a menace. The government began its transformation into a parental figure stepping in to help.

The Public Health Service Act of 1944, enacted near the end of World War II, streamlined and updated all legislation related to the Public Health Service. This law reinforced the PHS mission to promote public health and expanded its authority, further solidifying its role as a federally funded entity. With the influx of military personnel and European immigrants arriving in the US as WWII was winding down, the PHS assumed the critical responsibility of monitoring newcomers for signs of infectious diseases. Quarantine measures could be enforced and managed by a newly established branch, the Communicable Disease Center in Atlanta, Georgia. This agency was later renamed the Centers for Disease Control (CDC) in 1970 and, in 1992, became the Centers for Disease Control and Prevention, commonly known today as the CDC.

As federal agencies grew in size and number, several reorganization efforts arose to manage this expansion. Congress enacted **The Hill-Burton Act of 1946,** representing the first government-subsidized medical care legislation.[189] This act financed the construction of thousands of postwar hospitals, nursing homes, and other healthcare facilities nationwide. An amendment in 1954 provided funding to create long-term facilities, rehabilitation centers, and hospital outpatient departments.[190]

LEARN MORE

President Harry S. Truman signed **Executive Order 9708** on December 10, 1946. This EO was significant in that it transferred responsibility for public health and sanitation-related functions to various government agencies. It marked a shift in how health and welfare services were administered at the federal level.

Soon after Public Health Service Act was put in place, on January 27, 1951, Truman signed **Executive Order (E.O.) 10313**, "Specifying Communicable Diseases: for the Purpose of Regulations Providing for the Apprehension, Detention, or Conditional Release of Individuals to Prevent the Introduction, Transmission, or Spread of Communicable Diseases." The executive order provided the **legal framework for quarantine and isolation practices** in the US to control the spread of this list of communicable diseases that could be controlled using quarantines:

> Anthrax, Chancroid, Cholera, Dengue, Diphtheria, Favus, Gonorrhea, Granuloma Inguinale, Infectious Encephalitis, Leprosy, Lymphogranuloma Venereum, Meningococcus Meningitis, Plague, Poliomyelitis, Psittacosis, Ringworm of the Scalp, Scarlet Fever, Smallpox, Streptococcic Sore Throat, Syphilis, Trachoma, Tuberculosis, Typhoid Fever, Typhus, and Yellow Fever.

In 1983, the list was expanded by President Reagan's **E.O.12452** to include suspected Viral Hemorrhagic Fevers (Lassa, Marburg, Congo-Crimean, *Ebola*) and *others not yet isolated or named.* It wasn't changed again until 2003 when President George W. Bush revised the list under **E.O. 13295** to include Severe Acute Respiratory Syndrome (**SARS**), an infection with person-to-person transmission. This E.O. was updated to **E.O.13375** in 2005 to include "**novel or reemergent influenza viruses** that are causing, or have the potential to cause, a pandemic." And on September 17, 2021, through **E.O. 13674**, the Biden Administration added **measles** to the list of quarantinable illnesses.[188]

By 1968, Hill-Burton had helped to finance 9,200 new medical facilities in over 4,000 communities; by 1974, that number had ballooned to include almost one-third of all hospital projects in the US. Between 1980 and 1997, Hill-Burton had provided more than $6 billion to pay hospitals for the uncompensated services provided to eligible patients. By 2000, Hill-Burton had allocated more than $4.6 billion in grants and $1.5 billion in loans, **called federally matching funds,** to nearly 6,800 healthcare facilities in all 50 states.

As the agencies within the federal government continued to expand, several reorganizations took place in an attempt to better manage the increasing number of workers and policies. In 1953, the PHS became part of the Department of Health, Education, and Welfare (HEW). By 1979, HEW had grown so large that another government reorganization was necessary. This time, HEW was renamed the Department of Health and Human Services (HHS). The newly formed agency was given broad responsibility over several administrations: the Social Security Administration (SSA), the Family Support Administration, and the Public Health Service. This structure remained until 1995, when President Clinton restored the SSA to its original status as an independent agency, setting the stage for significant growth within HHS. Today, with more than 80,000 employees, HHS wields tremendous power and influence at the federal level and over state and local governments. The Secretary of HHS has administrative oversight of approximately 115 programs across 11 agencies, including the Food and Drug Administration (FDA), the Centers for Disease Control (CDC), the National Institutes of Health (NIH), and the Centers for Medicare and Medicaid Services (CMS).

> **HIGHLIGHT**
>
> Federally matching funds are how the federal government used – and continues to use – grants and contracts to tie the hands of state constitutions and legislatures so that constitutionally, the states have lost the sovereignty granted to them by the 10th amendment: "The powers not delegated to the US by the Constitution, nor prohibited by it to the States, *are reserved to the States respectively, or to the people.*"

MEDICARE AND MEDICAID, THE GAME CHANGERS

The framers of the US Constitution did not intend for the federal government to engage in matters of health. In fact, the word "health" does not appear anywhere in the document. The Constitution authorizes the government to "promote and provide for the general welfare," but it does not grant the federal government specific powers to be involved in health or healthcare. Therefore, as defined by the Constitution itself, "powers not expressly granted to the federal government are reserved for the states and the people." Public health regulations were established at the federal level to guard against periodic outbreaks of contagious illnesses associated with international commerce. However, in the nearly 75 years since the creation of the PHS, it has evolved into a massive and extraordinarily costly Nanny Agency, a significant division of government that interferes in every aspect of American life.

By far, the most significant legislative change that permanently altered the relationship between government, healthcare, and public health was the passage of the **Social Security Act Amendment,** signed into law in July 1965. This new program established **Medicare,** a supplemental insurance for individuals aged 65 and older. Funded by the federal government and partially financed through a payroll tax, Medicare serves as the government's health insurance that subsidizes payments to physicians and healthcare facilities for medical care provided to seniors while hospitalized. Concurrently, the Social Security Amendments established **Medicaid**, government insurance for low-income individuals. Both provisions promised to cover medical services for Americans of all ages. Combined, the two programs are in one agency called the Centers for Medicare and Medicaid, frequently referred to as simply CMS.

Medicare has created an enormous strain on public health initiatives and the federal budget, and this burden continues to grow year after year. As the US population aged, so did life expectancy. In 1900, life expectancy for men and women was 46 years and 48 years, respectively. When Medicare became law, with mandatory enrollment at age 65, life expectancy for American men was 67 years, while for women it was 74 years. The government deemed a few years of coverage for the baby boomer generation, those born between 1946 and 1964, to be reasonable and affordable. However, expanding access to prescription medications, advanced technologies, and better ways to maintain overall health has greatly increased both the life expectancy of seniors and the expenditures of Medicare.

On January 1, 2011, the first and oldest members of the baby boomers turned 65 years old. According to the Pew Research Center, nearly 10,000 boomers will turn 65 every day from that day forward for the next 19 years. By 2030, almost 72 million people – 18% of the nation's population – will be eligible for and receiving Medicare benefits. With life expectancy now at 76 years for men and just over 81 years for women, the longevity of boomers has significantly surpassed the ability of the payroll tax to cover the costs. The vision of providing health care for senior citizens for a few years between their retirement and their passing is on the verge of collapse. In fact, by 2024, the fastest-growing demographic in the US will be people over 100 years old, commonly referred to as **centenarians**.

To put these numbers into perspective, in 1960, national spending on healthcare services was 4.6% of gross domestic product (GDP). By 1985, this figure had risen to 9.5% of GDP and continued to climb to 16.4% by 2013. Medicare payments reached nearly $603 billion in 2014, surpassing defense spending of $594 billion and almost doubling the amount spent on Medicaid ($305 billion). Beginning in 2014, total outlays for Medicare and Medicaid were expected to increase by an average of about 5.2% each year. Specifically, the average annual growth rate for Medicare spending is projected to be roughly 6.5% from 2020 to 2030. Medicare alone was projected to exceed $1.1 trillion in 2023, and US healthcare spending was estimated to be approximately 17% of the country's Gross Domestic Product (GDP).

The demand for healthcare coverage for the elderly and infirm continues to grow. Healthcare costs have soared due to new, high-tech medical technologies and increased utilization of healthcare facilities. Consumer expectations have risen with these advancements, leading to demands that all lifesaving and life-extending tools be employed to save every life, regardless of the severity of injuries or the age of the patient. As a result, a significant portion of healthcare expenditures are spent in the final months or years of life. A commonly cited figure suggests that up to 30% of all Medicare spending occurs during the last two years of life.

The United States healthcare system is the most expensive in the world. How do we rank for all the money that is spent? In September 2024, The Commonwealth Fund released an updated report called "Mirror, Mirror." It is an economic analysis of 10 wealthy nations: Australia, Canada, France, Germany, the Netherlands, New Zealand, Sweden, Switzerland, the United Kingdom, and the United States. These countries were analyzed across 70 performance indicators within categories such as access to care, quality of care processes, efficiency, equity, and health outcomes. While all the countries have strengths and weaknesses, the **US ranks last** in nearly every category when compared to the other nine high-income countries.

As stated in the report, the US is not just an outlier on health system performance, it's an outlier on health care spending as well. While spending on healthcare in the US is by far the highest in the world, overall performance and outcomes are ranked the lowest by a significant margin. In fact, the US has a lower average life expectancy and higher avoidable mortality than the other nine middle- and high-income countries in the report.[191]

Sadly, this problem with the explosive costs of the CMS programs isn't new.

LEARN MORE

Medicaid is a jointly funded federal and state program. Its long-term sustainability is often discussed in light of rising healthcare costs, expanding enrollment, and state budget constraints. Any changes in federal contributions could prompt some states to make difficult budget decisions, potentially affecting the program's ability to meet rising demand in the future.

Medicare, on the other hand, is financed by the Hospital Insurance (HI) Trust Fund, established by the Social Security Act in 1965 and funded through payroll taxes. Employees and employers each contribute 1.45% of earnings to the fund, with higher earners (those making over $200,000 for individuals or $250,000 for married couples) paying an additional 0.9% due to provisions passed within the Affordable Care Act. The HI Trust Fund pays for Medicare Part A, inpatient hospital services, skilled nursing facility care, hospice, and some home health services. The Fund is projected to finally become completely insolvent by 2036.

On December 19, 2009 Senator Tom Colburn, an obstetrician from Oklahoma, read into the Congressional Record:

> "Medicare is broke, the State Medicaid Programs are broke, the census is broke. We heard this week that Fannie and

Freddie aren't going to require just $400 billion – that is a government-run mortgage insurance company that the Congress created – it is going to require $800 billion, almost $1 trillion to get us out of the [banking mess]. Social Security, we know, is going to be broke. It is fiscally unsustainable. The US Post Office business model is broke; cash for clunkers; the highway trust fund is broke. We can't even get the $8 billion we need to continue to run it. We have done a great job managing that. Now we are going to put another 20 percent of health care in this country under the auspices of the very people who run the broke programs that have created $1.4 trillion worth of deficits. It is broke in terms of methodology – because it is a Ponzi scheme. We have robbed the money. We have promised benefits for years and never raised the taxes to pay for them. We now manage 60 percent of the health care in the country."[192]

Keep in mind, this was in 2009. It is much worse in today's dollars.

Unfortunately, those dollars – your tax dollars – are not fully allocated to health services for the elderly and the poor. The Government Accountability Office (GAO) reported in March 2024 that the federal government issued nearly $236 billion in improper payments across entitlement programs in 2023 alone. Medicare was the largest individual program, responsible for $51.1 billion in improper payments, or 22% of the total. Medicaid closely followed at 21%, totaling $50.3 billion. Over the past 20 fiscal years, it is estimated that improper payments could have been as much as $2.7 trillion. According to the report, improper payments may include inaccurate recordkeeping, overpayments, or fraud.[193]

It seems obvious that stopping billions of dollars of fraud and improper payments would go a long way to shoring up Medicare financing. But government involvement has become more complicated than just paying the medical bills for the elderly and the poor. Data is the new gold and surveillance is the new priority, and the US government has devised technologies to maximize both.

LEARN MORE

In December 2009, while the Senate debated the passage of a trillion dollar healthcare bill, some of the costs that were projected were based on historical spending. The fiscal problems with CMS date back more than 15 years.

In 1963, the first year costs anticipated for Medicaid was $238 million; the actual costs were more than $1 billion. By 2009, Medicaid costs 37 times more than when it was launched, reaching more than $250 billion in 2009. In Fiscal Year (FY) 2023, total Medicaid spending was approximately $860 billion.

In 1963, the Medicare hospitalization program alone was supposed to cost $9 billion but the actual costs were around $67 billion. By 2003, Medicare spending was approximately $283 billion. By 2023, Medicare spending reached approximately $1.03 trillion, accounting for about 21% of total national health expenditures.

In 1973, the Medicare program for renal disease was estimated to cover approximately 11,000 participants. In 2009, 395,000 people were covered at a cost of $22 billion. As of 2019, there were approximately 534,000 Medicare beneficiaries diagnosed with End-Stage Renal Disease. Medicare expenditures for these patients were estimated at $36 billion.

What are Americans getting for these huge expenditures, aside from system-wide issues of redundancy, fraud and waste? It appears not much. What do we rank first in? Being one of the largest purchasers of drugs and vaccines in the world.

"Facebook is not your friend, it is a surveillance engine."

~Richard Stallman, the Free Software Foundation

CHAPTER 15

Tracking, Surveillance, and the Global Vaccination Agendas

THE BEGINNING OF TOTAL TRACKING: EHRS

Over the last several decades, public awareness and dissatisfaction have grown regarding the increasing reach of government into daily life. From NSA surveillance programs like PRISM that collect internet communications, to smartphones and car GPS systems that double as tracking devices, to the rise of 5G towers and biometric technologies like airport iris scanners, the message is clear: surveillance is everywhere, and privacy is shrinking. The government is tracking our every move.

Medical technologies add another dimension to the tracking landscape. Wearable devices allow individuals to monitor personal health metrics: weight, blood pressure, heart rate, and blood glucose. Physicians can remotely access this data through online patient portals, and these statistics can be trended and analyzed daily or even hourly, and stored in cloud-based systems for access. However, the most pervasive tracking mechanism may be electronic health records (EHRs), which are now standard in nearly all medical practices. EHRs serve not only as repositories of personal health data but also as tools for broader health surveillance systems.

In 2011, the CMS launched a program to incentivize doctors and hospitals to adopt electronic health records (EHRs). The carrot? Promises of greater convenience, improved care coordination, fewer medical errors, more efficient office visits, faster responses, and better access to patient records. The stick? Physicians were warned that payment for treating Medicare and Medicaid patients would hinge on converting to electronic billing systems. Physicians were told, "If you want to get paid for seeing Medicare and Medicaid patients, you must convert to electronic billing."

The main reason physicians resisted installing EHRs in their offices was straightforward: cost. Setting up and implementing an EHR system could run $30,000 or more *per physician*, with additional monthly and annual user fees. By 2008, only 10 to 15% of physicians were using basic EHR systems capable of tracking medical history, demographics, diagnoses, medications, and allergies. Some systems also offered features like electronic prescriptions and lab or X-ray result access. That same year, the housing market bubble burst, triggering a financial crisis known as The Great Recession, a collapse fueled by a surge in mortgage defaults. This collapse led to widespread bank failures and caused a severe recession. In response, the government enacted sweeping interventions to stabilize the economy, including the passage of the American Recovery and Reinvestment Act (ARRA) in 2009.

The HITECH Act was embedded in the massive ARRA; HITECH laid the groundwork for a nationwide IT framework aimed at promoting the sharing of health data to improve health outcomes. HITECH encompassed various initiatives, but its primary aim was to advance EHR adoption. The 2009 stimulus package followed shortly thereafter, allocating $27 billion to encourage hospitals and other health providers to implement EHR systems. Between May 2011 and September 2016, an additional $24.7 billion was funneled into Medicare and Medicaid EHR incentive programs. The legislation established two main financial incentive structures:

- **Medicare Incentives**: Providers could earn up to $44,000 over five years for adopting Medicare EHRs, with higher payments for early adopters and reduced incentives for those who joined later.
- **Medicaid Incentives**: Providers could receive up to $63,750 per physician over six years for adopting, implementing, or upgrading to EHR technology for Medicaid billing and demographic tracking. Incentives varied depending on individual state rules.

In exchange, providers had to prove they were using the EHRs in a "meaningful way," simply referred to as "meaningful use," or MU. As defined by the government, meaningful use was developed to:

- Improve quality, safety, efficiency, and reduce health disparities;
- Engage patients and family in their care;
- Improve coordination of care within a family;
- Institute public health policies throughout a population; and
- Maintain privacy and security of patient health information.

The financial incentives were quite enticing for small practices. Even better, this all sounded like a win for patients. But the government's offer came with a catch:

> "We'll cover the costs for hardware and software. We'll train you and your staff on how to use it. We'll even show you how to get paid faster, at higher rates, and more efficiently. All we ask in return is that you collect data on all your patients and report it back to us."

It seemed like a straightforward, reasonable trade-off, but once physicians adopted the EHR system, they were no longer just independent practitioners making treatment decisions based on their expertise and their patients' needs. Instead, many physicians became hospital employees, and thus bound by algorithm-driven medicine dictated by insurance companies, government agencies, and administrators. What began as a tool to improve care evolved into a multibillion-dollar data collection industry.

Like most government programs, the transition was gradual. Practitioners who chose to participate were required to meet Stage 1 criteria by 2014. This involved documenting 18 basic data points for all CMS patients, including vital signs, all medications, and all known allergies. Of these, 13 were mandatory, while the remaining 5 could be selected from a list of 9 optional criteria. By 2015, the number of core objectives had increased to 20, and physicians were required to report 9 out of 64 total clinical quality measures (CQMs). Here's a brief list of some CQMs reported to the government:[194]

- Asthma
- Adult Obesity
- Breast Cancer
- Childhood Obesity
- Coronary Artery Disease
- Diabetes
- Heart Failure
- Hypertension
- Ischemic Vascular Disease
- Smoking Cessation
- **Vaccination Status**

To further encourage adoption, providers who did not implement EHRs by 2015 faced reimbursement reductions, creating a financial penalty for non-adopters.

In 2017, the Meaningful Use (MU) program was absorbed into a new system called the Merit-based Incentive Payment System (MIPS). Under MIPS, providers are rewarded or penalized by downward adjustments in Medicare and Medicaid payments. This shift incentivized adherence to "standard protocols" and discouraged physicians from thinking independently. Since then, the reimbursement system for doctors and hospitals has become increasingly complex and difficult to navigate. Providers are now scored – and paid – based on a complicated set of performance criteria reported to CMS through the EHR system.

THE DARK SIDE OF EHR TRACKING

EHRs limit the physician's ability to provide the care they believe best suits their patients. EHR tracking also introduces significant ethical concerns as well as risks. As healthcare data became more centralized, a single breach could expose sensitive personal information and identifiable details, making it vulnerable to identity theft or fraud. A breach is defined as "an unauthorized access, use, or disclosure of protected health information that compromises the security or privacy of the information." The sheer volume of data in the HER systems increases the likelihood of security vulnerabilities that potentially affect millions of people.

In fact, this has already happened. From 2005 to 2019, healthcare data breaches affected a total of 249.09 million individuals. The largest known breach occurred in February 2015, the largest single breach that has occurred to date, was the network server for health insurance carrier Anthem, compromising the records of more than 78.8 million people. In 2019 alone, 41.2 million healthcare records were exposed, stolen, or illegally accessed across 505 healthcare data center breaches. According to the Data Breach Portal, managed by the US Office for Civil Rights within HHS, there have been breaches in 519 facilities, affecting the data security of more than 134 million people nationwide in the first eleven months of 2024. An IBM report noted that the average cost of a data breach in 2019 was $3.92 million, while a breach in the healthcare sector typically costs $6.45 million. Clearly, data privacy and confidentiality remain significant concerns for both individuals and organizations.[195]

LEARN MORE

The HITECH Act mandates that the Secretary of HHS post a list of breaches involving unsecured health information affecting 500 or more individuals. Personal health information secured only by a password and firewall is considered unsecured data.

Why would hospital systems and insurance companies allow unsecured data on their server networks? Several factors likely contribute to this. Legacy systems, which are still in use at many organizations, often lack modern security features, and upgrading them can be costly and disruptive. Smaller providers, with fewer resources, may not be able to afford advanced security measures like encryption or data destruction methods that render information unreadable, unusable, and indecipherable to hackers because they don't possess the encryption key. Smaller organizations also typically lack the expertise to implement proper data protections, which leaves the organizations more vulnerable to breaches. Human error, such as sending unencrypted emails or improper disposition of health records, can also lead to unsecured data.

While the law requires citizens to be notified of breaches involving unsecured data, no notification is required if the data has been securely encrypted. But can a patient know if their data is encrypted and protected from a hack? Why aren't patients or clients notified about the security status of their data either way?

A significant ethical dilemma arises with the commercialization of health data because use of personal information often happens without the patient's awareness and certainly happens without their consent. Companies share or sell or this data to third parties like pharmaceutical companies and marketing firms. The gaping lack of transparency raises serious privacy concerns and erodes patient trust in the healthcare system. Government involvement in the collection of sensitive health data – such as HIV status or vaccination records – has sparked fears of unwarranted surveillance. Many worry that their data will be used to implement even broader social control and infringe on personal freedoms.

HIPAA

A major concern for patients is the Health Insurance Portability and Accountability Act of 1996, or HIPAA. At every new patient appointment – whether with a doctor, dentist, or psychologist – patients are typically asked to sign a HIPAA form regarding the confidentiality of their medical records. Many believe this form and their signature guarantee the privacy of their health information, but this is far from the truth. Hidden within the 2009 financial stimulus bill was a provision that allowed many more entities and business associates to access a patient's health information without their consent. In reality, HIPAA does not protect medical privacy; rather, your signature on the form removes the need for additional consent to share any information entered into your EHR. HIPAA was intended to modernize the flow of health information, not to protect privacy.

In its original draft, HIPAA granted more than 600,000 health-related organizations access to information related to treatments, payment methods, and a broad range of activities categorized under "health-care operations." These operations include everything from quality assurance and customer service data to insurance tracking and protocol development. The requirements of HIPAA are outlined in a lengthy and complex document, often referred to as a "permissive rule," which allows extensive sharing of patient data within these broad parameters.

Current regulations allow more than **2.2 million organizations** and their business associates to legally access patient medical data. These entities include pharmacies, nursing homes, durable medical equipment suppliers, hospitals (both psychiatric and general), health insurers, and more. Patients are given no opt-out option and are often unaware it's even occurring. This vast unfettered access to records also poses serious security risks. Hackers seeking personal data for identity theft are seeking exploitable information; they are not interested in medical details like whether a person has hypertension or cancer, but granting millions of entities to access these sensitive medical records greatly increases the likelihood of data breaches and leaves individuals vulnerable to widespread criminal activity.

COMMENTARY

For a complete review and understanding of EHRs, CMS, HIPAA and more, I strongly recommend the award-winning book by Twila Brase, RN, PHN called *Big Brother in the Exam Room: The Dangerous Truth About Electronic Medical Records.* Written in 2018, it is more pertinent and important today than ever before.

VACCINE REGISTRIES

Since the early 1990s, states have been working to establish a nationwide electronic vaccine record system. On the surface, this seems practical – families often relocate, and retrieving medical records from a previous provider can be overlooked. Additionally, access to a centralized vaccination database could prove invaluable during emergencies, such as when an accident during a vacation necessitates an ER visit. However, enabling access to records across state lines has presented significant challenges.

By 2000, only 36% of states had enacted laws or regulations specifically addressing vaccine registries. By 2011, this number had risen to 66%, reflecting growing adoption of vaccine tracking systems. The participation rate in the national vaccine database has steadily increased, with 63% of children included in 2006, rising to 86% by 2012 – representing 19.5 million children under the age of six. Adult participation has also expanded, with 24.5% of adults (57.8 million individuals aged 19 and older) having their vaccine information entered by 2012, the latest year for which data is available. Notably, Connecticut and Rhode Island differ in their data collection practices. Connecticut limits tracking to children under six, while Rhode Island includes vaccine records for children and adolescents up to age 19, but excludes adults.

In an attempt to improve data capture, a plan to implement the Immunization Information System (IIS) was released in November 2013 as a joint effort between the CDC and the National Center for Immunization and Respiratory Diseases (NCIRD).[196] The Immunization Information System (IIS) is a population-based electronic database designed to track vaccine doses administered to individuals within a specific geographic area. State laws dictate what information is collected and entered into the IIS, leading to significant variability in requirements. While the primary purpose is to record vaccine information, many states mandate the inclusion of additional demographic data such as age, date of birth, race, sex, pregnancy status, employment status, and occupation. In some cases, the recipient's home address and zip code are also required. Notably, the information entered into the IIS is retained indefinitely; most states lack provisions for purging data once patients reach a certain age. This permanence raises questions about long-term data management and privacy protections.[197]

The IIS is designed to consolidate immunization data from individual providers and electronic health records (EHRs) into a centralized database, ensuring that clinical, administrative, and public health officials can access the information anytime and anywhere. According to the CDC's website, *parents must be allowed to choose whether to participate in the IIS.*[198] That's interesting because it is doubtful parents know anything about this database let alone its opt-out option. This is particularly significant because once a vaccination record is entered, it becomes a permanent part of the system, used for public health purposes. For those wishing to be removed, the process is nearly impossible, as there are no standardized provisions or clear mechanisms for opting out. As it stands, the IIS operates as a cradle-to-grave tracking system with limited flexibility for individuals who no longer wish to participate.

Progress toward achieving the goals of the 2014 IIS Strategic Plan has been gradual but steady. The number of children whose vaccination data is included in the IIS has steadily increased. By 2022, nearly 90% of children under the age of six were documented in the national immunization database.

While there are many concerns about IIS tracking, three key issues stand out:

1. **Data accuracy**: are records updated when individuals change their names due to marriage or divorce, or when families move across state lines or to another country? Inconsistent updates call into question the accuracy of the data, meaning the system is compromised.

2. **Data completeness**: maintaining these systems puts a heavy financial and administrative burden on providers. Small and rural practices with limited resources are particularly impacted. This raises concerns about whether all vaccination data is consistently and accurately entered into the system.

3. **Potential for misuse**: legitimate concerns exist regarding the IIS system being used for purposes beyond its original intent, such as enforcing vaccine mandates or enabling surveillance of individual healthcare choices, which could infringe on personal freedoms.

As tracking and data gathering of childhood vaccination statuses have been occurring in the US over the last 20 years, broader initiatives have been taking shape: ambitious plans to vaccinate every man, woman, and child worldwide.

THE NATIONAL VACCINATION PLAN

The Healthy People (HP) program, launched by the US government in 1979, aims to enhance the nation's health by establishing science-based, measurable goals for disease prevention and health promotion. Updated every decade, it focuses on a broad spectrum of health priorities and public health outcomes. Details of the HP programs will be explored in the next chapter.

Healthy People 2000 (HP2000) placed a significant focus on immunization and vaccine-preventable diseases as a key public health priority. The goal was to improve vaccination coverage and reduce the incidence of vaccine-preventable illnesses. By the time HP2010 came around, however, it became clear that a stronger push was needed to ensure broader compliance. Enter the Bill and Melinda Gates Foundation. On January 29, 2010, at the World Economic Forum, the Gates Foundation announced they would commit $10 billion over the next 10 years to research, develop, and deliver vaccines worldwide. Melinda Gates made it clear: "We've made vaccines our number-one priority at the Gates Foundation." This pledge was fueled by the success of Public-Private Partnerships, which had already made impressive strides in advancing vaccine development and delivery to transform vaccines into a profitable global enterprise. Spearheaded by the Gates Foundation, along with partners such as the WHO, UNICEF, and GAVI, the Vaccine Alliance, the "Decade of Vaccines" had officially begun.[199]

In the US, the Department of Health and Human Services (HHS) and the Centers for Disease Control and Prevention (CDC) quickly launched the 2010 National Vaccine Plan, with a comprehensive implementation strategy. Among the plan's lofty goals and priority recommendations were:

- Develop a catalog of priority vaccine targets for both domestic and global health needs.
- Strengthen the scientific foundation for the development and licensure of new vaccines.
- Increase awareness of vaccines, vaccine-preventable diseases, and the benefits and risks of immunization among the public, healthcare providers, and other stakeholders.
- Ensure a stable supply of, access to, and better utilization of recommended vaccines in the United States.
- Eliminate financial barriers for both providers and consumers to facilitate access to routinely recommended vaccines.
- Create an adequate and stable supply of vaccines for public health preparedness.
- Certify national standards for Electronic Health Records (EHRs) to ensure that eligible professionals and hospitals can meet required functions.

The 58-page document outlines detailed goals and objectives, as well as strategies for the enhancement of vaccine development, accessibility to vaccines, and public trust surrounding vaccines. The structure outlined in the document relied heavily on extensive surveillance and data collection techniques. This raised significant privacy concerns and eroded public confidence. The plan's emphasis on mandates and centralized control also sparked fears about individual autonomy. Critics voiced concerns that the prioritization of industry-driven innovation was overshadowing safety considerations. Ultimately, the National Vaccine Plan became a key tool in driving the COVID-19 vaccine mandates throughout 2020 and 2021.[200]

THE ADULT VACCINATION PLAN

Midway through the Decade of Vaccines, it became apparent to those at HHS and the CDC that the existing plans primarily focused on tracking children and the childhood vaccination schedule. The National Vaccine Advisory Committee (NVAC) and various stakeholder groups recognized the need to address adult vaccinations as well. In response to this gap, the National Adult Immunization Plan was launched on September 15, 2015.

The Adult Vaccination Plan had 4 primary goals, with 16 strategies (partially included here), starting with "this is a 5-year strategy to vaccinate *all adults* with *all currently approved vaccines* and "**any vaccine that is approved, now and in the future**." The 61-page plan's highlighted goals are concerning for several reasons. Here are the key points extracted from the document:

- **Goal #1:** Strengthen the Adult Vaccination Infrastructure, leveraging elements that already exist
  - Collect data for ALL approved, recommended vaccines
  - Rapidly assess safety to vaccinate more pregnant women
  - Develop "model agreements" to address legal issues and policy barriers that preclude data sharing between states and the IIS system

- **Goal #2:** Improve Access to Adult Vaccines
    - Create a funding mechanism for adults similar to the 1993 Vaccines for Children Program, providing free vaccines, delivery infrastructure, and education to providers
    - Devise methods to "encourage and incentivize" providers for recommending, providing, and recording adult vaccines
    - Expand the network of those who can vaccinate
        - Currently, more than 300,000 pharmacists are trained to administer vaccines and nearly 90% of Americans live within 5 miles of a pharmacy.[201]

- **Goal #3:** Increase the Community Demand for Adult Vaccines
    - Educate and encourage individuals, healthcare professionals, and leverage group influence (community and faith-based groups, etc.) to promote and then *to demand* access to adult vaccinations
    - Create more robust EHRs to include ***standing orders,*** reminder calls, and reminder mailings that vaccine boosters are due
    - Encourage development of "adult immunization champions" in communities and across all sectors

- **Goal #4:** Foster development of new vaccines and new vaccine technologies specifically for adults[202]
    - Ensure a steady supply of vaccines – critical for success
    - Develop new vaccines and make existing vaccines work better for adults
    - Develop new technologies for better distribution, storage, delivery, and shelf life

GLOBAL VACCINE ACTION PLAN AND BIG MONEY

The plan to vaccinate every person on the planet goes far beyond the US-focused National and Adult Vaccination Plans. Globalist agendas have much broader ambitions for implementing control.

In 2012, the WHO orchestrated the Global Vaccine Action Plan (GVAP), which was endorsed by all 194 member states of the World Health Assembly, the WHO's supreme decision-making body. The GVAP was a 10-year initiative designed to boost immunization coverage, eliminate diseases like polio and measles, and ensure vaccines reached the most vulnerable populations by 2020. The GVAP outlined six strategic objectives:

1. All countries commit to immunization as a priority.
2. Individuals and communities understand the value of vaccines and demand immunization as both their right and responsibility.
3. The benefits of immunization are equitably extended to all people.
4. Strong immunization systems are an integral part of a well-functioning health system.
5. Immunization programs must have sustainable access to predictable funding, quality supply, and innovative technologies.
6. Country, regional and global research, and development innovations will maximize the benefits of immunization across the entire spectrum of discovery, development, and delivery.

In addition to these six objectives, the GVAP called for research to identify and address resistance to vaccination, including strategies to overcome and influence those who refuse. The Plan also emphasized the need for social research to determine the most effective incentives for increasing vaccination uptake. Healthcare workers are to be trained in effective communication with the media, particularly when there are reports of serious adverse events, in order to allay fears and "tackle vaccine hesitancy."[203]

As the Global Vaccine Action Plan (GVAP) was nearing its conclusion, the Global Immunization Agenda (GIA) was introduced in 2021 to build upon the objectives of GVAP and tackle emerging challenges such as vaccine hesitancy. While both the GIA and GVAP focused primarily on vaccine delivery, the broader Global Vaccine Strategy, developed by the WHO, includes a comprehensive framework that extends well beyond the distribution of vaccines. This ambitious global plan also outlined a roadmap for global development and access, involving key partnerships with organizations such as UNICEF, the Global Polio Eradication Initiative, numerous non-governmental organizations (NGOs), and COVAX, which specifically focuses on ensuring equitable access to the COVID-19 vaccine. To finance these expansive and long-term initiatives, a new structure was necessary. That structure became the Geneva-based Global Alliance for Vaccines and Immunizations, known simply as GAVI.

THE GATES FOUNDATION AND GAVI

In 2000, GAVI was founded with an initial pledge of $750 million from the Bill & Melinda Gates Foundation. As a public-private partnership, GAVI has played a central role in uniting over 100 global governments, including the US, France, Saudi Arabia, and Japan. GAVI also involves the UN, and has financial arrangements that involve the WHO, the vaccine industry, and the private sector. These entities share a common goal to "improve childhood immunization coverage in poor countries and accelerate the development and access to new vaccines." Since its founding, the Gates Foundation has contributed or matched $5.1 billion to GAVI's efforts as of 2024, further cementing its influence in global vaccination initiatives.

While initial funding from the Gates Foundation played a key role in launching the initiative, GAVI required sustained and broader funding to advance its global vaccination efforts. According to GAVI. org, in addition to the Gates Foundation, the ELMA Vaccines & Immunization Foundation, operating under ELMA Philanthropies Services, has committed at least $10.3 million to GAVI's work. This private foundation is primarily funded by Clive Calder, a South African entrepreneur known for founding the Zomba Group, which he sold in 2002 to BMG, a German media conglomerate, for approximately $2.74 billion. Following this sale, Calder turned his focus to philanthropy, investing in vaccines for children and African community development by working closely with the Gates Foundation and GAVI.

Another significant source of funding for GAVI emerged in 2003 when the UK Treasury and the UK Department for International Development created the International Finance Facility (IFF), which allowed donor countries to provide immediate funding by issuing bonds. In 2006, the International Finance Facility for Immunisation (IFFIm) was established as a spin-off to specifically fund immunization efforts through its partnership with GAVI. IFFIm became the first and only entity to raise funds for vaccination initiatives by issuing vaccine bonds, with backing from the World Bank. In 2012, during a meeting of the G8 countries, leaders praised the success of these bonds in funding the global vaccination efforts, highlighting their pivotal role in advancing the worldwide vaccination agenda.[204]

IFFIm's success continued throughout the next decade, and the current financial base consists of grants from 11 countries. As of June 2024, these nations have pledged US$9.7 billion over 23 years from donors who make the payments on a specific schedule.[205]

Beyond these major backers, GAVI also receives funding from a range of sources, including NGOs, faith-based organizations, vaccine manufacturers, and research institutions. When you put it all together, it's clear why Big Pharma fiercely protects its vaccine sector. With billions at stake at the front end of the supply chain, and trillions to be made from vaccine-related injuries and illnesses, vaccines have become the central driver of the entire medical system. This financial network makes vaccines not just a public health tool or a matter of national concern, but a global endeavor with far-reaching implications, propelling not only the entire healthcare industry, but entire governments and institutions around the world.

In 2005, a separate initiative involving GAVI's resources was launched through a joint effort by the WHO, UNICEF, and other immunization partners, in consultation with many Member States. The Global Immunization Vision and Strategy (GIVS) outlined key goals, organized into four main strategies, designed to align with GAVI's mission and broader UN objectives.[206]

1. Vaccinate every person in the world.
2. Introduce new vaccines and delivery technologies so that immunization would become a **social value** and change demographics within economies.
3. Integrate **vaccination surveillance** into every country's health system. Immunization will become crucial for every country.
4. The global community will join together to guarantee funds so all people will have equal access to *all vaccines they need.*

The strategy set forth by GIVS, which ran from 2006 to 2015, aimed to expand vaccine coverage and ensure that vaccines were accessible to all children, particularly in low-income and underserved regions. GIVS was succeeded by the Global Immunization Agenda (GIA), which sought to further increase vaccine coverage and tackle new challenges in global health, such as vaccine hesitancy.

LEARN MORE

GAVI and **UNICEF** work closely together but their roles are distinct:

- **GAVI**, with its approximately 300 international employees, primarily handles **funding and purchasing** vaccines in bulk at lower costs. It then provides the vaccines to low-income nations.

- **UNICEF** is responsible for the **delivery and administration** of vaccines, using its expertise in supply chain management, logistics, and health systems in hard-to-reach areas. UNICEF employs over 13,000 staff globally, working in various roles from field offices to headquarters. UNICEF is responsible for National Immunization Days (NIDs) when campaigns are rolled out across entire countries, often vaccinating as many as 400,000 infants in less than a week.

In 2013, GAVI brought together 25 technical experts from across the globe to reach a consensus on strategies for expanding vaccination policies and collaborating on methods to achieve universal vaccination. The group's focus was on reviewing existing evidence regarding the "positive impact of vaccines on health outcomes, healthcare costs, productivity, and broader economic and social effects."

The problem is, the globalists only focus on the benefits of mass vaccination, such as "a healthier workforce leading to overcoming poverty," expanding tourism, and reducing mortality and morbidity. Nothing is ever mentioned about vaccine injuries, vaccine side effects, or vaccine-related deaths. Second and third world nations do not have a Vaccine Adverse Event Reporting System (VAERS). People do not have access to healthcare facilities if they, or their child, develops asthma, seizures or autoimmune conditions. And if a few people die? They have died for the Greater Good.

Understanding the scope of these vast plans is essential. Every individual must grasp the enormity of the global vaccination effort. It is a multinational operation – arguably one of the most lucrative cartels in existence. With decades of planning and many billions of dollars supporting their goals, the momentum behind this push to vaccinate is a formidable force, driven by money, influence, and power.

THE POWER OF THE GLOBALISTS

According to the Cambridge Online Dictionary, a globalist is someone who believes that economic and foreign policy should be planned at the international level and should supersede what independent governments believe is in the best interest of their citizens. The rise of the globalists driving the aforementioned expansive vaccination and healthcare initiatives has been a gradual, strategic process that spans many decades, marked by a combination of political maneuvering, financial investment, and alignment with major international organizations.

At the top of the globalist hierarchy, the World Economic Forum (WEF) brings together the wealthiest and most powerful individuals on the planet, many of whom come from long-established lineages of international bankers, aristocratic families, and royal bloodlines. Over generations, these elites have systematically consolidated control over nearly every aspect of modern society. Their reach spans the military, media, and major corporations, ensuring a dominant position in global governance. Individuals are strategically positioned within key organizations and institutions: religious organizations, foundation boards, and cultural strongholds like Hollywood and the music industry. From this perch, the globalists influence public perception, control the flow of information, and wield immense power, particularly over non-governmental organizations (NGOs), which the globalists fund through either private businesses or personal wealth. Their influence even extends to legal systems and political structures at every level, where they shape policies to serve self-interests.

HIGHLIGHT

GAVI targets low-income and lower-middle-income countries based on their **Gross National Income (GNI)** per capita. Countries that meet specific income thresholds are eligible for financial support. For example, the eligibility criteria are typically set for countries with a GNI per capita of $1,600 or less, though this threshold can change over time. As global standards of living have risen, the eligibility criteria for many countries have been tightened.

In response, in June 2021, GAVI introduced a new strategy for 2021-2025, known as "GAVI 6.0." This strategy aims to adapt to evolving global challenges and ensure long-term access to vaccines beyond childhood. Its new priority is to vaccinate people across their entire lifespan. The strategy also introduces innovative financing models to supplement existing funding methods. Additionally, GAVI is adjusting its eligibility standards to align with the improving GNI worldwide, while ensuring a sustainable way to utilize the promised funds for vaccination efforts. The full plan can be reviewed at https://www.gavi.org/our-alliance/strategy/phase-6-2026-2030

All of these actions further strengthen their grip on global affairs, and at the heart of their ambitions is a vision for a single global state led by the UN and financially fed by the WEF. The ultimate goal is to bring all of humanity under centralized control.

The crucial question is this: *why* do they continue to pursue such sweeping influence? The answer is that these globalists ultimately want control of literally everything: our planet's resources and even human behavior. The global policy serves as a means to an end, giving the elites what they want most – the ability to direct the future of nations and individuals alike. For them, the goal is not merely to increase their wealth, but to also create a system of total dominion over every aspect of life. With vast fortunes at their disposal, it's not about wealth – it's about power and control.

Most texts that explore the foundations of global control attribute its modern-time beginnings to Adam Weishaupt. He was a German philosopher, a professor of civil law, and later, a professor of Canon Law at Ingolstadt University in Bavaria. Weishaupt formed the Order of Perfectibilists in 1776, which later became known as the Illuminati. His goals were to promote enlightenment values like reason, secularism, and equality, and to combat superstition and clerical influence. The *Illuminati Manifesto* reflected anti-authoritarian and egalitarian ideals, aimed at reshaping society by influencing influential figures within secretive networks.

The Order was founded on the principle of providing free exchange of ideas, and Weishaupt's Jesuit background appears to have had an influence on the society's character. While scholars have written entire volumes about this group, the primary premise is that Weishaupt's theories formed the foundation of the Illuminati, seeking to undermine traditional structures of authority and influence. He argued that patriotism, religious devotion, belief in a Higher Power, and even the love of family had to be abolished for the good of society.

While the plan has been quietly expanded since his passing in 1830, his Weishaupt's premises were summarized in Ted Flynn's book, *Hope of the Wicked: The Master Plan for the World.*[207]

1. **Abolition of Religion and Traditional Values**: Abolish family life, family loyalty and the institution of marriage. Remove religious influence from society; particularly abolish Christianity, in favor of a secular, humanist worldview.

2. **Centralization of Power**: Abolish monarchies, patriotism, and nationalism to then consolidate power into the hands of

an elite few, eroding national sovereignty, and establishing a global government under their control.

3. **Social Engineering**: Abolish private property and inheritances. Change the structures of society, promoting universal education which is limited in scope and does not teach critical thinking skills. Gradually alter the moral and sexual values to align with ideals of control and power.

4. **Promotion of a New World Order**: Create a secret society that would infiltrate governments, institutions, and religions to effect global change, culminating in a "new world order."

5. **Manipulation of Economic Systems**: Use the power of money within financial institutions and economic systems to create dependency and to control populations.

6. **Control Through Crisis**: Orchestrate or exploit crises (such as wars, revolutions, and in modern times, pandemics) to advance the agenda of centralized control and social change.

COMMENTARY

Published on the WEF website was the first of three "sustainable developments." Rest assured, whenever you see the work "sustainable" or "sustainability" it represents the plans of the UN and the globalists:

> **"COVID-19 was the test of social responsibility"** – Billions of people across the world adopted a huge number of unimaginable public health restrictions. There are numerous examples: maintaining social distance, wearing masks, vaccinating mass groups and accepting contact-tracing.[208]

This summarizes how they gained power:

1. **Post-World War II Global Cooperation (1940s-1950s):** Following World War II, global cooperation and institutions like the UN, the WHO, and the World Bank were established. These institutions were initially aimed at fostering global peace and development, but over time, they expanded their influence into global health initiatives. The WHO, in particular, became a central player in organizing global health programs and began to shape policies around sanitation, disease eradication, and vaccination.

2. **Philanthropy and Global Health Partnerships (1990s-2000s):** In the late 20th century, prominent philanthropic foundations, most notably the Bill & Melinda Gates Foundation, became key players in the global health agenda. With massive financial resources, the Gates Foundation and others like it forged partnerships with the WHO, UNICEF, and organizations like GAVI to expand vaccine coverage worldwide. This era marked the beginning of a more structured and coordinated effort to influence global health policies, particularly regarding immunization.

3. **Public-Private Partnerships and Industry Influence (2000s-2010s):** The push for widespread vaccination was bolstered by the growth of public-private partnerships. The Gates Foundation, together with pharmaceutical companies and governments, played a key role in funding and promoting initiatives through GAVI. Through these partnerships, private entities gained significant influence over global health priorities. This also marked the beginning of the "Decade of Vaccines" and the establishment of global vaccination programs aimed at not just childhood vaccines but adults as well.

4. **The Expansion of Global Health Initiatives (2010s-2020s)**: As the reach of these global health initiatives grew, so did the financial commitments from governments and private organizations. The creation of structures like the GAVI and initiatives like the Global Vaccine Action Plan (GVAP) and the Global Immunization Agenda (GIA) solidified the role of global institutions in shaping vaccine distribution. These initiatives were further empowered by the rise of global health threats, both natural and created. Pandemics are but one example, showing both justification and opportunity for expanded global surveillance and vaccine mandates.

5. **The COVID-19 Pandemic (2020s)**: COVID-19 was the catalyst for the most extensive global vaccination campaign and power grab in history. The WHO, along with international organizations, governments, and pharmaceutical companies, mobilized unprecedented resources to develop and distribute the deadly vaccines worldwide. The pandemic reinforced the power of these global institutions.

Flynn's *Hope of the Wicked* was written in 2000, and it is striking in its eerie prediction of the widespread use of technologies like barcodes, QR codes, RFID tags, facial recognition scanners, and iris scans within the first 25 years of the 21st century. These tools, initially developed from the 1980s onward, were not just technological innovations – they were weapons designed to catalog and control every aspect of the human mind, body, and intellect. The blueprint behind this, disguised under the seemingly innocuous name of *Healthy People*, paved the way for the most destructive healthcare legislation ever passed against the American people: the PREP Act.

"A man who does not plan long ahead will find trouble at his door."

~Confucius

CHAPTER 16
The 40-Year March to 2030

Around the turn of the century, America began to shift in ways that subtly reshaped the fabric of personal freedom. Healthcare reforms transformed private health records into tools of surveillance, airport security systems expanded into invasive checkpoints, and the move toward incorporating the REAL ID into driver's licenses laid the groundwork for tight tracking and complete control. These were only the visible signs of deeper, more insidious changes. Beneath the surface, expansive plans were being crafted – plans of which most Americans remained blissfully unaware. While daily life seemed unchanged, the foundation of individual liberty was being systematically eroded, step by step, under the guise of safety and progress.

Before the government moved to consolidate personal data through electronic health records (EHRs), three earlier initiatives were quietly being implemented to monitor and influence public behavior. One of the most significant was the **Healthy People** program. At first glance, the name sounded innocuous – even ideal – when linked to public health goals. After all, agencies like HHS, CDC, and NIH promote health, right? However, the true scope of the program began to emerge following the introduction of 110 vaccine-related bills across 36 states in response to a minor measles outbreak in California in 2014. This sudden legislative push revealed a broader agenda behind Healthy People: a plan not merely to improve public health but to track and ultimately control nearly every facet of a citizen's life under the guise of health and safety. This marked a dramatic shift toward centralized oversight, cleverly disguised as public health advocacy.

THE HEALTHY PEOPLE GUIDELINES: 1990 TO 2030

In 1976, Congress created The Office of Disease Prevention and Health Promotion (ODPHP) to coordinate disease prevention and health promotion efforts across the United States. Three years later, Surgeon General Julius B. Richmond MD wrote a report on the state of health in America which came to be referred to as *Healthy People*. With the help of Assistant Surgeon General Michael McGinnis, a formal *Healthy People* publication was released in 1979, outlining six quantifiable goals to improve the health of Americans. The Surgeon General's goals for the decade from 1980 to 1990 were simple, reasonable, and succinct:

1. Eliminate cigarette smoking
2. Reduce of alcohol misuse
3. Moderate dietary changes to reduce intake of excess calories, fat, salt, and sugar
4. Increase moderate exercise
5. Periodic screening for disorders such as high blood pressure and certain cancers
6. Adherence to speed laws and use of seat belts[209]

At about that same time, a companion piece, *Promoting Health/Preventing Disease: Objectives for the Nation*, was released. This paper greatly expanded the six goals outlined by the initial Healthy People program.[210]

The first Healthy People guidelines became the foundation for future government intrusion into every area of our lives. The drafts began in 1987, and over the next two years, 157 organizations, including such divergent groups as the American Medical Association and the Girl Scouts, collaborated to create goals and objectives for the decade from 1990 to 2000. A final team of 500 individuals from both the private sector and public health boiled down the comments and concerns to 15 widespread diseases and created goals to reduce their morbidity and mortality. After all the papers had been reviewed by 167 medical experts, the recommendations were published in the Federal Register and circulated to more than 2,000 organizations for review and comment. After the "final-final" revisions, *Healthy People 1990* was released in the spring of 1980. The original Healthy People document submitted by Surgeon General Richmond, in combination with the HHS paper, are considered "landmarks" in the history of public health.

Keep in mind all of this back-and-forth during the 1980s was long before the days of a robust internet and email system!

By the mid-1990s, 43 states, Guam and the District of Columbia had adopted all of the original guidelines. Even though the HP plans were meant to establish national health standards, the States were free to determine the best way to deliver services and meet the goals. Near the end of the 1990s, the focus started to shift toward crafting a new set of goals for the *Healthy People 2000* guidelines.

The Healthy People Initiatives

Timeline	Named	Focus Areas	Objectives		
1980 to 1990	HP 1990	15		226	
1990 to 2000	HP 2000	22		319	
2000 to 2010	HP 2010	28		467	
2010 to 2000	HP 2020	42		1,200	
2020 to 2030	HP 2030	355 core objectives	40 new research objectives	115 developmental objectives	

Among the 15 focus areas and 226 objectives for HP1990 were lofty standards for nationwide vaccination, including the following:

- Develop a plan for mass vaccination in the event of an influenza pandemic, or other epidemic disease for which a vaccine may exist or be created;
- Vaccinate as least 50% of the population as soon as possible with all vaccines currently approved by the Advisory Committee of Immunization Practices (ACIP); all new vaccines should be administered to at least 50% of the population within 5 years of licensure;
- Enlist daycare centers, senior citizen centers, and churches to provide vaccination information regarding the importance of vaccination to parents and older people;
- Use of mass media to promote vaccination activities;
- Develop uniform and forceful implementation of school vaccination requirements to the point of exclusion from school for those who don't comply;
- Require vaccination as a condition of employment at health care institutions and for working in schools;
- Achieve a nationwide vaccination rate of least 60% for influenza and pneumonia vaccines in high-risk populations;

- Achieve complete vaccination of *at least* 95% of all children attending licensed day care facilities;
- Achieve complete vaccination of *at least* 95% of all children attending schools ages kindergarten through 12th grade with all approved vaccinations.

COMMENTARY

Keep in mind the *Healthy People 1990* recommendations were written in the 1980s. They sound suspiciously similar to today's vaccination agenda, and in fact, were the forerunners. But there is a big difference between the 1980 and the 2024 vaccine schedules. In 1980, only three vaccines were given to children: OPV (oral polio), DTwP (whole cell pertussis), and MMR (measles, mumps, rubella). No vaccines were given at birth, the five doses of the polio and the DTwP vaccines (replaced in the US with DTaP in 2001) were spread out between two months and five years of age. The MMR vaccine was given only once, around one year of age, with no other vaccines administered at the same time. Today, the total number of doses from birth to age 18 is 42 to 48 doses, depending on the brand of the meningitis B, rotavirus, HiB, human papillomavirus vaccines (HPV), and the specific recommendations for RSV (i.e., some brands are 2 doses; some require 3 doses). If an annual influenza shot is added, that increases the number of doses of vaccine to 67 to 72 by 18 years of age.

By the time ***Healthy People 2000*** was released in September 1990, more than 7,000 people and public health organizations at the local, state, and national levels had participated. The HP2000 plan had expanded the number of goals from 15 to 22 and the objectives from 226 to 319.[211]

The ***Healthy People 2010*** guidelines were released in January 2000, continuing the initiative of Healthy People 2000 that set specific US public health objectives to achieve by 2010. The new guidelines had a strong emphasis on improving access to care and reducing health disparities; key goals centered around education, disease prevention, and promoting healthier lifestyles. A new public health focus emerged as well: the role of the environment in public health.

Unlike previous versions, *Healthy People 2020,* with its 42 focus areas and more than *1200 objectives,* specific goals were integrated into the global health initiative from the **Decade of Vaccines** plan, also launched in 2010. HP2020 prioritized vaccine accessibility with the objective of increasing vaccination rates across all age groups. The release of HP 2020 also demonstrated the growing alignment of US national health goals with global health initiatives advanced by players like the WHO, WEF, and GAVI. This alignment also underscored the stronger US national and international efforts to expand vaccine mandates as an employment and requirement.

The data tracking metrics had changed by the time the *Healthy People 2030* plan was released. For Healthy People 2030, the objectives were categorized into three types: Core, Research, and Developmental objectives. The focus areas were divided into 355 Core, 115 Developmental, and 40 (newly added) Research objectives HP2030 also included a heavy focus on collecting data on the **Social Determinants of Health (SDOH).**

The concept of Social Determinants of Health (SDOH) was initially formed in the 1970s. At that time, there was a growing awareness that both social and economic factors had an influence on health outcomes. In 1978, the idea of SDOH gained traction at the International Conference on Primary Health Care, specifically with the Declaration of Alma-Ata. This declaration emphasized the critical role social conditions played in determining both the health of individuals and the community. The concept that became increasingly clear was that "health" encompassed more than biology. The realization that access to medical care directly related to social and economic factors also came to light. In the following decades, the initial SDOH framework was both formalized as well as widely adopted. By 2005, the WHO Commission on Social Determinants of Health had been established, and it solidified these social measures into a centrally focused public health research and policy.

The determinants – including economic stability, total income, education, housing, healthcare access, and neighborhood environment – were selected based on extensive research linking these factors to health outcomes such as life expectancy, disease prevalence, and quality of life. This shift redirected society's focus from merely ensuring affordable access to medical care and improving individual behaviors (such as smoking, obesity, and alcohol use) to understanding the systemic conditions that influence a population's overall health and well being.

Collecting data on SDOH raises significant concerns about government intrusion. Sensitive information about income, education, housing, and social circumstances increases the risk of data breaches, as previously discussed. These data could, at a minimum, be misused, and even worse, exploited to enable surveillance or enforce intrusive policies, both of which erode personal freedoms. Once these data are gathered and analyzed, the population's health could be controlled by a performance debit and credit system to achieve the government's desired outcomes.

Sound familiar?

Even more troubling is that SDOH data could be used to potentially discriminate regarding healthcare insurance coverage, or employment applications in which decisions may unfairly factor in socioeconomic status. Questions about accuracy also loom large, as self-reported personal data is often unreliable, and biased collection methods can cause systemic inequities.

Administrative burdens add to the challenges, because extensive resources are required to collect, manage, and protect the data – resources that smaller organizations often lack. Individuals often face ethical dilemmas when answering the questions asked by their provider or on a sterile questionnaire. Patients may not answer or may answer untruthfully because they are unsure how their information will be used or they may feel uncomfortable or even embarrassed about sharing sensitive information. Ultimately, the reasons for asking the SDOH questions needs to be explained at the time of the questioning and the focus should be on meaningful interventions, not just on amassing personal data that empower government overreach.

The National Center for Health Statistics (NCHS) is the principal federal entity responsible for collecting and analyzing the data gathered within the HP plans. Established in 1960, NCHS operates as a division of the CDC. NCHS provides the data infrastructure to monitor progress toward the HP initiative's goals. While implementing the HP plan goals and objectives across the country is the target, not all states have adopted the HP2030 guidelines, particularly when it comes to collecting the nosey SDOH. Some states with well-established public health infrastructures (e.g., California, New York, and Massachusetts), have shown strong alignment with the plan, including tracking SDOH factors like housing, employment, and education. States with fewer resources lag in implementation due to funding, data availability, or the political will to take on the monumental tracking. In more liberty-minded states, the guidelines may have been rejected outright, believing that the SDOH questions compromise personal rights to confidentiality.

MODEL STATE EMERGENCY HEALTH POWERS ACT

A second monumental shift occurred at the turn of the 21st century; it would suddenly and forever alter America. Of course, this was the collapse of the twin towers in New York City on September 11, 2001. Images from that day are seared into the memories of all who witnessed the horrific tragedy. The events of that day definitely left a permanent mark on the collective psyche. 9/11 was a tragedy that reshaped the NYC skyline by that also reshaped US policy and global relations for years to come.

At the same time as the nation was still reeling from the attack and still trying to understand its magnitude, the powerful Model State Emergency Health Powers Act (MSEHPA) was released on October 23, 2001, a mere six weeks after the event. The sheer extensive nature and painstaking detail of the legislation meant that the document had most likely been brainstormed and written months if not years prior to its release. In other words, the MSEHPA was a solidified plan waiting for an event. The plan was written by a collective, a collaboration of state governors, attorney generals and legislatures, with oversight provided by the groups like the CDC, Georgetown's Center for Law and the Public Health, and Johns Hopkins Universities. MSEHPA's stated purpose, outlined in the preamble, was to:

1. authorize the collection of data and records, the control of property, the management of people, and the access to communications;
2. facilitate early detection of a health emergency, and allow for immediate investigation … by gaining access to individuals' health information; and
3. grant state officials authority to use and appropriate property for care, treatment, and housing of patients, and for the destruction of contaminated materials (**including houses**).[211] (*emphasis added*)

The initial draft of the MSEHPA defined a "public health emergency" broadly and vastly expanded the powers of unelected officials during a declared emergency. The authority granted was so egregious that individual freedom activists, many freedom-advocating policy organizations, and, surprisingly, even the mainstream media and the American Civil Liberties Union (ACLU) spoke out loudly against the proposed legislation. Responding to public criticism, the wording was softened and the definitions made less vague, but there were very few substantive changes.

The updated, final version was released to the States two months later, on December 21, 2001.[212] The basic structure reflected 5 powers to be given to public health officials in the event of a declared emergency: *(emphasis added)*

1 **surveillance:** use all available measures to detect and track the emergencies;
2 **management of property;**
3 ensure adequate availability of resources: **vaccines, pharmaceuticals, and hospitals;**
4. *power to* **compel testing, treatment, isolation, vaccination, and quarantine;**
5 **control communication,** providing clear and authoritative information to the public, (e.g., power to **control the message** and **impose censorship**).[213]

This document from 2001, written twenty years ago, served as the original prototype for the tyrannical enforcement measures implemented in 2020 during the COVID-19 emergency.

Similar to the selective adoption of the HP program, by March 2023, 43 states had enacted at least some provisions of the MSEHPA, either through new legislation or updates to existing regulations. Alaska, South Dakota, and Wyoming have not adopted any of the initiatives, while New Hampshire has adopted only some of them.[214]

In 2023, the lead author of MSEHPA, Lawrence O. Gostin, published an article in the journal, *Health Affairs*, titled, "Public Health Law

Modernization 2.0: Rebalancing Public Health Powers And Individual Liberty In The Age Of COVID-19."[215] He explained that by May 2022, at least half of Americans believed public health had done only a "fair to poor job" responding to the pandemic. Rather than honestly evaluating the damage caused by the government's dictates, he attributed the growing public distrust to a failure to "understand the need to protect the overall population from a 'deadly' communicable disease."

HIGHLIGHT

COVID-19 had an overall death rate of less than 1.4%, meaning 1.4% of people infected with SARS CoV-2 have a fatal outcome, while 98.6% recovered.

Gostin expressed frustration over complaints that personal liberty was being "crushed." He argued that public health officials believe personal liberties should always be willingly sacrificed for the "greater good." Gostin's narrative largely ignored the devastating effects that poor government decisions have had on healthcare, education, and the economy. He also failed to acknowledge the catastrophic injuries and countless deaths attributed to the experimental COVID-19 vaccines, which has become a major driver of growing public distrust in bureaucratic institutions.

To date, more than 1,000 lawsuits have been filed since 2021 challenging the COVID-19 orders issued by public health officials, including the legitimacy of blocking public gatherings, mandating masks for Head Start program workers, "vaccinate or test to keep your job" orders, and "vaccinate or lose your job" mandates. Many rules set by HHS, CDC, governors, and large employers have been struck down. Many who refused vaccination have been reinstated to their jobs with back pay and/or awarded sizable judicial settlements for discrimination against their properly filed religious exemptions.

Hundreds of bills have been introduced in nearly every state calling for the "retrenching" or reduction of powers granted to unelected individuals and unaccountable health department officials. Laws introduced in 2021-22 sought to limit the authority and scope of governors, restrict the duration of orders, and define the scope of those orders. Interventions during a public health crisis must respect personal rights, and if decisions lead to disastrous outcomes, the public officials responsible must be held accountable. Gostin even admitted, "Emergency powers laws underwent a profound stress test during the COVID-19 pandemic. Designed primarily with bioterrorism in mind, they have proved to be ill-suited in some respects to the challenges presented by a multiyear pandemic." The problem is that the provisions outlined in the MSEHPA have been integrated into nearly every state and many national public health policies.

And what about those who were seriously injured by a COVID-19 vaccine? Fear drove the message, but now there is an avalanche of regret, as nearly everyone knows someone who was injured or died shortly after receiving the shot. Why can't pharmaceutical companies be broadly sued for the damages and deaths caused by their rushed-to-market, faulty products? The answer lies in legal protections also established two decades ago.

HOW THE PREP ACT BECAME LAW

As if massively expanding public health through Healthy People policies and threatening to seize private property during a declared emergency weren't alarming enough, the third transformative shift of the new century was the most disturbing: the passage of sweeping and permanent legislative protections for pharmaceutical products, particularly vaccines, during declared emergencies. These changes far exceeded the safeguards provided by the 1986 Childhood Vaccine Injury Compensation Act, marking a dramatic redefinition of accountability and a pivotal turning point in public health law for all Americans.

In fact, legislation passed 20 years ago laid the foundation for the broad protections the pharmaceutical companies enjoyed during COVID-19 and continue to benefit from today. It began on January 28, 2003, during President George W. Bush's State of the Union address.[216] On that fateful night, Bush revealed a new creation: the comprehensive effort to develop and make available the drugs and vaccines deemed necessary to protect against biological and chemical weapon attacks. It was called **Project BioShield,** and the initial program had a budget of $5.6 billion spread over ten years to purchase products for the national stockpile. Project BioShield was to form three major components: *(emphasis added)*

1. legislatively create a **permanent,** "indefinite funding authority" to spur the **development of medical countermeasures,** enabling the government to "purchase vaccines and other therapies as soon as experts believe that they are safe and effective."

2. confer **new authority to the NIH** to speed research, development, and release of drugs and vaccines that would block or mitigate bioterrorism threats and,

3. allow for the authorization of emergency **"fast track" provisions,** releasing treatments – drugs and vaccines – that would normally languish months to years waiting for FDA approval, when therapies were needed immediately "in the event of an emergency."[217]

Keep in mind these provisions were set in place in 2003-4.

As sweeping as the new authority seemed to be at the time, the BioShield legislation failed to include key provisions the drug companies were holding out for: **complete liability protection** for all present and future bioterrorism products. Many bills were introduced by both the House and the Senate throughout 2003, 2004, and 2005. In all, 13 bills were introduced in 2005 alone, in an attempt to secure protection for the industry through federal law. October 17, 2005, marked the most important date during this period. On that day, the Biodefense and Pandemic Vaccine and Drug Development Act of 2005 (known as BioShield II) moved the effort to the front burner so to speak, to "make good" for drug makers.[218]

Introduced by Senators Bill Frist (R-TN) and Richard Burr (R-NC), the bill was accelerated through the Senate Health, Education, Labor, and Pensions (HELP) Committee, *without hearings*. Its purpose, according to Burr's news release, was to create a partnership between the government and private corporations to "rapidly develop effective medical drugs and vaccines to protect the US from deliberate, accidental, or natural incidents involving biological pathogens." The introduction of BioShield II by the Senate raised the stakes to a new level. Named S.1873, the legislation was designed to give unprecedented advantages to the industry and to remove or severely weaken all of the safeguards to protect dangerous vaccines, drugs, and medical devices from reaching consumers.[219]

Public outrage began almost immediately. While websites, news outlets, and nationwide radio hosts began to decry the unbelievable benefits that passage of this bill would convey to the drug companies, dozens of activist groups representing thousands of constituents rallied a campaign to notify Congress of their dissatisfaction with S.1873. Faxes, emails, and phone calls conveyed message after message opposing the carte blanche promises about to be handed to the drug makers.

Because the outcry against S.1873 was so strong, the possibility of its passage appeared to be difficult at best. To circumvent the outraged public, Senate Majority Leader Frist attached a shortened version of the bill to the 2006 Department of Defense Appropriations Bill, HR 2863, literally at the eleventh hour. Known as **"Division E of the Public Readiness and Emergency Preparedness Act of 2005,"** or simply **the PREP Act,** this addition granted unprecedented immunity to drug companies. Sometimes referred to as Division E or the Frist addendum, the measure added 40 pages to an existing 423-page defense bill at 11:20 PM on Saturday night, December 17, 2005 – well after the House Appropriations Committee members had finalized and signed off on the defense bill, and most members had already left for home.

Division-E wields the power of the drug companies and allows them to function in a state of emergency with essentially no oversight. The HHS Secretary can deem a "disease, health condition, or threat" constitutes a public health emergency and therefore can accelerate the use, manufacture, testing, development, and *administration* of one or more *covered countermeasures*. These countermeasures are defined as a "pandemic product, vaccine or drug." Section (b)(7) of the document, "Judicial Review," states "no federal or state court will have jurisdiction to review *any action* taken by the Secretary." His ruling will *preempt any and all state laws* that are different from or in conflict with the declaration.

This distinct lack of checks and balances undeniably puts the public at risk and is indeed frightening. An appointed politician has been handed the power to order mandatory vaccination for everyone.

Appalled, Representative Dave Obey (D-WI), Ranking Member of the House Appropriations Committee, made the following statement on the floor of the House on December 22, 2005, laying out all the jaw-dropping provisions passed into law through Division E *without debate or without Congress ever reading the legal supplement*. Taken from the Congressional Record, this is his full objection:

> "... when the President requested nearly $7 billion to begin a much-belated crash program to develop a new generation of vaccines and antiviral drugs to combat a potential flu pandemic, the Republican Majority responded by cutting [that request] in half. When I asked Senator Ted Stevens (R-AK) in conference why we shouldn't fund the rest of

the Administration's request...he responded that *because liability protection language for manufacturers had not been adopted*, long-range funding should be withheld.

"The Conference Committee [on the Defense Appropriations Bill] ended its work with an understanding, both verbal and in writing, that there would be no – and *I repeat no* – legislative liability protection language inserted in this bill. And because the **Majority told us it** *did not want any compensation program for victims* **to come out of the discretionary portion of the budget,** no funding was provided for that either.

"But after the [Committee] finished at 6 p.m., Senator Frist marched over to the House side of the Capitol, about four hours later, and insisted 40 pages of legislation – which I have in my hand – *40 pages of legislation that had never been seen by Conferees* be attached to the bill.

"Speaker [Dennis Hastert R-IL] joined Frist's insistence, and **without a vote** of the Conferees, the legislation was unilaterally and arrogantly inserted into the bill, after the Conference was over. [This was] a blatantly abusive power play by two of the most powerful men in Congress.

"We then discovered that this language provided all sorts of insulation for pharmaceutical companies and that this insulation applied not just to drugs developed to deal with the [avian] flu, but in fact applied to a far broader range of products." In essence, the provisions allowed the Secretary of HHS to issue a declaration that has the effect of almost completely prohibiting lawsuits in State or Federal courts by people whose health was injured against manufacturers and various others for compensation for injuries caused by the use of covered countermeasures.

"That determination would bar lawsuits against a wide range of covered persons involved with the countermeasures including manufacturers and their suppliers, their distributors, State and local governments and their employees involved with the use of the countermeasures, medical personnel both prescribing and administering the countermeasures, and so forth. **That is indeed very broad power to ban lawsuits.** Unlike the language requested by the administration, the Division E language is not limited to products to combat a flu pandemic. Rather, it applies to **any drug, vaccine, medical device, or other products** useful in dealing with anything the Secretary considers to constitute a health emergency or that could constitute an emergency in the future.

"Although a rationale often offered for lawsuit protection is that it is needed to encourage manufacturers to develop and produce new treatments, the protections of Division E are not limited to new or experimental products. Rather, nothing in the language would prevent the Secretary from providing protection against lawsuits to drugs that have been on the market for decades. Further, **the language explicitly prohibits any judicial review in either federal or state court of the Secretary's decisions to grant immunity from lawsuits.**

"If anyone believes that the power is being exercised too broadly, or even in violation of the law, they apparently would have **no remedy** other than asking the Secretary to change his mind or asking Congress to amend the law.

"Although proponents point to provisions of this language that make an exception and allow lawsuits in *cases of willful misconduct*, that exception is so narrowly drawn as to be almost meaningless. First, the provision defines 'willful misconduct' as acts taken intentionally to achieve a wrongful purpose, knowing there is no legal or factual justification, and in disregard of known or obvious great risk. Basically, Mr. Speaker, the only conduct that would permit a lawsuit **under this definition is probably conduct so egregious as to be criminal in nature.**

"However, even this highly restrictive definition of 'willful misconduct' doesn't seem to have been enough restriction on lawsuits to satisfy the authors of Division E. They added yet another provision that allows the Secretary of HHS to promulgate regulations further narrowing the scope of actions that could give rise to a right to sue. Then there is yet another provision that says that if the conduct in question is regulated under the Food and Drug Act or Public Health Service Act, *a lawsuit for willful misconduct can be brought only if the Federal Government has taken enforcement action against that conduct.*

"Finally, the language makes various changes to the normal rules of civil procedure to add further obstacles and difficulties in front of a potential plaintiff. In short, as a practical matter, there is virtually no right for anyone to sue about anything covered by a secretarial determination under this language.

"In summary, the administration asked for some very broad liability protections for manufacturers and others involved with countermeasures against pandemic flu, and the administration's proposal was widely criticized as going too far. With Division E of the Defense appropriations conference report, Congress would be providing even broader protection, potentially covering a wide range of drugs, vaccines, and devices far beyond what is needed to deal with flu. **Further, this denial of the right to sue is**

more sweeping than provided in the case of childhood vaccines or in the case of smallpox vaccine. In the smallpox case, manufacturers were protected by basically substituting the Federal Government as defendant, with the scope of potential lawsuits against the Federal Government narrowed, but not eliminated.

"The result of this legislative action was a provision in the pending bill that *prevents anyone who is a victim of a faulty vaccine from being able to obtain compensation in the courts.* It says, in effect, that if you become seriously ill because of mistakes in manufacturing, you lose your right to sue for compensation, but you can as an alternative seek compensation from the government. **The problem is that _a fund was not set up_, or no money was provided, for that fund.** So anyone who gets sick would have to lobby Congress to put money in the fund before they can collect. Thus, people injured lose their right to sue. *They are not guaranteed any alternative means of covering their medical bills, lost earnings, and other costs.*

"Mr. Speaker, the Committee system was created years ago to protect the public interest, so legislation would be carefully reviewed before it was placed before the body for consideration. But that protection was arbitrarily by-passed by the Leadership in both Houses. This is the second time that this Congress has supinely done the bidding of the pharmaceutical industry in the dead of night. The first time, a vote was held open for three hours while the Republican Majority twisted arms to create the complex and ridiculously confusing [Medicare] prescription drug bill that our seniors are now so desperately trying to understand – a bill that was ushered through this institution by over **600 lobbyists that protected [drug] companies** by preventing the government from even attempting to negotiate lower drug prices.

"If I thought that denying unanimous consent on this bill would force the Majority to eliminate that language I would object. But, Mr. Speaker, it has also been made quite clear to me that the Majority *will not relent on the language that insulates drug companies.* So Mr. Speaker, I want it to be clear that the action to insert this special interest language in the bill is in my view a **corruption of the legislative practices of the House**. When Congress returns in January, I intend to raise a question about the privileges of the House, highlighted by this action, because it has brought discredit to the House and should disturb every Member who serves here. No Member of Congress, no matter how powerful, should be able to unilaterally insist that provisions never discussed and never debated in the Conference should not be slipped into that Conference report without a vote of that same Conference.

"This is what happens when there are no checks and balances, when one party controls the White House, the Senate, and the House and respects no limits on its own use of power. We have been placed in this position because the House Republican leadership had sent Members home for the Christmas holidays with the message to the Senate that we would not be here even if the Senate changed the legislation the House sent. **That was irresponsible and the country will pay the price.** This institution will pay a price as well, in terms of diminished respect from the people we were elected to represent. Members on both sides know it and it is time to have a modicum of respect for the way we do the people's business.

"This is a shameful and shabby way to end the worst session of Congress I've experienced in 36 years in Congress. I most reluctantly withdraw my reservation because lodging an objection at this point would simply delay the shameful inevitable."[220] *(emphasis added throughout)*

The nefarious language that Congressman Obey objected to in the Division E addendum deserved every bit of his tirade. Even Senator Ted Kennedy (D-MA) commented, "Generally around here we measure who the winners are and who the losers are, and we have seen over the period of the last year, year and a half, how the drug companies come out [winners] time and time again, **but never, never, ever, ever like they have with this sweetheart deal.**" *(emphasis added)*

LEARN MORE

This is how the PREP Act, originally introduced as controversial, stand-alone legislation, became law: by adding an unread addendum called Division E to essential defense legislation literally in the dead of night. The final version of the PREP Act emphasized sweeping liability immunity for those involved in the production, distribution, and administration of declared "medical countermeasures" during declared emergencies. This is the legislation that provided the legal shield that protected Pfizer, Moderna, and others during the distribution of their damaging and deadly experimental products released during COVID-19. In one of the final sections of the PREP Act, participants are assured that the plan will include education with respect to contraindications, and it mentions briefly that the program is "voluntary." The idea of "voluntary participation" was obviously left out of the Covid-19 shot rollout, when many were coerced into being injected with an experimental product to keep a job or a lifetime career.

Senator Kennedy sought to address issues within the PREP Act, particularly its lack of funding for injured parties and the extreme immunity granted to manufacturers, distributors, and administrators of medical countermeasures, especially vaccines and drug treatments. He and twenty colleagues sent a letter to the Speaker of the House and Majority leader urging its repeal, arguing that the PREP Act **"could be used to allow manufacturers of virtually any drug or vaccine to escape responsibility for gross negligence or even criminal acts."**[221] *(emphasis added)*

The letter gained no response.

In 2006, Kennedy co-sponsored an amendment aiming to ensure compensation for those injured by medical countermeasures and to establish a Vaccine Injury Table to compensate injuries, disabilities, illnesses, and other conditions caused by the countermeasures, including death. Note that the PREP Act specifically excluded funding to be set aside for an injury compensation program. Kennedy's legislation, S. 2291, passed out of committee but with the death of Sen. Kennedy in 2009, the work to revise or repeal the PREP Act stopped and no other member of congress in the House or the Senate has attempted to move forward funding to cover injured parties.

In the end, Senator Frist (a medical doctor) handed the drug companies (a special interest group) more immunity for their products than any bill that has ever been introduced and passed by Congress. The legislation provides several sweeping provisions:

1. Immunity from liability for **all drugs, vaccines, or biological products deemed as a "covered countermeasure"** in the event of an outbreak of any kind. The proposal is so broad that it could include drugs like Tylenol and Advil... and would have applied to the deadly anti-inflammatory drug, Vioxx.

2. Immunity for **any product used for any public health emergency declared by the Secretary of HHS.** As explained

below, the authority to declare an emergency now rests in the hands of the Secretary of HHS – an appointed, often non-medical person who has no accountability to the general public. The president's person, hand-picked to be part of his "inner circle," will have the power to mandate vaccines and other medications to the American people. In the event of a public health crisis, the Sec. of HHS holds the power of mandates over every person in America, making him or her the most powerful person in the Administration.

3. Immunity from accountability, **no matter what a drug company did wrong.** Even if the company's dirty facility created a batch of contaminated vaccines or research and quality assurance on a new, rushed product was essentially non-existent, leading to injury or death of thousands of people, the drug company remains immune from liability.

4. **Protection from lawsuits.** A person who has suffered any type of loss will be *legally prohibited from suing* the drug companies. Pharma was given immunity from almost everything, perhaps even murder. The bill's provisions provide a mechanism for filing a lawsuit, but the language explicitly protects frivolous suits by setting a standard for liability more rigid than any known standard of negligence. In fact, according to the American Trial Lawyers Association, the PREP Act contains language never before seen in *any* proposal. In simple terms, if a plaintiff files a claim, it can only proceed if the injured party proves that the drug company committed an "act of willful misconduct" resulting in injury or death. In other words, the injured party would need to demonstrate that the vaccine manufacturer intentionally designed the product to cause harm.

5. **Lack of funding.** The legislation actually **prohibited** funding for the Countermeasure Injury Compensation

Program (CICP). As we'll see, this program exists mostly in name only. The provisions to care for the injured are meager and essentially nonexistent.

Unbelievably, even if a pharmaceutical company **knowingly harms people**, it remains immune from legal prosecution unless the US Attorney General initiates an "enforcement action" against the company on behalf of the claimant. This means the US government would need to go to bat for the injured party against the drug company for the lawsuit to proceed, a very difficult and unlikely event.

Keep in mind that the person who rammed this bill through to completion is a *medical doctor* who at one time in his life took an oath to "do no harm."

PREP ACT UPDATE

The PREP Act was unequivocally the legal cover used for the release of the untested, unapproved COVID-19 jabs that have been defined by many as bioweapons. In 2020, former HHS Secretary Alex Azar issued a declaration invoking the PREP Act's immunity provisions nationwide for COVID-19-related treatments, including vaccines. The Act's protections covered all aspects of the pandemic response, from manufacturing to administration and effectively shielding healthcare providers from liability.

The Secretary of HHS is authorized to issue updated declarations for the purpose of maintaining the **liability protection** for injuries caused by the countermeasures. In this case, the harm being seen early on in the plan to vaccinate everyone in the US and around the world was ignored. On December 11, 2024, the current HHS Secretary, Xavier Becerra, signed the 12th in a series of amendments to update the PREP Act for the COVID-19 Medical Countermeasures.

- **Amendment 1** - February 4, 2020 - SARS CoV-2 and COVID-19 was declared a public health emergency; the PREP Act **liability protection** was expanded to include vaccines, diagnostics, and other treatments associated with COVID-19
- **Amendment 2** - April 10, 2020 - **Liability protection** was extended to cover pharmacists and other "non-traditional" vaccinators to facilitate the rapid administration of the vaccines
- **Amendment 3** - August 10, 2020 - The list of covered countermeasures was extended and **liability protection** was applied to all
- **Amendment 4** - November 13, 2020 - **Liability protection** was applied to all vaccines released under the emergency use authorizations (EUAs) and protection was assured for all individuals administering these vaccines
- **Amendment 5** - December 3, 2020 - **Liability protection** was extended to more medical products
- **Amendment 6** - January 8, 2021 - Expanded **liability protection** and increased vaccine distribution strategies for pregnant women and children
- **Amendment 7** - March 11, 2021 - **Liability protection** was extended to non-traditional vaccination locations, such as long-term care and assisted-living facilities
- **Amendment 8** - July 8, 2021- Ensured l**egal protection for boosters**
- **Amendment 9** - December 6, 2021 - Provided updated vaccination recommendations for children and **ensured comprehensive liability protection**
- **Amendment 10** - March 7, 2022 - Clarified **legal protection** to updated COVID-19 countermeasures
- **Amendment 11** - May 9, 2023 - **Extended legal** protection for COVID-19 countermeasures to December 31, 2024

- **Amendment 12** - December 11, 2024 - Extended the **legal protection** duration for COVID-19 countermeasures until December 31, 2029

The PREP Act, designed and signed into law twenty years ago, has been greatly expanded to give even broader protection to unapproved products labeled as "countermeasures," which includes any antiviral, any other drug, any biologic, any diagnostic, any other device, or any vaccine, used to treat, diagnose, cure, prevent, or mitigate COVID-19.

LEARN MORE

Who made the decisions to activate the PREP Act protections during COVID-19?

Alex Azar graduated from Yale Law School in 1994. He joined HHS in 2001 and later became the Deputy Secretary of HHS under President George W. Bush from 2005 to 2007. From 2009 to 2017, Azar held senior positions at Eli Lilly, a major pharmaceutical company. During COVID-19, Eli Lilly produced two products, the monoclonal antibodies bamlanivimab and etesevimab, both protected by the PREP Act. Under the Trump Administration, Azar was Secretary of HHS from January 29, 2018 to January 20, 2021.

Xavier Becerra earned his law degree from Stanford Law School in 1984 and worked for about 3 years as a Deputy Attorney General for California before entering politics. He served 12 terms in the US House of Representatives from 1993 to 2017, representing California's 30th, 31st, and later 34th congressional districts. He also held leadership roles, including as Chair of the House Democratic Caucus. While Becerra did not work directly in the pharmaceutical industry, unlike Azar, his work as a public official has included significant engagement with pharmaceutical companies in regulatory, legal, and consumer protection contexts.

This is a comprehensive list of products that were protected during the COVID-19 declared pandemic:

1. **Vaccines**
   - All COVID-19 vaccines authorized for Emergency Use (EUAs) or FDA-approved (e.g., Pfizer, Moderna, Johnson & Johnson, Novavax).

2. **Therapeutics and Treatments**
   - Antiviral drugs (e.g., remdesivir).
   - Monoclonal antibody treatments (e.g., Regeneron, and other Eli Lilly products).
   - Many other authorized medications used to treat COVID-19 symptoms or complications.

3. **Diagnostics**
   - Polymerase Chain Reaction (PCR) tests.
   - Rapid antigen tests.
   - Antibody (serology) tests.
   - Home testing kits authorized for COVID-19.

4. **Personal Protective Equipment (PPE)**
   - N95 respirators and other approved face masks.
   - Surgical masks.
   - Disposable and reusable gloves.
   - Isolation gowns and coveralls.
   - Face shields and goggles.

5. **Medical Devices and Supplies**
   - Ventilators.
   - Oxygen equipment (e.g., concentrators, tanks).
   - Infusion pumps for medication delivery.
   - Pulse oximeters for monitoring oxygen levels.

6. **Drugs and Biologics**
   - Antibiotics such as Azithromycin and Ceftriaxone.
   - FDA-approved drugs repurposed for COVID-19 treatment such as Olumiant (baricitinib), a drug

    generally used for rheumatoid arthritis. One pill of this medication costs approximately $100.

- Various biologics used to mitigate severe symptoms of COVID-19.

7. **Distribution and Administration Supplies**
   - Syringes, needles, and alcohol swabs.
   - Vaccine storage materials (e.g., ultra-cold freezers, temperature monitoring devices).
   - Vials, stoppers, and other vaccine packaging materials.

8. **Testing and Laboratory Supplies**
   - Swabs and viral transport media for sample collection.
   - Reagents and chemicals used in COVID-19 testing.
   - Equipment used for laboratory-based diagnostics.

9. **Public Health Tools and Technology**
   - Mobile health applications for COVID-19 exposure notification or health tracking.
   - Digital platforms for vaccine scheduling and tracking.

10. **Supportive Equipment**
    - Emergency medical tents and portable shelters.
    - Equipment for temporary hospital expansions.

11. **Sanitization and Disinfection Products**
    - EPA and CDC approved hand sanitizers.
    - EPA approved disinfectants for surfaces.

12. **Other Countermeasures**
    - Any product or technology designated by HHS as necessary to prevent, mitigate, treat, or diagnose COVID-19 during the public health emergency.

These countermeasures are all protected under the PREP Act. However, time was running out on this protection, making Amendment 11 most interesting. It was added to allay any concerns about liability risks arising from the continued manufacture, distribution, administration or use of the countermeasures while they are still authorized for use under the EUA. Not to miss a beat protecting their pharma overlords, Amendment 12 was added on December 11, 2024 to extend the protection from civil and criminal lawsuits until December 31, 2029, past the end of the current Trump Administration.

This date change technically extends the Countermeasures Injury Compensation Program (CICP), but in practice, its one-year statute of limitations for filing a claim limits its accessibility. Without the PREP Act's legal shield, vaccine-injured individuals could potentially sue manufacturers, including Pfizer and Moderna, for damages under state tort laws. Congress could address these gaps by transitioning COVID-19 vaccines to the National Vaccine Injury Compensation Program (NVICP) or creating a new framework to ensure fair compensation and accountability for damages caused by the COVID-19 response. Neither is likely to happen.[222]

Even with the PREP Act's liability protections extended by another amendment, the law's ability to shield manufacturers, distributors, and healthcare providers from liability is under growing scrutiny. Documented evidence of harm and negligence – highlighted in *The Pfizer Papers*, thousands of research studies, numerous congressional hearings, and calls to remove the mRNA vaccines from use by a core group of physicians – suggests that the Act's liability shield and limited compensation mechanism have enabled negligence while leaving injured individuals with little recourse.

As the millions of individuals struggling to recover from injuries and those grieving loved ones lost to these jabs continue to share their stories through books, documentaries, social media, and activist organizations, public pressure may compel policymakers to modify or even eliminate blanket liability protections of the PREP Act. The 1986 NVICP offers a well-established pathway for vaccine injury claims, but COVID-19 vaccines fall outside its scope. The next chapter explores the Countermeasures Injury Compensation Program (CICP) which has utterly failed to serve the population.

"The most dangerous untruths are truths moderately distorted."

~Georg Christoph Lichtenberg, physicist

CHAPTER 17
Sacrificed for the Greater Good

Senator Frist wasn't acting alone in his zeal for drug company protection. The push to pass this protective legislation was actually started within the Bush Administration. At a press conference held November 1, 2005, President Bush pushed for increased financial benefits for the drug companies and "relief from the burden of litigation" for the vaccine manufacturers, stating:

> "I'm also asking Congress to remove one of the greatest obstacles to domestic vaccine production: the growing burden of litigation. In the past three decades, the number of vaccine manufacturers in America has plummeted from 26 to 5, **as the industry has been flooded with lawsuits.** Today, there is only one manufacturer in the United States that can produce influenza vaccine. That leaves our nation vulnerable in the event of a pandemic. We must increase the number of vaccine manufacturers in our country, and improve our domestic production capacity. **So Congress must pass liability protection for the makers of life-saving vaccines.**" *(emphasis added)*

President Bush and his advisors should have been held accountable for the misinformation spewed onto the under-informed general public. To begin with, in 2005, there were two flu shot manufacturers, Aventis and Chiron, not one. And as far as the industry retreating due to "being flooded with lawsuits"?

That wasn't factual either.

A study published that same year in the *Journal of the American Medical Association* (JAMA) examined jury verdicts and judicial decisions involving flu vaccines and identified only 10 reported cases over the 20 years from 1985 to 2005. The researchers found little evidence of significant litigation over flu vaccines. They concluded that pharmaceutical companies were withdrawing from influenza vaccine manufacturing due to factors such as high regulatory compliance costs, cumbersome production processes, low profit margins, and unpredictable demand – *not liability concerns*.[223] In addition, protective legislation for the vaccine industry had been in place for nearly 20 years at this point. Distorted narratives were used to justify pushing for complete indemnity for the vaccine makers.

In the 1980s, drug companies were indeed opting out of the vaccine business due to skyrocketing legal costs from defending lawsuits over vaccine injuries, particularly those linked to the whole-cell pertussis vaccine. By convincing government officials that the nation's vaccine program was essential to US public health, industry advocates persuaded government officials to act. As a result, President Reagan was pressured into signing the National Childhood Vaccine Injury Act (NCVIA) of 1986, a law designed to shield drug manufacturers from lawsuits stemming from injuries caused by childhood vaccines.

The number of covered vaccines has increased significantly since the program's inception. Initially, it covered three vaccines – MMR, DTP, and polio – but now includes multiple doses of 17 vaccines. All vaccine claims are managed and adjudicated by the Federal Court of Claims.

By statute, eight judges, known as Special Masters, are appointed by the Chief Judge of the Court to serve four-year terms. Other federal judges may recommend candidates with significant legal expertise, particularly in tort law, administrative law, and medical injury claims. Over the years, the exponential growth in the number of vaccines – and injuries – added to the program has caused the workload of the Special Masters to explode. According to testimony given to Congress in 2024 by Renee J. Gentry, a vaccine injury attorney with over 20 years of experience in the National Vaccine Injury Compensation Program (NVICP), the typical wait times for vaccine-injured petitioners in 2023 were reported as follows:

- Initial Review by HHS: 12-16 months
- Trial Dates: 18-24 months, or longer
- Decisions of Special Masters on Compensation awards: 12-18 months to multiple years

…which amounts to three to four years from filing to adjudication. She added that "the system is collapsing under the caseload of the large backlog of petitions caused by the failure of Congress to update the vaccine injury compensation program's infrastructure."[224] As of May 2023, more than 3,800 cases were pending review.[225] Those who "did the right thing," were vaccinated, and then harmed or killed, are left to languish for years.

In an attempt to address this overwhelming issue, **H.R. 3655, the Vaccine Injury Compensation Modernization Act of 2021**, was introduced by Representatives Lloyd Doggett (D-TX) and Fred Upton (R-MI), along with eight bipartisan co-sponsors. The bill aimed to update the program's infrastructure, adjust compensation rates to reflect inflation since 1986, and swiftly add new vaccines and injury profiles, including the COVID-19 vaccine, to the compensation program. However, the bill stagnated and was never passed out of the House Energy and Commerce Subcommittee on Health.

On August 4, 2023, Representative Lloyd Doggett reintroduced the bill as **H.R. 5142**, titled the **Vaccine Injury Compensation Modernization Act of 2023**. The bill was co-sponsored by Lloyd Smucker (R-PA), Earl Blumenauer (D-OR), and received bipartisan support from representatives of five other states and the District of Columbia. The last action on the bill occurred on August 11, 2023, when it stalled once again in the **House Energy and Commerce Committee**. As of this writing, it has not progressed. Vaccine-injured individuals were once again denied fair and just compensation through the government's program.

TRACKING THE INJURIES

Since the swine flu debacle in the 1970s, the law has required health professionals and vaccine manufacturers to report adverse events to HHS if they occur after the administration of routine vaccines. Unfortunately, many providers have not complied, often due to a lack of knowledge on how to file the report, reluctance to take the time for the tedious manual process, or an unwillingness to admit that the vaccine may have caused the reaction. The efforts to improve filing an adverse event report was facilitated by the establishment of the Vaccine Adverse Event Reporting System (VAERS) by statute in 1990 as part of the National Vaccine Childhood Injury Act. According to the CDC:

> VAERS is a national early warning system to detect possible safety problems in US licensed vaccines. VAERS is co-managed by the CDC and the FDA. It is a surveillance program, required by law, to collect information about adverse events that occur after a person is vaccinated. The VAERS data are updated monthly and the data are made **available to the public for review and analysis.**[226] *(emphasis added)*

On June 30, 2017, **VAERS** released a new reporting form, known as **VAERS 2.0**, which replaced the outdated VAERS Reporting Form that had been in use from July 1, 1990 to June 29, 2017. The updates included the collection of additional data elements, revisions to existing questions, and the removal of some older questions.[227]

That sounds easy enough and very transparent, except that's not how it works.

To search VAERS, one must be familiar with a query system called WONDER, which stands for Wide-ranging ONline Data for Epidemiologic Research.[228] The program is used to search many different datasets within the CDC's massive website including population centered data, the mortality data, issues with the environment, such as land surface temperature data to days of sunlight, and more. It is also used to search VAERS. The CDC describes WONDER as an "easy-to-use, menu-driven tool." I can assure you that unless you are familiar with vaccine abbreviations and how to use similar tools, it is not "easy" to use. In addition, the data retrieved is not complete.

As it turns out, when reports are filed with VAERS, the CDC records and stores everything submitted. However, certain fields are removed, hidden, or simply not posted, making them inaccessible through the WONDER search engine. In a 2023 report by *The British Medical Journal's* investigative arm, *The BMJ*, it was uncovered that physicians and advocates held several meetings with the FDA between 2021 and 2022 regarding missing data and concerns that the VAERS system wasn't functioning properly, leading to missed signals of adverse events.[229] Further investigation revealed that VAERS actually has two separate databases: a *public-facing* database that only contains initial reports, and a *private system* that holds all data fields, updates, and corrections – such as formal diagnoses, stages of recovery, or whether the injury resulted in death. This follow-up information is hidden from WONDER searches and the public. It also was discovered that the CDC has been scrubbing data records filed by petitioners, removing updates, and concealing additional fields that they apparently don't want researchers or the public to see. This is literally keeping two sets of books. What are they hiding… and *why?*[230]

> ## HIGHLIGHT
>
> A new vaccine gains liability protection when it is approved by the Advisory Committee for Immunization Practices (ACIP) and added as a requirement to the routine **pediatric** vaccination schedule. Once approved for babies, not only does the vaccine gain liability protection the manufacturers also gain an immediate market share for the product (recall there are approximately 77,000 live births per week in this country).

REACT 19

An independent organization, **React 19**, has challenged the VAERS reporting system. React 19 is a nonprofit that began as a small community of medical professionals who experienced adverse reactions after receiving one or more doses of a COVID-19 vaccine. Although members were previously healthy, the group shared a long list of similar adverse reactions. The group collectively offers financial, physical, and emotional support for those suffering from long term COVID-19 vaccine adverse events.

According to their website:

> React19 reviewed 126 VAERS reports filed by 103 independent COVID vaccine-injured individuals in November 2022. The audit was conducted because members never received their VAERS report Identification Number, could not find their personally published VAERS

reports, and/or their reports had been altered, combined with previous reports, or removed. Of the 126 reports, they found:

- 61% has been filed correctly
- 22% did not have a permanent ID, therefore could not be seen publicly
- 12% of reports had been deleted
- 5% could not file their report due to "system errors"

In all, the audit found that one in 3 reports was either not processed for public review *or deleted.* This is another example of VAERS keeping two sets of books. Again, what are they hiding… and *why?*[231]

THE TABLE

Injury claims filed under the VAERS program are not lawsuits, rather they are no-fault claims for compensation. The program is supported administratively by the Health Resources and Services Administration (HRSA) within HHS which pays compensation to claimants. The intent of the 1986 injury compensation legislation was to create an alternative to civil litigation, meaning that if an injury occurred following a vaccine, negligence would not have to be proven by legal standards and compensation would automatically be paid by the government for the "personal sacrifice" that had been made by that individual who agreed to be vaccinated for the "good of the whole."

Recall that claims filed in the US Court of Federal Claims in Washington DC, commonly referred to as the Vaccine Court, are overseen by the Office of Special Masters. Like trial judges, the Special Masters hear the evidence then determine whether or not the individual was injured by the vaccine. Approximately 80% of litigants agree to a settlement, 10% of cases are dismissed, and 20% of the remaining cases are litigated either about the facts of the case or about the amount of the compensation entitlement. If it is determined that the vaccine did indeed cause the injury, the Special Masters (lawyers, not medical experts) determine the amount of the award to be paid. Injury claimants must exhaust the processes within Vaccine Court before they can attempt to bring a civil lawsuit against a vaccine manufacturer.

As straightforward as it seems – *or as it was intended to be* – there are serious flaws in the program. The most glaring issue is that only certain vaccine injuries are eligible for compensation. The lynchpin of the program is a list referred to as the "Vaccine Injury Compensation Table," or simply "**The Table**," which limits the types of injuries eligible for compensation. In other words, even sustaining a life-altering, permanent injury doesn't automatically trigger compensation. The Table's definitions are set by statute and determined *by the government* to be a "presumption of causation" (remember that term) or not. Simply put, the definitions on The Table determine whether an injury can be assumed to be caused by the vaccine – the connection between a vaccine and an injury are not established by the doctor who cared for the injured person and certainly not by the person who experienced or witnessed the adverse event. The "diagnosis" is made by a table created by politicians and medical bureaucrats at the CDC and HHS.

The Table also clearly defines the time frames in which the injury must occur to be a qualified claim. If the time sequence – the time between when the shot was given to the onset of the reaction – does not match those set by The Table, the "burden of proof" is placed back on the injured party. This means the person must go against the government and the pharmaceutical industry to prove that the vaccine caused their injury. Obviously, with the deck stacked against the injured party, compensation for damages not defined by The Table is challenging to prove and nearly always denied.[232]

For example, an "allowed definition" for a reaction to the DTaP vaccine is anaphylactic shock. According to The Table, the time interval from the shot to the onset of shock must be no more than four hours. If a child develops a delayed anaphylactic reaction, say, five or six hours after receiving the shot, it is considered "off Table," and the government will rule that the anaphylaxis was not caused by the DTaP vaccine. Another example is an injury caused by the hepatitis B vaccine, added *to* The Table in 1997. The only events eligible for government compensation are anaphylaxis or death from anaphylactic shock, which must occur within four hours of receiving the vaccine. Despite the large number of medical literature reports of autoimmune and neurological complications following hepatitis B vaccination in both children and adults, anaphylaxis remains the only injury that qualifies for compensation. All other complications are considered a "coincidence" and deemed "off Table," meaning they are not considered caused by the vaccine.

These are two examples of the thousands of serious side effects reported after vaccination to VAERS. Reports can be filed electronically by a parent, a doctor, or any concerned observer or caretaker. VAERS reports are a chronicle of adverse events thought by the petitioner to be caused by vaccines. But unfortunately, most researchers at the CDC and the FDA view the reports as merely "points of interest." The CDC and the drug companies claim that vaccine injuries are rare, occurring in no more than one or two people per million shots given. If The Table is used as the measure for the number of "approved reactions," that is an accurate statement. There are relatively few cases of anaphylaxis and immediate death following vaccines. However, if all types of reactions are considered, including those published in and supported by the medical literature, the actual number of injuries caused by, or associated with, vaccines is staggering.

COMMENTARY

Another problem with The Table and the compensation program is that certain vaccines **cannot** be covered. For a vaccine to be part of the NVICP, there are three exacting criteria: 1) the vaccine must be recommended and approved for routine administration to children or pregnant women; 2) by federal law, the shot must be subject to an $0.75 per dose excise tax (paid by parents); and 3) the vaccine must formally be added to the program by the Secretary of HHS. All three steps are essential for an injured party to apply for compensation.

For example, if an adverse event occurs in association with yellow fever, shingles, adult pneumonia, rabies, and a few other vaccines, the injury is not covered by the program. The primary reason the flu shot and the COVID-19 jab were recommended for infants starting at six months of age, wasn't because babies were highly susceptible to these infections, it was so that manufacturers would have liability protection by adding the shot to the childhood vaccination schedule. **Remember, always follow the money.**

VAERS BEFORE COVID

Prior to COVID, the VAERS database received around 30,000 reports per year. That number has grown steadily since 2005, when only about 12,000 reports were filed each year. Of these, at least 15 percent of the reports were considered "serious" (i.e., necessitated a trip to the emergency room, required a hospitalization, or resulted in a permanent disability).

However, most people even today – including most doctors – aren't aware of VAERS and underreporting remains a substantial problem. Dr. David Kessler, FDA Commissioner from 1990 to 1997, had expressed an oft-quoted concern about the underreporting of vaccine injuries to VAERS. Overall, it is estimated that less than one percent of all adverse events from vaccines are reported. Based on that estimate, the number of vaccine-related adverse events occurring each year could actually be more than 3,000,000 instead of the 30,000 reported, a truly jolting number.

Language written into the 1986 NCVIA legislation granted the Secretary of HHS broad discretionary authority to alter the Table. The latitude was given to introduce flexibility into the system, allowing the list of Table conditions to *increase,* to give *more options* for compensation and to include *additional injuries* as they became apparent with existing vaccines and vaccines in the future. However, the exact opposite came to pass. Former Secretary Donna Shalala, the Secretary of HHS serving under President Bill Clinton from 1993 to 2001, used her discretionary authority to *remove compensable events* from the Table and redefine permanent injuries, placing a greater burden upon petitioners to prove that vaccination caused the injury or a death.

HIGHLIGHT

While petitioners grapple with overwhelming medical debt and endure heart-wrenching social challenges, waiting years to see if they will be granted some compensatory relief from the Federal Court of Claims, salaried court officials, government bureaucrats, and seasoned trial attorneys – supported by administrative staffs – all receive steady paychecks funded with taxpayer dollars. These public employees are not tasked with helping injured citizens but with protecting the defendant, their bosses at HHS. This is an uneven, often demoralizing battle for struggling parents, injured individuals, and their determined attorneys. How can a system claim to deliver justice when it wields the vast resources of the government to oppose the very citizens it was created to help?

Since the beginning of the compensation program in 1989 through November 2024, only 23,788 petitions have been filed with the compensation program; 12,766 were dismissed and 11,022 received compensation from the court. The total amount paid out by the program to injured parties and their attorneys has been more than $5.245 billion, with $4.725 billion going to injured parties. This deceptively appears to work out to approximately $427,000 per claimant, an inaccurate number because only a few settlements were very large while most were a pittance in comparison. Recall that up to 70 percent of all compensation is paid as a negotiated settlement with the injured parties. This is done to get to a settlement quickly and to minimize the risk of losing their case. These payments are not included in the data of paid claims because the decisions and the amount of compensation are usually sealed so the exact amount each claimant receives is unknown. In addition, legal fees are reimbursed, whether or not the petitioner is awarded compensation by the Court. By statute, attorneys are not allowed to collect a contingency fee if a large settlement is awarded.[233] (For more detail about the VAERS system and the intended and unintended consequences of the Federal Court of Claims, referred to as Vaccine Court, I direct readers to the well-documented and somber book by Wayne Rohde, *"The Vaccine Court 2.0: Revised and Updated: The Dark Truth of America's Vaccine Injury Compensation Program."*)

VAERS has become increasingly more difficult to use despite the WONDER search tool. To file a complaint, the petitioner needs to know the name of the vaccine AND the abbreviation used in the VAERS system. In addition, beginning in 2002, vaccine manufacturers started to combine multiple vaccines into one shot, claiming it would "streamline the schedule." Actually, there was a deeper motivation. Parents were becoming more informed and increasingly resistant to giving their infant four or more shots during a single office visit. In addition, parents were refusing all of the many vaccines in ever-higher numbers. Parents who questioned the vaccine's ingredients, and even its necessity, were disparagingly labeled "vaccine hesitant" or worse, "vaccine resistant." By combining multiple vaccines into one shot, parents could be falsely reassured that their baby was only getting "one vaccine today" at the office visit. Additionally, manufacturers were cagey in another way: by combining several vaccines into one injection, it was impossible to tell which antigen had caused the reaction (e.g., was it the pertussis fraction or was it hepatitis b that had caused a reaction?) This has made filing a VAERS report nearly impossible.[234]

The beginning of the deception was the release of **Pediarix** in 2002, a combination of DTaP (diphtheria, tetanus, and pertussis), IPV (inactivated polio vaccine), and Hepatitis B into a single shot. If there was a side effect after the injection, such as a seizure, which vaccine was to be blamed? In the pre-release clinical trials for **Pediarix**, 400 children were divided into four groups to compare immune responses. Three groups received the individual vaccines given in different limbs (called the "comparator" groups), while those in the fourth group received a single combination dose of Pediarix. Researchers measured the antibody levels produced in response to the vaccines given individually versus all vaccine antigens injected at one time, in one shot. They found that the antibody levels in the comparator groups were nearly identical to those in the Pediarix group. Based on these findings, researchers concluded that Pediarix could reduce the number of injections needed in a child's first two years of life, streamline the immunization schedule, improve compliance, and encourage acceptance of additional vaccines.

They proved *convenience*, but not safety.

LEARN MORE

Several combination vaccines are currently available in the US. There are similar combination vaccines in other countries. usually offered under different names:

- **Kinrix**: DTaP and IPV (diphtheria, tetanus, pertussis, and inactivated polio)

- **Pentacel**: DTaP, IPV, and Hib (diphtheria, tetanus, pertussis, inactivated polio and H. influenzae type b)

- **Quadracel:** DTaP and IPV (diphtheria, tetanus, pertussis, and inactivated polio)

- **Twinrix**: Hepatitis A and Hepatitis B

- **Vaxelis:** DTaP, IPV, Hib and Hep B (diphtheria, tetanus, pertussis, inactivated polio, H. influenzae type b and Hepatitis B

- **ProQuad**: MMRV - Measles, mumps, rubella, and varicella (chickenpox). *Note: This vaccine has been on and off the market several times due to serious side effects from injecting four live, attenuated viruses at the same time.*

OPENVAERS

Out of the frustration of trying to file VAERS reports for themselves or their children, a small group of tech savvy people collaborated in 2021 to form a truly easy-to-use database called OpenVAERS. The OpenVAERS team does not change, modify or vet the data and there is zero monetization of the site.

OpenVAERS is particularly focused on COVID vaccine injury reports. Researchers downloaded the data gathered into VAERS, which is open source and publicly available, then parsed the data into groupings that are easy to use and understand. The results are posted on their website in "red box summaries," dividing the data into categories such as myocarditis, hospitalizations, doctor office visits, heart attacks, and deaths. The website was last updated on November 29, 2024 at the time of this writing. As of that date, 1,656,138 injury reports had been filed with VAERS associated with the COVID-19 injection. OpenVAERS also reported more than 219,000 hospitalizations, more than 50,000 cardiac events, more than 38,000 deaths, and 72,492 had become permanently disabled.[235] Those are staggering numbers, especially since government institutions and their mainstream media mouthpieces continue to deny any association between the shots and injury or death.

When the CDC and FDA were gearing up for routine surveillance of the COVID -19 jabs through VAERS, a very explicit planning document was released on February 2, 2022, by the CDC's VAERS Team. The weekly reports were to include the following:

- Tables summarizing data from fields on the VAERS form (e.g., age of vaccinee, COVID-19 vaccine type, adverse event)
- Enhanced surveillance implemented with **any reports** of the following occurrences of adverse events of special interest such as:
  - Guillain-Barré Syndrome (GBS), seizure, stroke, narcolepsy/cataplexy, anaphylaxis, acute myocardial infarction, myopericarditis, coagulopathy (including thrombocytopenia, disseminated intravascular coagulopathy [DIC], and deep venous thrombosis [DVT]), Kawasaki's disease, multisystemic inflammatory syndrome in children (MIS-C), multisystemic inflammatory syndrome in adults (MIS-A), thrombosis with thrombocytopenia syndrome (TTS), transverse myelitis, and **death**

A 37-page document, *Vaccine Adverse Event Reporting System (VAERS) Standard Operating Procedures for COVID-19* was given to CDC employees. It had detailed instructions on what to look for in early reports. Workers were also given detailed instructions on how to record and report the injuries, when follow up inquiries were to occur, and more.[236]

However, the VAERS teams at the CDC and the FDA were completely unprepared for the unprecedented number of reports that soon followed at the beginning of 2021. The staff was literally buried in the avalanche of reports. *The BMJ* report further detailed the problem:

> "Faced with an unprecedented number of adverse event reports that came pouring in shortly after the rollout of COVID-19 vaccines, most of which were labeled 'serious,' the VAERS' staffing was woefully inadequate and could not review even a fraction of the reports submitted, including reports of death. While other countries acknowledged deaths were 'likely' or 'probably' related to mRNA vaccination, *the CDC* – claiming to have reviewed nearly 20,000 VAERS preliminary reports of death (far more than other countries) – as of 2023, had *not acknowledged a single death linked to mRNA vaccines.*"[237]

THE V-SAFE DATABASE

Originally launched in December 2020, the V-safe database was designed to monitor people receiving a COVID-19 jab in real time. After enrolling, the V-safe system would send confidential check-ins via text message or email to ask the person how they felt after the vaccination; they were to respond, even if they experienced no side effects. In all, 10.1 million people participated in V-safe, completing more than 151 million V-safe surveys about their experiences following a COVID-19 injection. Data was collected from 12/13/2020 to 9/25/2022. The V-save website admits the data is incomplete and the last time the data on the site was updated was July 25, 2023, therefore, ongoing injuries and deaths are not being tracked. Why did they stop collecting data points? The expression, "you can't find what you're not looking for" comes to mind.[238]

The CDC bragged that the roll out of the COVID-19 jabs was part of "the most intensive safety monitoring effort in US history" which we have learned four years later, was a completely fabricated statement. For example, a critical part of V-safe data was hidden from the public and public searches: the free-text fields, areas where claimants are able to use up to 250 characters to describe their symptoms, injury, and medical care.

The Informed Consent Action Network (ICAN) wanted to know what they were hiding. In June 2021, a FOIA request was filed to obtain the data. When the CDC did not provide the requested information, ICAN sued. It took two lawsuits to force the CDC to release the information that was critical to understanding the injuries caused by the COVID-19 jabs. The first lawsuit, in 2023, garnered the release of the "check-the-box" portion of the V-safe data. In January 2024, a second legal action was filed. District Court Judge Matthew Kacsmaryk forced the CDC to release 7.8 million "free text" entries over 12 months, critical information that V-safe had collected but had hidden.

ICAN was ultimately able to obtain 144 million data entries from the V-safe system. To analyze the vast amount of data, ICAN developed a specialized software to filter, sort, and visualize the data by race, gender, timing of symptoms, health impacts, and vaccine type (e.g., Pfizer, Moderna, etc.). Out of approximately 10 million user entries, more than 782,000 individuals (7.7%) reported health events requiring medical attention, emergency care, or hospitalization. Additionally, more than 25% of participants reported events severe enough to interfere with daily activities such as work or school. Identifying trends and patterns, the program enabled ICAN to make significant observations, such as the higher rate of adverse events with Moderna vaccines and the disproportionate impact on women. The data can be downloaded and reviewed from ICAN's website for all independent investigators to explore. It has been slow, but the truth and the extent of government coverup is being exposed through *The Pfizer Papers*, V-safe lawsuits, OpenVAERs, and other books and documentaries which are continuing to roll out the horror stories of how the COVID-19 shots destroyed health and lives.[239]

According to USAFacts.org, at least 270 million people, or 81%, of the population have received at least one dose of a COVID-19 shot and, overall, about 70% of the population is considered fully vaccinated, defined as two shots and at least one booster. Edward Dowd, author of *Cause Unknown*, said in April 2024 in an interview on Epoch Times' show, *American Thought Leaders*: "There were a tremendous amount of excess deaths that really peaked in 2021, then started coming down in 2022 and 2023. There have been 1.1 million excessive deaths in America since the roll out of the shots, with about 300,000 of those deaths occurring in working aged people, aged 15 to 64."[240]

With over 1.6 million vaccine injury reports submitted to VAERS, a fundamental misunderstanding endures: VAERS is not equipped to handle countermeasure compensation claims. Attempting to do so is as futile as visiting the Bureau of Motor Vehicles to buy a plane ticket: it's the wrong agency to do the needed job. VAERS serves solely as a reporting system, not a venue for adjudication or compensation. Additionally, since the COVID-19 vaccine is not listed on the VAERS Injury Table, claims filed through the Vaccine Court are automatically dismissed without review. This bureaucratic gap leaves injured individuals in limbo. Most people had never heard of VAERS before COVID-19, and even fewer were aware of the Countermeasures Injury Compensation Program (CICP) – the sole option for COVID-19 vaccine-related claims, which is notoriously limited, complex, and rarely provides substantial relief. 342

THE CICP

Authorized within the 2005 PREP Act, the Countermeasures Injury Compensation Program (CICP) was designed to "provide compensation to individuals who sustained a serious physical injury, significant side effects, or death as a direct result of the administration or use of a covered countermeasure." The CICP was activated in 2010, when the 2009 H1N1 vaccine was determined to be a covered countermeasure for the swine flu pandemic.[241]

The vaccines on the list of countermeasures include:
- Anthrax
- Botulinum Toxin
- Ebola
- Marburg
- Pandemic Influenza for H1N1
- Smallpox and other orthopoxviruses (e.g., monkeypox)
- Zika
- COVID-19

As previously discussed, countermeasures under the PREP Act during COVID-19 included any drugs or medical devices used "to diagnose, mitigate, prevent, treat, or cure" COVID19. We have also seen that the language of the PREP Act prohibits Congress from funding the CICP to assist countermeasure-injured people.

FILING A CLAIM

Filing an injury compensation claim with the CICP can be a daunting process, particularly for individuals already burdened by disabling medical conditions. The CICP enforces rigid rules and deadlines, and demands extensive documentation and medical records. Managing these bureaucratic obstacles would be no small feat, even for a healthy individual, For those grappling with severe neurological impairment, cardiac injuries, or other significant health issues, trying to meet these requirements would be insurmountable. The complexity of the requirements is of course designed to act as a barrier, and naturally defeats the program's intended purpose to deliver relief to those harmed by countermeasures. The injured party has the option to appoint a legal or personal representative to help compile and submit the required documentation for a claim, but if a lawyer assists, the legal fees are not reimbursed. This places an additional financial strain on the injured party. In cases where the claimant has died, the estate may qualify for compensation, but only if it can be proven that the death was a direct result of one of the covered countermeasures. This process adds another layer of difficulty to an already burdensome system, making it difficult for families to seek relief.

The filing requirements include:

- The **"Request for Benefits" form** needs to be completed and returned with the packet of required medical records
- A list of *all doctors* and *all healthcare providers* seen for the injury and their contact information
- *All* medical records, test results, procedure results, hospital records, physician and nursing notes
- A list of *all* medications, supplements, over-the-counter meds, and other conventional or alternative therapies
- **Proof of use** - such as a copy of COVID-19 vaccination card or medical documentation to prove when the shot was administered

The most disturbing aspect of filing a CICP claim is the **strict one-year deadline** to submit a claim. The Code of Federal Regulations on the CICP is very firm with this deadline:

If the Secretary determines that a Request Form or Letter of Intent was not filed by the set deadline, (one year), the Request Form (or Letter of Intent) **will not be processed** and the requester **will not be eligible** for benefits under this Program.[242]

The unreasonably short timeframe poses a significant obstacle for injured individuals. In the first year following a severe medical event, most are preoccupied with seeking treatment, undergoing tests, and trying to understand their sudden and complex health challenges. By the time they realize their condition was likely associated with or caused by the COVID-19 jab or specific drug, such as remdesivir, the statute of limitations has already passed. Missing the deadline results in the outright denial of their case, leaving them without any recourse. Such a rigid deadline fails to consider the practical realities of post-injury diagnosis and recovery, further harming those the program is designed to assist.

HIGHLIGHT

By comparison, under the NVICP, if a claim is filed for a person who died as a result of the vaccine injury, the petition must be filed within two years of the death. For a vaccine injury claim, there is a three-year statute of limitations that begins at the date the symptoms become associated with the vaccine, which may actually be years after the vaccine was injected. Successful petitioners may receive reimbursement for medical expenses, lost income, and reasonable attorney costs and fees. Petitioners who are dissatisfied with the compensation awarded may opt to pursue actions in civil court.

The CICP system was set up to move quickly. A staff person was to review the package of materials from a petitioner within weeks. But like many government initiatives, the CICP has not only failed to meet these expectations, it has failed miserably. According to HRSA, the case backlog awaiting review is substantial. It currently takes the agency **approximately 12 months** just to complete the initial review of each petition. This significant delay undermines the program's purpose of timely relief and compounds the frustration for petitioners, many of whom are grappling with serious medical and financial challenges while awaiting a decision.[243]

THE CICP TABLES

Similar to the VICP, the CICP has its own Injury Compensation Tables. The first Table was set up for problems associated with the smallpox vaccines given to first-responders and military members after the 9/11 attacks in 2001. However, the list of Table Injuries – the injuries given the designation of "presumption of causation" – weren't published and didn't become effective until September 15, 2021. Anyone injured twenty years prior, even if their injury had met the criteria set forth by the table, would no longer be eligible for compensation because the claim would be long past the *one year* application limit from the day the shot was received.[244]

A second Countermeasure Injury Table, finalized in 2016, was officially published in the Federal Register for the H1N1 pandemic vaccine used widely in 2009. The Table listed injuries eligible for presumptive compensation, including anaphylaxis, Guillain-Barré Syndrome, and certain ventilator-associated injuries. However, injured individuals were still subject to the standard one-year filing deadline from the date of vaccination. As a result, many claims were excluded, regardless of the severity of the harm suffered, because the Table was published five years after the vaccine was administered. This delay effectively barred injured parties from accessing compensation, undermining the program's intent to quickly provide relief.

Establishing the Injury Table is central to the process of filing for and obtaining compensation through the CICP. Petitioners must either:

1. Demonstrate that their injury matches one listed on the Injury Table within the government-specified time frame, or
2. Prove causation independently, showing that the vaccine or countermeasure was the sole direct cause of the injury.

However, the government explicitly states that a "temporal association" – the timing of an adverse event occurring shortly after the vaccine or drug – is not sufficient evidence by itself to prove causation. For example, even if someone experiences a seizure or a heart attack within minutes of receiving a COVID-19 vaccine, this temporal link alone does not meet the program's burden of proof.

According to a report by the Congressional Research Service:

> CICP claimants must prove their eligibility for compensation by **demonstrating their injury was on the Countermeasure Injury Table**, a distinct problem for COVID-19 injuries. The existing Table was established for the H1N1 pandemic influenza vaccine; *no such table has yet been promulgated for any COVID-19 countermeasure, including vaccines.*[245]

That was published in March 2023. As of the time of this writing, nothing has changed. Without a table of predefined, presumptively compensable injuries, claimants must present extensive medical documentation, expert testimony, and scientific evidence to establish a direct causal link. This process is costly, complex, and often unattainable for most injured parties. However, a person may attempt to pursue a claim as long as the injury is based on "compelling, reliable, valid, medical and scientific evidence," in accordance with the rules set forth by 42 CFR 110.42(f). This is a long and expensive process, especially when faced with PREP Act protections given to the drug companies.

CLAIMS FILED TO DATE

The Countermeasures Injury Compensation Program (CICP) has received a meager 14,126 claims since its establishment in 2010, when it was administratively set up to address injuries arising from the countermeasures during the H1N1 (swine flu) pandemic. Of these, only 4,057 claims (29%) have been adjudicated. Since the program's inception, only **50 claims have been compensated over the last 14 years**, a strikingly low number given the total claims filed.

When the data regarding the COVID-19 vaccine is examined more closely, an analysis of the table compiled by the CICP program reveals that over **75% of claims** involve injuries or deaths attributed to the COVID-19 vaccine. The remaining claims pertain to injuries or deaths caused by other COVID-19 countermeasures.[246] HRSA is careful to pepper the word "alleged" on all its forms, pages, and tables.

Further, as of December 1. 2024, **only 13 COVID-19 claims** have been compensated, with an average payout of $30,769. For example, an individual who experienced an anaphylactic reaction received $2,020, while the highest compensation for a myopericarditis injury was $8,962. Five others were compensated at roughly half that amount, the remaining claims for even less.

Let that sink in.

Only **13 injured people** have been compensated while more than 1.6 million injury reports have been filed incorrectly with VAERS (instead of with CICP). In addition, the compensation is extremely limited. It will only cover:[245]

1. reasonable medical expenses that are not already covered by the petitioner's private health insurance (e.g., unreimbursed hospitalization costs);
2. income lost from inability to work due to disability – *capped at $50,000/year* with a lifetime cap yet to be determined; and

3. a standard death benefit that ranged from $370,000 to $422,000.

Under the current CICP, injured individuals receive no justice. The program does not cover attorney fees nor does it compensate individuals for pain-and-suffering damages. In essence, it deprives claimants of essential financial support for legal representation or health recovery. Most troubling, decisions made by HRSA are final and cannot be challenged. The PREP Act *explicitly prohibits* any legal or judicial review of CICP determinations, leaving victims with no avenue for appeal of inadequate compensation awards in cases where claims are denied.

This lack of oversight ensures that HRSA's decisions remain unchecked, effectively shutting the door on those harmed by government-designated countermeasures. In practice, the CICP offers the vaccine-injured "little more than the right to file and lose," further compounding their suffering.

THE BOTTOM LINE

The above discussion regarding the CICP may have sounded like a bunch of dry legal explanations but what this lays out is hard to swallow.

Here's the summary:

1. Since no CICP Table has been created for the COVID-19 jab, there are no injuries or side effects that have been given the designation of *presumption of causation*. No conditions, not even myocarditis, have been assigned to an Injury Table.

2. Without an injury table for the COVID-19 jab, all injuries or side effects are considered "off table" injuries and must be proven by "compelling, reliable, valid, medical and scientific evidence." More than 3,000 peer-reviewed articles and the analysis of 450,000 pages of documentation summarized

in *The Pfizer Papers* expose the cardiovascular, neurologic, oncologic, autoimmune, and reproductive injuries and harm that have been caused by the COVID-19 shots.[247] Even with all of this highly researched documentation, as of this writing, the government continues to deny the association between the COVID injection and injury, and has done nothing to create an injury table or further fund the CICP program. We don't need more research; we need to use the documentation that is already done to force the government to act.

3. All injury reports filed with the Vaccine Adverse Event Reporting System (VAERS) will be denied. Yes, all 1,656,138 injury reports filed (to date) will be tossed out unless the COVID-19 jab is moved under the NVICP for compensation. The injury reports were filed with the wrong agency; they should have been filed with CICP.

4. The injury reports will also be denied because the one-year filing limitation has expired. Most injuries occurred when the roll out began, which started at the beginning of 2021 and continued into 2023. Injury reports must be filed within one year of the date of the injection or usage of the countermeasure. If the filing deadline is missed, a request for reconsideration can be submitted to HRSA within 60 days of the denial, but as previously explained, they are routinely denied. Since the time of this writing (end of 2024), all early injuries have missed filing and reconsideration deadlines.

5. All decisions made by the case reviewers at HRSA are **final.** Injured parties are not entitled to counsel. They have no right of appeal and there is no judicial oversight. There are no pain and suffering damages and awards are a pittance compared to actual economic damages. Section (b)(7) of the PREP Act, under "Judicial Review," states that *"no federal or state court will have jurisdiction to review any action taken by the Secretary."*

This ruling will preempt all state laws that are different from, or in conflict with, the declaration. The distinct lack of checks and balances undeniably puts the public at risk and is indeed frightening. It appears that an appointed politician has been handed the power to order mandatory vaccination for everyone. This lack of due process is being challenged in court as being unconstitutional. Let's hope the legal petition will change this provision.

6. At this point in time, lawsuits against Pfizer and other manufacturers are prohibited by the PREP Act. As discussed previously, even if a pharmaceutical company **knowingly harms people**, the company will be immune from legal prosecution *unless* the US Attorney General initiates "enforcement action" against the company in the name of the claimant. However, the protection the PREP Act gives the COVID-19 countermeasures could come to a screeching halt if the PREP Act amendments are reversed or eliminated by a new HHS Secretary before the December 31, 2029 expiration.

Can you now see that this lack of response and compensation has all been by design, starting in 2005 with the passage of the PREP Act? The public has a right to know about this terrible program, which will fan the flames of anger and frustration, and that will rightfully further drive vaccine hesitancy.

An additional government restriction was implemented during COVID-19 that deserves to be addressed because it is part of a separate template that will be used again in the event of another pandemic scare. Many restrictions we were forced to endure came from many years ago, including the inappropriate use of quarantines.

*"A lie can travel halfway around the world while
the truth is still putting on its shoes."*

~Mark Twain

CHAPTER 18

Quarantines vs Shutdowns:
Then and Now

With the passage of the PREP Act in 2005, drug companies were handed a whole new level of unparalleled liability protection that continues to this very day. There remains no incentive to ensure safety of any product made for a pandemic. All the manufacturers have to do is label a product a "countermeasure" and it has no liability worries for releasing faulty or untested products during a declared emergency. As an aside, vaccine injuries increase product sales – which are good for shareholders. And when a person is injured, more tests, procedures, doctor's visits, and drugs are needed to treat their injury.

Almost before the ink had dried on The PREP Act, often called the Frist Addendum, it was announced that Fluarix would be the first vaccine to receive "FDA accelerated approval." Looking back, this was a test run for things to come. Widely touted as an "effective government/ industry collaboration to bolster the flu vaccine supply," Fluarix was approved in the US in 2005, even though it had been approved in 1998 in the EU and Canada. A quadrivalent version was approved in 2009 for adults and for infants in 2013. The FDA gave accelerated approval based on four clinical studies done in Europe involving approximately 1,200 adults. FDA Commissioner Lester Crawford crowed that the "accelerated approval has allowed us to evaluate and approve Fluarix in record time." NIAID Director, Anthony Fauci, MD, added, *This effort is a model for the type of effective collaboration that will be needed to quickly produce vaccines in the event of a pandemic.*"

Definitely a sign of things to come.

HIGHLIGHT

Lester Crawford was the 2005-2006 acting FDA commissioner. He was forced to resign after the discovery of an undisclosed ownership of pharmaceutical stocks, including GlaxoSmithKline (GSK). Crawford's stock ownership and some other financial holdings raised concerns about potential conflicts of interest, given his role in overseeing drug approvals and regulatory matters at the FDA. Of note, GSK is the manufacturer of Fluarix.

MODERN DAY QUARANTINES

Using quarantine, as previously mentioned, was a disease-prevention tool that began during the fourteenth century in an effort to protect coastal cities from plague epidemics. Ships arriving from infected ports were required to sit at anchor for 40 days before landing. Therefore, the practice of quarantine acquired its name from the Italian words *quaranta giorni* which means, "40 days."

In 1944, with the passage of the Public Health Service Act, the federal government's authority to quarantine was clearly established for modern times. In 1953, the Public Health Service became part of the Department of Health, Education, and Welfare (HEW), which later morphed into the Department of Health and Human Services (HHS). In 1967, the role of quarantine was transferred to the National Communicable Disease Center, now known as the Centers for Disease Control and Prevention, the CDC.

About the same time that the US Public Health Service was established, a list of communicable diseases that could be corralled using quarantines was declared through Executive Order 9708, issued by President Truman. This list has been periodically updated over the last 60 years. Title 42 of the Public Health Service Act has many subsections. The regulations contained in Chapter 6A, Section G, called, "**Quarantine and Inspection**," give the public health service full responsibility for preventing the transmission of communicable diseases.[248]

Prior to 2002, the steps for ordering a national quarantine were clearly defined:

> On the recommendation of a **consensus of the National Advisory Health Committee** and in agreement with the Surgeon General, the president would be notified of a disease thought to cause significant risk to the general population. The name of that disease would be added to the list of risky communicable diseases by a presidential Executive Order.

However, this chain of command changed with the passage of the "Public Health Security and Bioterrorism Preparedness and Response Act of 2002," also referred to as **The Bioterrorism Act.**[249] Signed into law June 2002, H.R. 3448, gave HHS and the Dept. of Agriculture new authorities to regulate the possession, unlawful use, and unauthorized transfer of biological agents and toxins. The law gave the Sec. of HHS the ability to assess civil and/or criminal fines up to $500,000 and attach penalties could include up to 5 years in prison. The Congressional Budget Office (CBO) estimated that spending to implement the legislation would increase by $10 million over the 2003-2012 period.[250]

Section 142 of the Bioterrorism Act was revised to "streamline and clarify" quarantine provisions, shifting significant authority to the President to impose quarantines through Executive Orders. This power now rests solely on the recommendation of the Secretary of HHS, in consultation with the Surgeon General, eliminating the need for a consensus opinion from the 12-member National Advisory Health Committee.

This change is critical. Instead of drawing from the collective expertise of a full medical committee, decisions now rely on the input of just two individuals. While the Surgeon General is a medical doctor, the Secretary of HHS is most often a politician, neither of whom is accountable to the public, as both are political appointees. In effect, these revisions concentrated enormous power in the hands of unelected officials, significantly altering the balance of decision-making during public health emergencies.

Other key provisions of the 2002 Bioterrorism Act included:

A. National Preparedness and Response Planning, Coordinating, and Reporting
   - Developing and maintaining medical countermeasures;
   - Developing non-overlapping plan for coordinating Federal, State, and local efforts in the event of an outbreak; and
   - Enhancing the readiness of hospitals to respond effectively to such emergencies

B. Development of the Strategic National Stockpile and Priority Countermeasures
   - To maintain a stockpile of drugs, vaccines and other biological products, medical devices, and other supplies; and

- To provide for the emergency health security of the US in the event of a bioterrorist attack or *other public health emergency*

C. **Improving State, Local, and Hospital Preparedness for and Response to Bioterrorism and Other Public Health Emergencies (7 of 18 points)**
    - Develop statewide plans for responding to bioterrorism and *other public health emergencies;*
    - Conduct exercises to test the capability and timeliness of response activities;
    - Enhance public health laboratories;
    - Provide training for safety of workers and workplaces in the *event of bioterrorism;*
    - Prepare a plan for triage and transport management of people, products, and specimens;
    - Enhance training for healthcare professionals to provide appropriate health care for large numbers of individuals exposed to a bioweapon;
    - Develop, enhance, and coordinate with existing telemedicine programs

One of the most unnerving changes in the 2002 Bioterrorism Act is the new definition of who can be detained. Previously, only those "reasonably thought to be infected" could be quarantined. In the revised Act, Section 142(b)(2)(B) was changed. People thought to be in a "pre-communicable state", meaning the disease "would be likely to cause a public health emergency if transmitted to other individuals", can now be mandatorily confined.

The combined effect of the bioterrorism legislation and E.O. 13295 is that the Secretary of HHS can issue a directive for a person to be quarantined under the "suspicion" of exposure or the "possibility" that he *may* become sick. A cough, a sneeze, or a fever could put a person at risk of being quarantined without recourse and for an extended period of time. Penalties for violating the quarantine law "without permission of the quarantine officer in charge" can be a fine of up to $1,000 or imprisonment for up to one year or both.[251]

The **Bioterrorism Act of 2002** and the **PREP Act of 2005** together established the framework for implementing quarantines, expanded the power of **Executive Orders**, and allocated funding to bolster planning for bioterrorism events. These measures streamlined government responses, creating a centralized and expedited process for handling public health emergencies.

COMMENTARY

That's a lot of power. This is akin to quarantining a person who coughs or sneezes because they are "pre-sick" and they just might infect others. What if they just have allergies? Can you see where the groundwork for lockdowns, social distancing, and implementation of fear-based behaviors, such as forced use of worthless masks started twenty years ago? All of these laws and Executive Orders have taken power away from elected officials, who are accountable to We the People, and have given massive authority to an unelected, appointed political figure: the Secretary of HHS.

Notably, these foundational plans were put in place **long before COVID-19**, underscoring that the infrastructure for such actions was not a reaction to the pandemic but rather a result of years of preemptive policy-making.

When President Bush added "influenza caused by novel or re-emergent influenza viruses that are causing, or have the potential to cause, a pandemic" to the list of quarantinable diseases with E.O. 13295 in 2003, another template was created. The public laws were gradually expanded in scope and power over the ensuing 20 years to give more and more control to the government and to suppress resistance. The template's implementation was tested with relatively mild pandemics, bird flu in 2005, and then swine flu in 2009. The culminating event was the COVID-19 exploding out of control in 2020.

The template has now been perfected for future pandemics:

1. create an emergency;
2. pump fear into people about it;
3. develop the countermeasure – they will have full liability protection – drugs, tests, vaccines;
4. declare rules such as masks, distancing, quarantines to remove freedoms;
5. make vaccine and medication compliance "seem" mandatory;
6. medicate people with the countermeasures, making them sick and providing no compensation for their permanent illnesses and injuries.

Rinse and repeat.

COVID ANALOG

Within the PREP Act, participants are assured that the plan to administer or use a covered countermeasure would include education regarding the pros, cons, and contraindications of the countermeasure. The legislation mentions briefly that the program is "voluntary." Where is the section on informed consent and the right to refuse? The program was "voluntary" but consequences for not volunteering to be injected were harsh: loss of job, loss of status, loss of freedom to travel, loss of pension, etc. A quote by previous US Representative Ron Paul (R-TX) says it all:

> "When we give the government the power to make medical decisions for us, we, in essence, accept that the state owns our bodies."

The templates were set in place for the next pandemic, such as the current bird flu, monkeypox, ebola, or Disease X. The "X" really means "fill in the blank for things to come."

LEARN MORE

After the passage of The Bioterrorism Act, formally known as the Public Health Security and Bioterrorism Preparedness and Response Act of 2002, the law was updated and amended several times. The key updates and related legislative actions are:

1. **The Pandemic and All-Hazards Preparedness Act (PAHPA)**: Passed in 2006 and reauthorized in 2013 and 2019, the Act improved the management and distribution of the Strategic National Stockpile of medical supplies and pharmaceuticals. It furthered the development of medical countermeasures with funding provided through the legislation for vaccines, drugs, and diagnostic tools needed for emergencies and more extensive electronic medical records.

2. **The Food and Drug Administration Amendments Act (FDAAA) of 2007**: This Act gave more authority to the FDA for fast approval and expedited review of new medications and vaccines viewed to be "essential."

3. **The 21st Century Cures Act**: Enacted in 2016, this law further accelerated the approval process for drugs and medical devices. It helped bring new treatments to market more quickly by giving the FDA more flexibility in evaluating and approving them.

MANDATED AT A HIGH LEVEL

The pressure to pass protective legislation for the benefit of drug companies didn't just come from drug company lobbyists. A plan was underway to vaccinate the entire world. From the WHO to local newspapers, the same message was repeated over and over: a pandemic is near. Get ready.

At a global meeting held at the WHO in November 2005, the Director General of the WHO was quoted as saying, "It is only a matter of time before an avian flu virus – *most likely H5N1* – acquires the ability to be transmitted from human-to-human, sparking an outbreak of human pandemic influenza. We don't know when this will happen. *But we do know that it will happen*." *(emphasis added)* That's a really strong statement.[252] Stating emphatically that "it will happen" sounds like they knew the outcome had been predetermined.

First published in 1999, the WHO Global Pandemic Planning document demonstrated that preparedness meetings had been ongoing for a long time. Undoubtedly, the US Congress and President Bush were not operating independently in their urgency to protect the pharmaceutical industry and shovel a massive amount of tax dollars into their already overflowing financial coffers.

The next WHO global planning document, released early in 2005, contained step-by-step guidelines of how a human H5N1 infection was to be handled at the international level when the pandemic was declared. The plan listed detailed instructions, with objectives and action items, that were to be followed at both national and global levels. On examination, it becomes clear that the WHO "game plan" was followed precisely by our government.[253]

According to the WHO plan, conditions representing **Phase 1** were called the "Inter-pandemic Period." The overarching goal during this period was to "strengthen influenza pandemic preparedness at the global, regional, national, and sub-national (local) levels." On page 23, Item 5 under "all countries" were the following instructions:

"**Resolve liability and other legal issues** linked to use of the pandemic vaccine for mass or targeted emergency vaccination campaigns, if not yet done." *(emphasis added)*

The WHO preparedness plan has a long list of items compiled into a checklist, streamlining the process for manufacturers of the countermeasures – drugs, vaccines, and other products. The lists were designed to help all countries in the world to get their local processes in place before the (bird flu) pandemic occurred. Getting the liability issues in place was a specific line item. The intimations were very clear: mass vaccination programs would begin as soon as the liability issues were resolved and the vaccine became available.

These are some of the overarching goals in **Phase 5** of the Pandemic Alert period: *(emphasis and explanations added in brackets)*

- **Implement all interventions identified by the WHO** during the contingency planning phase.
- Implement **real-time monitoring** of essential resources (medical supplies, pharmaceuticals, infrastructure, vaccines, hospital capacity, human resources, etc.).
- Consider use of antivirals and other drugs for early treatment.
- Support preparations **for large-scale pandemic vaccine production** and licensing, and prepare for deployment as supplies become available.
- Provide public and private health-care providers with updated case definitions, protocols, and algorithms for **case-finding,** management, infection control, and surveillance. [**precursor for contact tracing**]
- Adjust priority lists of people to be vaccinated. [**Elderly first, then add pregnant women and children**]
- Consider deploying prototype pandemic vaccines, if available. [**precursor to vaccine release under EUA**]

- If agreements are in place with manufacturer(s), consider **recommending cessation of seasonal vaccine production** and initiation of full-scale pandemic vaccine production.
- Plan for vaccine distribution and accelerate preparations for **mass vaccination campaigns [Operation Warp Speed]**
- Information exchange with global vaccine manufacturers **[determine who has the capability to manufacture mRNA vaccines]**
- When a pandemic vaccine has been developed, **activate emergency procedures** for rapid licensing and use of pandemic vaccines (all countries).
- Implement **corpse management** procedures.
- Review lessons learned.

Look closely at the above list.

The points highlighted were drawn from pages 31 to 37 of a 49-page document *written in 2005*. The plan contains many more goals and objectives beyond those included here. Interestingly, it reads as though it could have been written in 2019, just before the onset of the COVID-19 pandemic in March 2020.[253]

=*"The truth brings with it a great measure of absolution, always."*

~R.D. Laing

CHAPTER 19

Tying It All Together: The Activist Playbook

What do sick cows, sick chickens, sick people, and sick wild animals, particularly wild birds, all have in common? An unhealthy immune system better described as an unhealthy terrain.

THE HEALTH OF THE TERRAIN

We have all been taught that germs are bad and they are everywhere, lurking around every corner, waiting for the opportunity to invade defenseless humans. Some don't believe that viruses exist, but bacteria, fungi, and parasites certainly do. Many go to great lengths to combat these potential invaders; we employ frequent handwashing with copious amounts of soap, lather our skin with hand sanitizers, wear masks that don't work, and grimace at the thought of eating a morsel of food quickly retrieved after falling on the floor.

Doctors and the media alike discuss the flu season as though "getting the flu" is inevitable without the flu shot. But similar to other concepts in modern medicine that have been unquestioningly accepted, perceived immunological frailty is a medical myth. A better understanding of the relationship between humans, animals, and microbes is necessary to create optimal health.

The immune system is the name given to the complex interaction between white blood cells, hormones, proteins, enzymes, antibodies, and inflammatory molecules called cytokines, all dancing together in synchrony to maintain health. Every moment, the body is exposed to billions of microbes living on the skin, in the mouth, in the digestive tract, and on everything we touch. Microbes that coexist with humans and animals are called symbionts – organisms that have developed a mutually beneficial relationship with our body and are considered to be part of the body's normal flora. The immune system recognizes organisms that aren't part of a person's microbiome, the ones that "don't belong" in or on the body and effectively eliminates them. This process occurs thousands of times per day with little or no fanfare. However, it is not the invasion of external microbes that leads to symptoms known as an infection; it is the compromise of the immune system due to the contamination of the terrain that allows this to occur.

One of the fundamental differences between conventional (allopathic) medical practitioners and those who embrace alternative or integrative medicine lies in their perspectives on the **Germ Theory of Disease**, credited to **Louis Pasteur**, and its impact on health. Discussions about the validity of the Germ Theory often provoke divisiveness and hostility among both medical professionals and laypersons, as it serves as the cornerstone of much of modern medicine.

Pasteur's mechanistic view of disease – matching a specific "cure" (drug) to each germ – laid the foundation for the pharmaceutical industry and its dominance in medical care today. Unfortunately, this premise was accepted to the exclusion of other perspectives, becoming the sole narrative about health and disease. This singular focus has overshadowed alternative approaches that offer a more holistic understanding of the human body and its relationship to illness.

By most mainstream historical accounts, **Louis Pasteur** is regarded as a towering figure in science. His discovery of microbes revolutionized our understanding of disease transmission, laying the groundwork for improved hygiene in hospitals. His work with rabies marked the early days of the study of viruses. Pasteur is also credited with inventing **pasteurization**, a process designed to destroy harmful microbes in food and drink using heat – supposedly without degrading their quality. However, the broader implications of pasteurization remain a contentious topic, deserving a deeper discussion at another time.

Rewriting history is a monumental task, especially when critically assessing figures like Pasteur. However, an alternative view of disease challenges Pasteur's 150-year-old premise: Health is determined by the condition of the body's "terrain" or "soil," the interacting cells. Only when the terrain is disrupted can invasive pathogens take hold.

The debate between the germ theory and the terrain theory has been central to medical history. While many prominent figures in the late 1800s and early 1900s contributed to this discussion, the most vocal were Pasteur and his contemporaries, Claude Bernard and Antoine de Béchamp. Bernard, a physiologist regarded as the Father of Experimental Medicine, famously declared, "The terrain is everything; the germ is nothing," sparking a debate that persists to this day.

What is little known about germ theory is that Pasteur himself had doubts about his own conclusions. Throughout his career, Pasteur and Claude Bernard frequently debated whether germs caused disease or whether the body's resistance was more crucial. Pasteur emphasized the microbe, while Bernard focused on the environment – the terrain – and the body's ability to maintain balance. On his deathbed, Pasteur is said to have acknowledged Bernard's view: *"Bernard avait raison. Le germe n'est rien, c'est le terrain qui est tout."* ("Bernard was right. The germ is nothing, the soil is everything.") Yet, by then, the germ theory had become so entrenched and profitable that modern medicine dismissed Pasteur's final confession as the ramblings of a dying man.

It bears repeating: The money is in the medicine – not the cure.

Bernard's view was that disease is an "inside-out job." He argued that when the body's physiological functions are disrupted by the toxicities prevalent in industrialized societies – vaccines, chemicals, heavy metals, preservatives, processed food, and more – disease follows. As the body's acid-base balance shifts toward acidity, healthy tissue becomes compromised. Intracellular acidity impairs the cell's ability to utilize oxygen, leading to enzyme dysfunction and the accumulation of cellular waste.

For those in the medical field, this disruption affects critical systems like the Krebs cycle and the cytochrome P450 system in the liver, both of which operate less efficiently in an acidic environment. According to Bernard, when cells begin to die, disease begins. This concept is supported by Guyton's *Textbook of Medical Physiology*, which states that one of the key factors in maintaining health is normalizing pH or balancing the acid-alkaline ratio. When cells become acidic, homeostasis is disrupted, and nearly all body functions are affected.

Once the body's defenses are compromised, pathogens can find a favorable environment in which to thrive. Contrary to popular belief, germs are attracted to diseased tissues – they are not the primary cause of disease. Dr. Rudolph Virchow, known as the Father of Modern Pathology, supported this idea: "If I could live my life over again, I would devote it to proving that germs seek their natural habitat – diseased tissue – rather than being the cause of the diseased tissue; in other words, mosquitoes seek stagnant water, but do not cause the pool to become stagnant." Symptoms commonly associated with the flu or pneumonia – fever, chills, cough, and excess mucus – are actually secondary illnesses. The initial "illness" is the loss of health in the underlying tissues.

If everything on planet Earth is here for a reason and for a stated purpose, it may be that microbes are here to trigger the body's highly reactive inflammatory response – essentially a modified cytokine storm – helping to detoxify. It would be interesting to test the secretions expelled during a bout of "the flu" for chemicals and heavy metals. Rather than being the problem, viruses and bacteria might actually be part of the solution, acting as the "clean-up crew" to help clear the body of toxins such as chemicals, pharmaceutical drugs, metals such as aluminum, mercury, cadmium, and other environmental pollutants. It's important to recognize that humanity evolved because of the relationship with microbes, not despite them.

For example, if a person reportedly died from pneumonia, it's possible the body was trying to expel a large amount of chemical-laden mucus. If the person was too immunologically weak to mount an adequate response or if their lymphatic system was too congested to clear the accumulated toxins – and more chemicals were introduced during the acute episode, such as antibiotics, anti-inflammatories, and steroids – the body might become overwhelmed, leading to death. The death was attributed to the microbe, but the real cause could be the person's inability to detoxify. This is a completely novel perspective that would require a massive paradigm shift to accept, but it's certainly worth considering.

People who are rarely sick may have lower levels of toxicity in their bodies, perhaps because they eat mostly organic food, avoid refined foods, don't smoke or drink alcohol, and stay hydrated with fresh, filtered water. They may undertake frequent, rigorous exercise, do daily saunas, use red light therapy, and take high quality supplements to strengthen their body's ability to eliminate environmental toxins. In cases of faulty detoxification, "toxic overload" can occur. Microbes might actually play a helpful role by "inflaming" the system and clearing out accumulated waste. An episode of "the flu," with symptoms such as a productive cough, diarrhea, and nasal drainage, could be the body's way of cleaning out the internal dross.

Supporting the body through this elimination process with herbs, vitamin D, C, and A, and perhaps homeopathy and Chinese medicine rather than suppressing symptoms with conventional Western treatments, may hold the key to health and longevity.

OSTEOPATHIC MEDICINE

One of the systems of medicine that is parallel with, but separate from, conventional medicine, is osteopathic medicine. Founded by Dr. Andrew Taylor Still, the son of a Methodist minister, osteopathy emphasizes the body's self-healing capacity. Dr. Still earned his medical degree from the College of Physicians and Surgeons in Kansas City, Kansas, in 1870. In the early years of his career, Dr. Still served as a state legislator and achieved the rank of major during the Civil War. However, after the war, he grew increasingly disillusioned with the medical practices of the time, such as bloodletting, blistering, and the use of toxic substances such as mercury, antimony, arsenic, and other purgatives, which were believed to act as "tonics." These treatments caused more harm than good, resulting in many fatalities. In contrast, Dr. Still believed that instead of poisoning the body, the primary role of the physician was to facilitate the body's inherent ability to heal itself.

Although Dr. Still's intent was to improve the existing medical system, not to create a new one, his ideas were met with strong opposition from his peers. The American Medical Association (AMA), founded in 1847, had little tolerance for therapies that didn't rely on drugs and chemicals. The AMA's original charter outlined three main goals:

1. The establishment of medical licensing laws to limit the number of physicians in each state, thereby reducing competition and ensuring a more "stable economic climate."
2. The dismantling of existing medical schools in favor of fewer, non-profit institutions that would train a "smaller and more select student body."

3. The elimination of "heterodox medical sects," which included homeopathy, Chinese medicine, herbology, and other alternative practices.

In essence, the AMA was formed to eliminate competing medical philosophies. Although less overt in its tactics, little has changed in this regard to the present day.[254]

Nonetheless, he was convinced that his theories of health and healing were in the best interest of patients. Armed with a deep understanding of human anatomy and physiology, Dr. Still founded the Kirksville College of Osteopathic Medicine in 1874 based on five foundational tenets 1) the body is a unit; 2) the person is a unit of body, mind, and spirit; 3) the body is capable of self-regulation, self-healing and health maintenance; 4) structure and function are interrelated; and 5) the rule of the artery is supreme.

Osteopathic medicine was designed to support natural healing by identifying and correcting structural abnormalities that could hinder the free flow of blood and lymph. Simple, manual techniques, such as lymphatic drainage, were used with patients to normalize fluid flow, eliminate toxins, and restore health. The core principles of osteopathy – assisting the immune system and facilitating the body's healing processes – remain relevant but are often underutilized. This approach to healthcare should be considered mainstream, not "alternative" medicine.

Investigating methods to restore health is rarely a focus for researchers. For instance, the large number of people who have been exposed to others with influenza symptoms but either didn't get sick or fully recovered have received little attention. In our fear-driven, drug-focused society, the emphasis is placed on the death rate, not the survival rate. This small shift in focus alters the entire narrative. For example, when discussing smallpox, the death rate was relentlessly highlighted to be a staggering 30 percent, while the 70 percent survival rate was seldom mentioned. The same can be said for the hysteria surrounding bird flu.

If 30 children are in a classroom and five become ill, such as with strep throat or a cold, what is it about the innate health of the other 25 that allows them to remain well? Shouldn't we be studying those who are healthy rather than focusing solely on those who are ill? What is it about the immune systems of those who stay healthy during outbreaks that, if identified, could be replicated in others to create a healthier world?

In the end, THAT discovery would be true science.

But it's unlikely to happen any time soon. The money lies in ongoing treatments, not cures, or even in promoting health itself. This concept was highlighted by Goldman Sachs when analyzing Gilead Sciences' decline in revenues – from $12.5 billion in 2015 to $4 billion in 2018 – from the sale of direct-acting antivirals (DAAs) for hepatitis C. These drugs boast a cure rate of over 90%, short treatment durations, and minimal side effects. In April 2018, analysts from Goldman Sachs raised the provocative question, "Is curing patients a sustainable business model?" Analyst Salveen Richter wrote in a report to clients, "While this proposition [gene therapy] carries tremendous value for patients and society, it could represent a challenge for genome medicine developers looking for sustained cash flow."[255]

GETTING INVOLVED

Pharmaceutical, chemical, and agribusiness companies, along with Big Gas and Big Oil, are not truly separate industries. Instead, they operate more like "sister enterprises," collaborating for mutual benefit, power, and profit. These industries act as synergists, generating massive wealth by creating drugs to address health problems that often stem from their own products. The intricate connection between these industry giants is both deliberate and masterful. Here's one intricate example:

The pharmaceutical company AstraZeneca was created through a merger between UK-based Zeneca, a major producer of industrial chemicals and pesticides, and the Swedish drug giant Astra. In 1997, the year before the merger, Zeneca reported total sales of $8.62 billion, with 49% stemming from pesticides and industrial chemicals and another 49% from pharmaceuticals – primarily cancer treatments.

Notably, Zeneca's pesticide acetochlor was linked to several cancers, including lung, skin (melanoma), pancreatic, and **breast cancers**. The pesticide was licensed in the US through a co-registration agreement with Monsanto. In 1994, the Environmental Working Group highlighted that multiple herbicides in the triazine family – atrazine, simazine, and cyanazine – had been repeatedly shown in studies involving female rats to cause **breast cancer,** with evidence suggesting a similar increased risk in women. The primary manufacturer of atrazine and simazine is **Syngenta**, a company formed through the merger of Novartis' agribusiness division and Zeneca's agrochemical division. Interestingly, two drugs are produced by Novartis Oncology – Femara, used to treat **breast cancer,** and Zometa, used to treat **breast cancer** that has spread (metastasized) to the bones.

In 1985, when still owned by Imperial Chemical Industries, **Zeneca** founded **National Breast Cancer Awareness Month**, a campaign that has since become synonymous with pink ribbons and events like "Run for the Cure." After the merger that created AstraZeneca, the company continued its significant role in shaping the campaign, funding materials such as leaflets, posters, and ribbons. AstraZeneca also held the original patent for **tamoxifen,** a drug widely prescribed to prevent breast cancer recurrence. However, tamoxifen is a known carcinogen. It has been linked to an increased risk of two types of cancer: endometrial cancer, which develops in the lining of the uterus, and uterine sarcoma, which arises in the uterine muscle. According to the NIH and The Cancer Information Network, women taking tamoxifen are twice as likely to develop uterine cancer compared to those taking a placebo. Despite these risks, the drug remains a cornerstone of **breast cancer treatment,** underscoring the complexities and contradictions of the industry's approach to health care. **Adriamycin,** a drug commonly used to treat endometrial cancer, is manufactured by Pharmacia, Inc., a former owner of **Monsanto,** the company behind **Agent Orange.** Similarly, **Syngenta's Bt 176™** technology was first introduced to genetically modify (GM) corn and has since been applied to modify thirteen different fruits and vegetables. Despite the widespread presence of GM foods, independent research into their potential health risks remains sparse.

Animals, however, appear to sense something humans overlook. During their annual migration, geese in Illinois avoided consuming rows of soybeans planted with Monsanto's GM soya. In 1999, *The Washington Post* reported that rodents refused to eat GM tomatoes. When researchers force-fed the tomatoes to the animals via stomach tubes, 17% died within two weeks. The instinctive behavior of animals might serve as a warning we should heed.[256]

These examples underscore the complex and troubling relationship between agribusiness and pharmaceuticals. The same industries that produce chemicals linked to the development of cancer also manufacture the drugs used to treat the very diseases their products may have helped cause.

WHAT YOU CAN DO

After coming this far, exposing the international plans for global compliance with "pandemic preparedness," the question becomes, what can be done? What can I do? For those encountering this information for the first time, it's natural to feel a mix of anger, frustration, and even helplessness.

My suggestion is to get involved. Choose an issue discussed in this book – one that resonates with you – whether it's stopping mandatory vaccination, educating friends and family about vaccine ingredients, advocating to repeal the PREP Act, or helping the vaccine-injured recover. You don't have to tackle everything at once, so pick one cause that speaks to your heart and dedicate yourself to it. Commit to it for six months, and if it still matters to you after that time, continue. If not, choose a new focus, roll up your sleeves, and dive in.

For every issue, there are organizations tirelessly working to combat corporate greed and demand greater accountability. These groups need your financial support, but even more, they need your time. They need you to spread the word, stuff envelopes, distribute flyers, make phone calls, and petition Congress. In fact, Congress must be pressured by concerned citizens to fund and overhaul the **CICP program**, making it fair, fast, and accessible to compensate the millions injured by the COVID-19 shot or other countermeasures like remdesivir or PCR nasal swabs.

On a personal level, start eliminating as much toxicity from your life as possible. By improving your overall health, you'll strengthen your immune system. Clean up your diet by minimizing, or ideally, eliminating, refined white sugar, refined white flour, food additives, and other harmful ingredients. Invest in a good water filtration system. There are many well-written books on these topics – pick one and get started. The key is not which one you choose, but that you simply begin and expand as you have time and money to do so.

Choose a form of healing for yourself and your family outside the Western paradigm, which often relies on chemicals labeled as "drugs" for "medicine." Conventional treatments view illness as an "outside-in" issue, where something external causes the body to become sick. While prescription drugs may be necessary for acute or critical health problems, they are often used inappropriately for chronic conditions as "suppressive medicine." These drugs control or eliminate symptoms but fail to address the root cause of the problem. Health is defined as being well in the absence of medications. Health is *not defined* as the *absence* of symptoms in the *presence* of pharmaceuticals.

Learn the truth about vaccines – they will not protect you and carry serious consequences for everyone who receives even one. Every person who gets vaccinated suffers some level of cellular damage from the injection of foreign substances into the body. The mRNA vaccines, in particular, increase the risk of serious illness. Vaccines are not the solution to bird flu in chickens or cows either; in fact, they only serve to further disrupt the immune systems of these animals. The real solution lies in cleaning up the terrain – in humans and in farm animals.

What is it going to take for you to engage?

- You were methodically stripped of your right to refuse a mandatory medication; your religious exemptions were ignored.
- Dangerous vaccines, funded by the DoD, were forced on you by governments and employers.
- Our food supply has become contaminated and genetically manipulated into commodities that are making you sick.
- Vaccines have never been safe, effective, or protective.
- The PREP Act has given Big Pharma jaw-dropping protections and they have no incentive to make a time-consumingly safe product. Their mRNA products will make us sick or kill us.
- Animals – the cornerstone of our food supply – are being killed mercilessly for profit.

There are 330 million Americans across this great land, yet only about 1,000 politicians and bureaucrats in Washington, D.C. They are our employees, we pay their salaries, but they give themselves outrageous raises and benefit packages without our consent – raises we can't afford. And with the hundreds of thousands of government workers, what are they really doing? What value are they adding for this country or for you personally? They are stealing from our nation and giving us orders. We should be marching in the streets, demanding accountability, and firing them all.

WHERE IS YOUR OUTRAGE?

For those seriously harmed by any vaccine, especially the COVID-19 jab, unite and raise your voices together, demanding answers and restitution. Join React19 or other activist groups committed to seeking justice. Demand that Congress take action to rectify these flawed programs and return to the original intent of the 1986 Injury Compensation Act: providing non-litigious, full compensation for all medical bills resulting from the injection of the experimental, non-approved COVID-19 gene therapy bioweapon.

You were lied to; they need to pay.

Speaking out does not mean you are a zealot or a fanatic. George Washington, Thomas Jefferson, and Patrick Henry were all labeled as extremists and radicals by agents of the British Crown. If your friends call you such, you are in good company. We must make our voices heard. Our "representatives" must stop wasting our money on toxic and ineffective vaccines, stockpiling worthless drugs, and granting drug companies, chemical companies, and agribusinesses complete liability protection for their harmful products and practices. It is crucial for citizens worldwide to unite and put an end to the devastation of our planet and its inhabitants, caused by the combined effects of global businesses and war.

We must stop GAVI's lavish yearly spending to eradicate the last traces of polio in remote, war-torn villages. Those global funds should be directed toward buying books for education, building safe homes, promoting hygiene, providing non-genetically modified grain to farmers, offering electricity, providing adequate food, and digging wells for clean water.

By reallocating time and resources to projects that directly improve the lives of the world's poorest populations, we can create lasting, positive change. Helping clean up the planet and protecting personal rights is crucial. If we don't act now, the next pandemic could be the first of many more to come.

You can continue to sit on the sidelines, or you can choose to make a difference. The time for complacency has passed – each of us must step outside our comfort zones and get involved. Unlike the Puritans and Pilgrims, who left a society they could no longer tolerate, we have no place to escape as the Earth's basic resources – soil, water, food, air, our children – become irreparably contaminated. What is happening is both a physical and spiritual battle. What is happening is both a temporal and spiritual battle. We must clean up the planet, protect our food supply, restore our health, and return to God. We must stop relying on drugs as "health" and vaccines as "help."

If you are anti-vaccine, wear the label proudly. It signifies that you are informed, capable of critical thinking, and willing to question the *status quo*. It means you care about the well-being of children and do not support harming them by injecting them with toxic chemicals and foreign matter repeatedly during the first year of their lives. In contrast, being pro-vaccine often means blindly following the prevailing narrative without considering the potential risks and consequences.

The time is **now** and the urgency is **real** – but not for the reasons you are being told.

ACRONYMS AND ABBREVIATIONS

5G	Fifth Generation
AAFP	American Academy of Family Practice
AGES	Austrian Agency for Health and Food Safety
ALV	Avian Leukosis Virus
APHIS	Animal and Plant Health Inspection Service
ARRA	American Recovery and Reinvestment Act
ASPR	Administration for Strategic Preparedness and Response
BARDA	Biomedical Advanced Research and Development Authority
BSE	Bovine Spongiform Encephalopathy
BVDV	Bovine Diarrheal Virus
CBER	Center for Biologics Evaluation and Research
CDC	Centers for Disease Control and Prevention
CDFW	California Department of Fish and Wildlife
CEO	Chief Executive Officer
CHIP	Children's Health Insurance Program
CICP	Countermeasures Injury Compensation Program
CIDRAP	Center for Infectious Disease Research and Policy
CJD	Creutzfeldt-Jakob Disease
CMS	Centers for Medicare and Medicaid Services
CMV	Cytomegalovirus
COVID	Coronavirus Disease

COVID-19	Coronavirus Disease-19
CQM	Clinical Quality Measures
CSL	Commonwealth Serum Laboratories
DAA	Direct-Acting Antivirals
DHS	Department of Homeland Security
DHHS/HHS	Department of Health and Human Services
DNA	Deoxyribose Nucleic Acid
DoD	Department of Defense
DTaP	Diphtheria, Tetanus, and acellular Pertussis
DTP	Diphtheria, Tetanus, and Pertussis
DTwP	Diphtheria, Tetanus, and whole cell Pertussis
EAV	Endogenous Avian Retrovirus
EMA	European Medicines Agency
EMF	Electromagnetic Frequency
EO	Executive Order
EPA	Environmental Protection Agency
ER	Emergency Room
EU	European Union
EUA	Emergency Use Authorization
FAERS	FDA Adverse Event Reporting System
FAO	Food and Agriculture Organization of the United Nations
FAR	Federal Acquisition Regulation
FDA	Food and Drug Administration
FDAAA	Food and Drug Administration Amendments Act
FOIA	Freedom of Information Act
FOX	Fox Broadcasting Company
GAVI	Global Alliance for Vaccines and Immunization
GBS	Guillain-Barré Syndrome
GDP	Gross Domestic Product
GIVS	Global Immunization Vision and Strategy
GNI	Gross National Income

GSK	GlaxoSmithKline
GVAP	Global Vaccine Action Plan
H1N1	Hemagglutinin (H1) Neuraminidase (N1) subtype of avian influenza A
H2N2	Hemagglutinin (H2) Neuraminidase (N2) subtype of avian influenza A
H3N2	Hemagglutinin (H3) Neuraminidase (N2) subtype of avian influenza A
H3N8	Hemagglutinin (H3) Neuraminidase (N8) subtype of avian influenza A
H5N1	Hemagglutinin (H5) Neuraminidase (N1) subtype of avian influenza A
H5N2	Hemagglutinin (H5) Neuraminidase (N2) subtype of avian influenza A
H5N6	Hemagglutinin (H5) Neuraminidase (N6) subtype of avian influenza A
H6N1	Hemagglutinin (H6) Neuraminidase (N1) subtype of avian influenza A
H6N4	Hemagglutinin (H6) Neuraminidase (N4) subtype of avian influenza A
H7N2	Hemagglutinin (H7) Neuraminidase (N2) subtype of avian influenza A
H7N3	Hemagglutinin (H7) Neuraminidase (N3) subtype of avian influenza A
H7N4	Hemagglutinin (H7) Neuraminidase (N4) subtype of avian influenza A
H7N7	Hemagglutinin (H7) Neuraminidase (N7) subtype of avian influenza A
H9N2	Hemagglutinin (H9) Neuraminidase (N2) subtype of avian influenza A
H10N3	Hemagglutinin (H10) Neuraminidase (N3) subtype of avian influenza A

HA	Hyaluronic Acid
HAV	Hepatitis A Virus
HBV	Hepatitis B Virus
HCSO	Health Communication Science Office
HCV	Hepatitis C Virus
HEW	Health, Education and Welfare Office
HGV	Hepatitis G Virus
HIPAA	Health Insurance Portability and Accountability Act
HIV/AIDS	Human Immunodeficiency Virus/ Acquired Immunodeficiency Syndrome
HPAI	Highly Pathogenic Avian Influenza
HRSA	Health Resources and Services Administration
IBV	Infectious Bronchitis Virus
ICU	Intensive Care Unit
IFF	International Finance Facility
IFFIm	International Finance Facility for Immunisation
IIS	Immunization Information System
ILI	Influenza-Like Illness
ISCOM	Immune-stimulating complexes
LNP	Lipid Nanoparticle
M1	Matrix Protein 1
M2	Matrix Protein 2
MD	Medical Doctor
MDCK	Madin-Darby Canine Kidney
MERS	Middle East Respiratory Syndrome
MHS	Marine Hospital Service
MIPS	Merit-based Incentive Payment System
MMA	Medicare Modernization Act
MRC	Medical Research Council
MS	Multiple Sclerosis
MSEHPA	Model State Emergency Health Powers Act
MU	Meaningful Use

NA	Not Applicable
NAPAPI	North American Plan for Animal and Pandemic Influenza
NBC	National Broadcasting Corporation
NCHS	National Center for Health Statistics
NCIRD	National Center for Immunization and Respiratory Diseases
NCVIA	National Childhood Vaccine Injury Act
NEP	Nuclear Export Protein
NGO	Non-governmental Organization
NIAID	National Institute of Allergy and Infectious Disease
NIBSC	National Institute of Biological Standards and Control
NIC	National Influenza Center
NIH	National Institutes of Health
NIP	National Immunization Program
NNT	Number Needed to Treat
NNV	Number Needed to be Vaccinated
NVIC	National Vaccine Information Center
NVICP	National Vaccine Injury Compensation Program
ODPHP	Office of Disease Prevention and Health Promotion
OIE	Office International des Epizooties
OTA	Other Transaction Agreements
OTC	Over The Counter
PAHPA	Pandemic and All-Hazards Preparedness Act
PCR	Polymerase Chain Reaction
PEG	Polyethylene Glycol
PhD	Doctor of Philosophy
PHMPT	Public Health and Medical Professionals for Transparency
PHS	Public Health Service
PPN	Partial Parenteral Nutrition
PREP	Public Readiness and Emergency Preparedness Act

RCT	Randomized Controlled Trial
RNA	Ribonucleic Acid
RRPV	Rapid Response Partnership Vehicle
RSV	Respiratory Syncytial Virus
RSV	Rous Sarcoma Virus
SARS	Severe Acute Respiratory Syndrome
SARSCo-V2	Severe Acute Respiratory Syndrome Co-Variant 2
SDOH	Social Determinants of Health
SPF	Specific Pathogen-Free
SSA	Social Security Administration
SV40	Simian Virus 40
TPN	Total Parenteral Nutrition
TSE	Transmissible Spongiform Encephalopathy
TV	Television
UK	United Kingdom
UN	United Nations
UNICEF	United Nations International Children's Emergency Fund
US	United States
USDA	United States Department of Agriculture
WEF	World Economic Forum
WHO	World Health Organization
WI	Wistar Institute
WOAH	World Organization for Animal Health
WONDER	Wide-Ranging Online Data for Epidemiologic Research
WSP	World Sanitation Program
WWI	World War 1
VAERS	Vaccine Adverse Event Reporting System
VITT	Vaccine-Induced Immune Thrombotic Thrombocytopenia

REFERENCES

FOREWORD

1. Duesberg, P. Inventing the AIDS Virus, Gateway Books, 2016.
2. Bookchin D, Schumacher J. The virus and the vaccine: The true story of a cancer-causing monkey virus, contaminated polio vaccine, and the millions of Americans exposed. New York: St. Martin's Press; 2004.
3. Humphries, Suzanne, and Ronald Bystrianyk. Dissolving Illusions: 10th Anniversary Edition, Chapter 4, "Menagerie Roulette," 2024.

CHAPTER 1

4. The Bodyguard. Stanford Medicine Magazine, Stanford University School of Medicine, Summer 2011. Available from: https://sm.stanford.edu/archive/stanmed/2011summer/article7.html
5. Humphries, Suzanne. Vaccination and Renal Patients: A Critical Examination of Assumed Safety and Effectiveness. 2015. Available from: https://drsuzanne.net/2015/03/vaccination-and-renal-patients-a-critical-examination-of-assumed-safety-and-effectiveness-suzanne-humphries-md/.
6. Paul, J. R. History of Poliomyelitis. Yale UP, 1971.
7. Humphries, Suzanne, and Ronald Bystrianyk. Dissolving Illusions: 10th Anniversary Edition Companion and Reference Book, "Menagerie Roulette," 2024.
8. Morens, David M., Jeffrey K. Taubenberger, and Anthony S. Fauci. "Rethinking Next-Generation Vaccines for Coronaviruses, Influenza Viruses, and Other Respiratory Viruses." Cell Host & Microbe, vol. 31, no. 1, 2023, pp. 146–157, https://doi.org/10.1016/j.chom.2022.11.016.

9. Chen, H., et al. "Avian Flu: H5N1 Virus Outbreak in Migratory Waterfowl." *Semantic Scholar*, 2005. Available from: https://www.semanticscholar.org/paper/Avian-flu%3A-H5N1-virus-outbreak-in-migratory-Chen-Smith/fabc850efb3227541ea7b9b85974224e5adc01a1.

10. **Reuters**. "Chile Detects First Case of Bird Flu in a Human." *Reuters*, 30 Mar. 2023. Available from: https://www.reuters.com/world/americas/chile-detects-first-case-bird-flu-human-2023-03-29/.

11. **CDFW News** | Avian Influenza Detected in Deceased Mountain Lions. California Department of Fish and Wildlife. Available from: https://wildlife.ca.gov/News/Archive/avian-influenza-detected-in-deceased-mountain-lions.

CHAPTER 2

12. Chapman, J., and J. Arnold. "Reye Syndrome." *NCBI Bookshelf*, 2020. Available from: https://www.ncbi.nlm.nih.gov/books/NBK526101/.

13. Ku, A. S., and L. T. Chan. "The First Case of H5N1 Avian Influenza Infection in a Human with Complications of Adult Respiratory Distress Syndrome and Reye's Syndrome." *Journal of Paediatrics and Child Health*, vol. 35, no. 2, Apr. 1999, pp. 207–209. Available from: https://onlinelibrary.wiley.com/doi/abs/10.1046/j.1440-1754.1999.t01-1-00329.x.

14. de Jong MD, Hien TT. "Avian Influenza A (H5N1)." *J Clin Virol.*, Jan. 2006, vol. 35, no. 1, pp. 2-13, doi: 10.1016/j.jcv.2005.09.002. Epub 2005 Oct 6. PMID: 16213784; PMCID: PMC7108344. Available from: https://www.ncbi.nlm.nih.gov/pmc/articles/PMC7108344/.

15. "Influenza (Flu)." Centers for Disease Control and Prevention, 2024, Available from: https://www.cdc.gov/Flu/Index.htm.

16. "H5N1 Bird Flu: Current Situation." Avian Influenza (Bird Flu), Centers for Disease Control and Prevention, 12 July 2024. Available from: https://www.cdc.gov/bird-flu/situation-summary/index.html.

17. **Centers for Disease Control and Prevention.** "President's Budget FY 2023." 2023. Available from: https://www.cdc.gov/budget/documents/fy2023/FY-2023-CDC-Budget-Detail.pdf.

18. Nowak, G., and National Immunization Program. "Planning for the 2004-05 Influenza Vaccination Season: A Communication Situation Analysis." Children's Health Defense, 2004. Available from: https://childrenshealthdefense.org/wp-content/uploads/2004_flu_nowak.pdf.

19. "Misinformation: Seeing Is Believing." *EurekAlert!*, 17 May 2005. Available from: https://www.eurekalert.org/news-releases/741586.

20. Begley, Sharon. "People Believe a 'Fact' That Fits Their Views Even If It's Clearly False." *Science Journal*, p. B1, 2005. Available from: http://www.honolulutraffic.com/WSJ020404.pdf.

CHAPTER 3

21. Koehler CSW. Epidemics and wars. Condensed from "Camp followers." J Mod Drug Discov. 2001. Available from: https://pubsapp.acs.org:6443/subscribe/journals/mdd/v04/i04/html/MDD04DeptTimeline.html

22. Billings M. The influenza pandemic of 1918. Stanford (CA): Stanford University; June 1997. Available from: https://virus.stanford.edu/uda/

23. Rivers TM, The Rockefeller Institute for Medical Research. Viruses and Koch's postulates. J Bacteriol. 1936;33(1). Available from:https://www.ncbi.nlm.nih.gov/pmc/articles/PMC545348/pdf/jbacter00773-0005.pdf

24. Walker, Larry et al. "Koch's postulates and infectious proteins." Acta neuropathologica vol. 112,1 (2006): 1-4. doi:10.1007/s00401-006-0072-x. Available from: https://pubmed.ncbi.nlm.nih.gov/16703338/

25. De Gascun C, Carr M, Hall W. Influenza viruses. In: Infectious Disease. 3rd ed. St. Louis: Mosby Press; 2010:1590. Available from: https://www.sciencedirect.com/sdfe/pdf/download/eid/3-s2.0-B9780323045797001611/first-page-pdf

26. Gwartney A. Home. Virology Blog. 2023 Aug 1. Available from: https://virology.ws/

27. Kuhn JH. Virus taxonomy. In: Elsevier eBooks. 2021:28-37. doi: 10.1016/b978-0-12-809633-8.21231-4. Available from: https://www.ncbi.nlm.nih.gov/pmc/articles/PMC7157452

28. Jones RaC. Global plant virus disease pandemics and epidemics. Plants. 2021;10(2):233. doi: 10.3390/plants10020233. Available from: https://www.ncbi.nlm.nih.gov/pmc/articles/PMC7911862

29. **FA180/FA180**: Viral nervous necrosis (Betanodavirus) infections in fish. Ask IFAS - Powered by EDIS. Available from: https://edis.ifas.ufl.edu/publication/FA180

CHAPTER 4

30. Taxonomy. Taxonomy browser (root). Available from: https://www.ncbi.nlm.nih.gov/Taxonomy/Browser/wwwtax.cgi

31. Davison S, Laboratory of Avian Medicine and Pathology, Penn Vet. Testimony to the House Agriculture and Rural Affairs Committee informational meeting on highly pathogenic avian influenza outbreak. 2015. Available from: https://pasenategop.com/aument/wp-content/uploads/sites/69/2015/06/AI-Testimony.pdf

32. **BBC News | ASIA-PACIFIC.** Bird flu hits Hong Kong. BBC News. Available from: http://news.bbc.co.uk/2/hi/asia-pacific/1334053.stm

33. Lee C, Swayne DE, Linares JA, Senne DA, Suarez DL. H5N2 avian influenza outbreak in Texas in 2004: the first highly pathogenic strain in the United States in 20 years? J Virol. 2005;79(17):11412-11421. doi: 10.1128/jvi.79.17.11412-11421.2005. Available from: https://www.ncbi.nlm.nih.gov/pmc/articles/PMC1193578/

34. Hundreds of thousands of chickens killed. UPI. 2004 Mar 7. Available from: https://www.upi.com/Archives/2004/03/07/Hundreds-of-thousands-of-chickens-killed/6678001303465/

35. Lederman Z. One Health and culling as a public health measure. Public Health Ethics. 2016 Apr;9(1):5-23. doi: 10.1093/phe/phw008. Available from: https://academic.oup.com/phe/article-abstract/9/1/5/2362775?redirectedFrom=fulltex

36. HPAI detections in mammals. USDA-APHIS. Available from: https://www.aphis.usda.gov/livestock-poultry-disease/avian/avian-influenza/hpai-detections/mammals

37. Taubenberger J, Reid AH, Lourens RM, et al. Characterization of the 1918 influenza virus polymerase genes. Nature. 2005;437(7056):889-893. doi: 10.1038/nature04230.

38. Tumpey TM, Basler CF, Aguilar PV, et al. Characterization of the reconstructed 1918 Spanish influenza pandemic virus. Science. 2005;310(5745):77-80. doi: 10.1126/science.1119392.

CHAPTER 5

39. Starko KM. Salicylates and pandemic influenza mortality, 1918–1919: pharmacology, pathology, and historic evidence. Clin Infect Dis. 2009 Nov 15;49(9):1405-1410. doi: 10.1086/605559.

40. Shanks GD. How World War 1 changed global attitudes to war and infectious diseases. Lancet. 2014;384(9955):1699-1707. doi: 10.1016/s0140-6736(14)61786-4.

CHAPTER 6

41. Gleason S. FBI, CDC investigating several vials labeled 'smallpox' found at vaccine research facility. USA Today. 2021 Nov 17. Available from: https://www.usatoday.com/story/news/health/2021/11/17/smallpox-vials-found-philadelphia/8649685002/

42. **Fox News.** Dr. Deborah Birx says she "knew" COVID vaccines would not "protect against infection." Fox News. 2022 Jul 22. Available from: https://www.foxnews.com/media/dr-deborah-birx-knew-covid-vaccines-not-protect-against-infection

43. Schmeck H. US calls flu alert on possible return of epidemic virus. The New York Times. 1976 Feb 20;69.

44. Jones C. Trump-appointed judges revive lawsuit against L.A. schools' COVID vaccine mandate. CalMatters. 2024 Jun 11. Available from: https://calmatters.org/education/2024/06/covid-vaccine-mandate-schools/

45. Maria Zeee: Part 1 -- Top ten media blackout stories | Part 2 -- Dr. David E Martin. BitChute. Available from: https://www.bitchute.com/video/itEyieCiJpuG/

46. **Swine Flu Act**. Pub. L. 94-380; 42 U.S.C. 247b(j)-(l). 1976.

47. Neustadt RE, Fineberg HV. The Swine Flu Affair: Decision-making on a Slippery Disease. DHEW; 1978. Available from: LSU Law Center's Medical and Public Health Law Site, https://biotech.law.lsu.edu/cphl/history/books/sw/

48. **Swine Flu Vaccine Injury Compensation** - Unthank v. United States, 732 F.2d 1517 (10th Cir). Available from: http://biotech.law.lsu.edu/cases/vaccines/Unthank.htm

49. One Hundred Heroes and Icons of the 20th Century. Time Magazine. 1999 Jun 14.

50. **Working Group on Civilian Biodefense.** Smallpox as a biological weapon: Medical and public health management. JAMA. 1999;281:2127-2137.

51. Beigel JH. Avian influenza A(H5N1) infection in humans. N Engl J Med. 2005; 353:1374-1385.

52. Ungchusak K, et al. Probable person-to-person transmission of avian influenza A (H5N1). N Engl J Med. 2005;352:333-340.

53. **Johns Hopkins Center for Health Security.** Tabletop Exercises. Available from: https://centerforhealthsecurity.org/our-work/tabletop-exercises

54. Mack T. A different view of smallpox and vaccination. N Engl J Med. 2003;348(5):460-463. doi: 10.1056/nejmsb022994. Available from: https://www.nejm.org/doi/full/10.1056/NEJMsb022994

55. Roos R. Relatives of avian flu patients have asymptomatic cases. CIDRAP News. 2005 Mar 9.

56. Del Giudice G, Podda A, Rappuoli R. What are the limits of adjuvanticity? Vaccine. 2001;20:S38-S41. Available from: http://www.gphealth.org/covid-19-resources/covid-19-antigen-test/

57. **National Academies of Sciences, Engineering, and Medicine.** The Smallpox Vaccination Program: Public Health in an Age of Terrorism. Washington, DC: The National Academies Press; 2005. Available from: https://nap.nationalacademies.org/read/11240/chapter/1

CHAPTER 7

58. **Smallpox 2002:** *Silent Weapon. IMDb. Available from:* https://www.imdb.com/title/tt0320482/

59. **American Lung Association.** *Trends in lung disease: A report of the American Lung Association. [Internet]. American Lung Association; 2024 [cited 2024 Dec 3]. Available from:* https://www.lung.org/getmedia/98f088b5-3fd7-4c43-a490-ba8f4747bd4d/pi-trend-reportpdf

60. **Massachusetts Institute of Technology.** *The Impact of Technological Change on Industry and Society. [Internet]. Cambridge (MA): Massachusetts Institute of Technology; 2013 [cited 2024 Dec 3]. Available from:* https://dspace.mit.edu/handle/1721.1/69811

61. **Statista.** *COVID-19, pneumonia, and influenza deaths reported in U.S. 2023. Statista. 2023 Aug 22. Available from:* https://www.statista.com/statistics/1113051/number-reported-deaths-from-covid-pneumonia-and-flu-us/

62. **Notice to Readers:** *Considerations for distinguishing influenza-like illness from inhalational anthrax. MMWR Morb Mortal Wkly Rep. 2001 Nov 9. Available from:* http://www.cdc.gov/mmwr/preview/mmwrhtml/mm5044a5.htm

63. **WebMD.** *Common cold causes. [Internet]. New York (NY): WebMD LLC; [cited 2024 Dec 3]. Available from:* https://www.webmd.com/cold-and-flu/common_cold_causes

64. **Centers for Disease Control and Prevention.** *Human coronavirus types. CDC. Available from:* https://archive.cdc.gov/www_cdc_gov/coronavirus/types.html

65. **Pan American Health Organization (PAHO).** *The health sector's response to the mental health needs of the migrant population in the Americas. [Internet]. Washington (DC): Pan American Health Organization; 2017 [cited 2024 Dec 3]. Available from:* https://www3.paho.org/english/dd/pin/Number22_article1d.htm

66. *Gupta R, Sharma A, Agarwal P, et al. Development of AI-based diagnostic models for predicting disease outcomes in cardiology. Comput Methods Programs Biomed. 2023;241:107648. doi:10.1016/j.cmpb.2023.107648.*

67. *Klein A. Fauci admits to Congress that certain COVID social distancing guidelines lacked scientific basis: 'Sort of just appeared'. New York Post. 2024 Jan 10. Available from:* https://nypost.com/2024/01/10/news/fauci-admits-to-congress-that-certain-covid-social-distancing-guidelines-lacked-scientific-basis-sort-of-just-appeared/

68. **Expose News.** *20 million dead as a result of COVID vaccination, claims report. Expose News. 2022 Oct 1. Available from:* https://expose-news.com/2022/10/01/20milllion-dead-covid-vaccination/

69. *Wu Y, Zhang Q, Liu X, et al. Characterization of the antimicrobial resistance profile of Listeria monocytogenes in food production environments in China. Microorganisms. 2024;12(7):1343. doi:10.3390/microorganisms12071343.*

70. **Public Health Policy Journal.** *A systematic review of autopsy findings in deaths after COVID-19 vaccination. Public Health Policy J. 2023 [cited 2024 Dec 3];Volume(Issue). Available from:* https://publichealthpolicyjournal. com/a-systematic-review-of-autopsy-findings-in-deaths-after-covid-19-vaccination/

71. **U.S. Department of Health and Human Services.** *National Action Plan for Artificial Intelligence and Public Health. [Internet]. Washington (DC): U.S. Department of Health and Human Services; 2021 [cited 2024 Dec 3]. Available from:* https://www.phe.gov/Preparedness/international/Documents/napapi.pdf

72. **United Nations.** *The Pact for the Future: A Transformative Agenda for the United Nations. [Internet]. New York (NY): United Nations; 2024 [cited 2024 Dec 3]. Available from:* https://www.un.org/sites/un2.un.org/files/sotf-the-pact-for-the-future.pdf

CHAPTER 8

73. **U.S. Department of Health and Human Services.** *Press release from Secretary of HHS regarding the avian influenza A (H7N9) virus. [Internet]. Washington (DC): U.S. Department of Health and Human Services; 2024 [cited 2024 Dec 3]. Available from:* https://public-inspection.federalregister.gov/2024-16247.pdf

74. **World Health Organization (WHO).** *New initiative launched to advance mRNA vaccine development against human avian influenza (H5N1). [Internet]. Geneva (Switzerland): World Health Organization; 2024 Jul 29 [cited 2024 Dec 3]. Available from:* https://www.who.int/news/item/29-07-2024-new-initiative-launched-to-advance-mrna-vaccine-development-against-human-avian-influenza-(h5n1)

75. **Reuters.** *Finland to start bird flu vaccinations for humans, in world first. Reuters. 2024 Jun 26. Available from:* https://www.reuters.com/business/healthcare-pharmaceuticals/finland-start-bird-flu-vaccinations-humans-2024-06-25/

76. **U.S. Food and Drug Administration (FDA).** *Package insert for Sanofi Pasteur Influenza Virus Vaccine H5N1. [Internet]. Silver Spring (MD): U.S. Food and Drug Administration; [2007]. [cited 2024 Dec 3]. Available from:* https://www.fda.gov/media/74534/download?attachment

77. **U.S. Food and Drug Administration (FDA).** *Package insert for Influenza A (H5N1) Virus Monovalent Vaccine. [Internet]. Silver Spring (MD): U.S. Food and Drug Administration; [2013]. [cited 2024 Dec 3]. Available from:* https://www.fda.gov/media/87479/download?attachment

78. **U.S. Food and Drug Administration (FDA).** *AUDENZ (Influenza A (H5N1) Monovalent Vaccine) Information. [Internet]. Silver Spring (MD): U.S. Food and Drug Administration; [cited 2024 Dec 3]. Available from:* https://www.fda.gov/vaccines-blood-biologics/audenz

79. **U.S. Food and Drug Administration (FDA).** *FDA Briefing Document: VRBPAC Meeting. October 10, 2024. HPAI (H5) Virus Vaccines. [Internet]. Silver Spring (MD): U.S. Food and Drug Administration; 2024 [cited 2024 Dec 3]. Available from:* https://www.fda.gov/media/182543/download

80. **CIDRAP News.** *HHS awards Moderna $176 million to develop mRNA H5 avian flu vaccine. CIDRAP News. 2024 Jul 2. Available from:* https://www.cidrap.umn.edu/avian-influenza-bird-flu/hhs-awards-moderna-176-million-develop-mrna-h5-avian-flu-vaccine

CHAPTER 9

81. **Antiviral Drugs Advisory Committee.** *Relenza (Zanamivir for inhalation) GlaxoWelcome Incorporated, for the Treatment of Influenza A and B. Food and Drug Administration, Center for Drug Evaluation and Research. 1999 Feb 24.*

82. *Willman D. RELENZA: Official Asks If One Day Less of Flu Is Worth It? Los Angeles Times. 2000 Dec 20. Available from:* https://www.latimes.com/nation/la-122001relenza-story.html

83. *Jolson HM. Relenza® (zanamivir for inhalation) for treatment of influenza. Food and Drug Administration, Center for Drug Evaluation and Research. 1998 Oct 26.*

84. *Hayden FG, Treanor JJ, Osterhaus ADME, et al. Use of the oral neuraminidase inhibitor oseltamivir in experimental human influenza randomized controlled trials for prevention and treatment. JAMA. 1999;282(13):1240-1246. doi:10.1001/jama.282.13.1240.*

85. *Hayden FG, Treanor JJ, Schooley RT, et al. Use of the selective oral neuraminidase inhibitor oseltamivir to prevent influenza. JAMA. 1999;341(15):1336-1343. doi:10.1001/jama.1999.30122270085029.*

86. *Kiso M, Iida S, Furusawa I, et al. Resistant influenza A viruses in children treated with oseltamivir: descriptive study. Lancet (London, England). 2004;364(9436):759-765. doi:10.1016/S0140-6736(04)16934-3.*

87. **University of Washington.** *East Asia: No new evidence of Tamiflu-resistant H5N1. [Internet]. Seattle (WA): University of Washington; 2005 Oct 7 [cited 2024 Dec 3].*

88. **U.S. Food and Drug Administration, Center for Drug Evaluation and Research.** *TAMIFLU® 3 (oseltamivir phosphate) information. [Internet]. Silver Spring (MD): U.S. Food and Drug Administration; 2004 Jun 28 [cited 2024 Dec 3]. Available from:* https://www.fda.gov/media/76542/download

89. **CIDRAP News.** *Tamiflu may pose risk of mental side effects. [Internet]. Minneapolis (MN): Center for Infectious Disease Research and Policy, University of Minnesota; [cited 2024 Dec 3]. Available from:* https://www.cidrap.umn.edu/influenza-general/tamiflu-may-pose-risk-mental-side-effects

90. Maxwell SR. *Tamiflu and neuropsychiatric disturbance in adolescents.* BMJ. 2007 Jun 16;334(7606):1232-1233. doi:10.1136/bmj.39131.545708.47.

91. **CIDRAP News.** *FDA panel: Children's deaths unrelated to Tamiflu.* [Internet]. Minneapolis (MN): Center for Infectious Disease Research and Policy, University of Minnesota; 2005 Nov 18 [cited 2024 Dec 3]. Available from: https://www.cidrap. umn.edu/avian-influenza-bird-flu/fda-panel-childrens-deaths-unrelated-tamiflu

92. **DataBridge Market Research.** *Tamiflu Global Market.* [Internet]. Pune (India): DataBridge Market Research; [cited 2024 Dec 31]. Available from: https://www.databridgemarketresearch.com/reports/ global-tamiflu-oseltamivir-phosphate-drugs-market

93. Kaiser LA, Popovich J, Jacobs MR, et al. *Impact of oseltamivir treatment on influenza-related lower respiratory tract complications and hospitalizations.* Arch Intern Med. 2003;163(14):1667-1672. doi:10.1001/archinte.163.14.1667.

94. Gupta YK, Meenu M, Mohan P. *The Tamiflu fiasco and lessons learnt.* Indian J Pharmacol. 2015;47(1):11-16. doi:10.4103/0253-7613.150745.

CHAPTER 10

95. A complete review of the history of vaccination is far beyond the scope of this text. For more information, consider the book Bodily Matters by Nadja Durbach (2005) and the two-volume Tenth Anniversary edition, Dissolving Illusions by Dr. Suzanne Humphries and Roman Bystrianyk (2024). Older books such as Vaccine and Serum Evils by Herbert M. Shelton (1935), The Case Against Vaccination by Dr. Walter Hadwen (1896) and many others written in the 1800s are important and interesting recounts of the early use of the smallpox vaccine may be found at www.Archive.org.

96. **Advisory Committee on Immunization Practices (ACIP).** *Personal transcript of ACIP meeting, Atlanta, Georgia, June 19 and 20, 2002.* [Internet]. Atlanta (GA): Centers for Disease Control and Prevention.

97. **Fierce Pharma.** *The top 10 vaccine companies worldwide.* [Internet]. LinkedIn; 2024 Dec 31 [cited 2024 Dec 3]. Available from: https://www. linkedin.com/posts/fierce-pharma_the-top-10-vaccine-companies-worldwide-activity-6987787759880957953-_Kwe

98. Clabaugh J. *Popular Science crowns FluMist.* Washington Business Journal. 2003 Nov 7. Available from: https://www.bizjournals.com/washington/ stories/2003/11/03/daily36.html

99. Pollack A. *The media business: advertising; anatomy of a failed product introduction: How a nasal spray flu vaccine flopped in the marketplace.* New York Times. 2003 Nov 19. Available from: https://www.nytimes.com/2003/11/19/business/media-business-advertising-anatomy-failed-product-introduction-nasal-spray-flu.html

100. Prabhala A, Alsalhani L. *Pharmaceutical manufacturers across Asia, Africa and Latin America with the technical requirements and quality standards to manufacture mRNA vaccines.* [Internet]. 2021 Dec 10 [cited 2024 Dec 3]. Available from: https://accessibsa.org/mrna/

101. **Human Rights Watch.** *Experts identify 100 plus firms to make COVID-19 mRNA vaccines.* [Internet]. 2021 Dec 15 [cited 2024 Dec 3]. Available from: https://www.hrw.org/news/2021/12/15/experts-identify-100-plus-firms-make-covid-19-mrna-vaccines

102. **The New York Times.** *Coronavirus vaccine tracker.* [Internet]. New York (NY): The New York Times; [cited 2024 Dec 31]. Available from: https://www.nytimes.com/interactive/2020/science/coronavirus-vaccine-tracker.html

103. Cuevas E. *Bird flu vaccine development funds awarded to Moderna amid multistate outbreak.* USA Today. 2024 Jul 3. Available from: https://www.usatoday.com/story/news/health/2024/07/02/moderna-bird-flu-vaccine-outbreak/74277961007/

104. Becker Z. *CSL Seqirus scores $30M government contract to produce and test avian flu vaccine candidate.* Fierce Pharma. 2022 Oct 10. Available from: https://www.fiercepharma.com/pharma/were-machine-csl-seqirus-scores-301-million-barda-contract-test-avian-influenza-vaccine

105. **ClinicalTrials.gov.** *Study to evaluate safety and immunogenicity of different priming and booster regimens with adjuvanted H5N8 and/or H5N6 influenza vaccine in adults.* [Internet]. Bethesda (MD): National Library of Medicine; 2023 Jun 6 [cited 2024 Dec 3]. Available from: https://www.clinicaltrials.gov/study/NCT05874713

106. **CSL Seqirus.** *CSL Seqirus, a proud champion of pandemic preparedness, announces U.S. government award in response to avian influenza.* [Internet]. 2024 May 30 [cited 2024 Dec 3]. Available from: https://www.cslseqirus.us/news/csl-seqirus-announces-us-government-award-in-response-to-avian-influenza

107. **Department of Health and Human Services, Administration for Strategic Preparedness and Response (ASPR).** *Organizational chart.* [Internet]. Washington (DC): U.S. Department of Health and Human Services; [cited 2024 Dec 3]. Available from: https://aspr.hhs.gov/AboutASPR/ProgramOffices/Documents/ASPR-Organizational-Chart.pdf

108. **U.S. Congress.** *Title 42, Chapter 6, Subchapter II, Part B, Funding.* [Internet]. Washington (DC): U.S. Government Publishing Office; [cited 2024 Dec 3]. Available from: https://uscode.house.gov/view.xhtml

109. **Rapid Response Vaccine Platform (RRPV).** *Current members.* [Internet]. [cited 2024 Dec 3]. Available from: https://www.rrpv.org/current-members/

110. **Rapid Response Partnership Vehicle (RRPV).** *OTA. [Internet]. [cited 2024 Dec 3]. Available from:* https://www.rrpv.org/ota/

111. **OpenSecrets.org.** *Money to Congress per election cycle. [Internet]. Washington (DC): Center for Responsive Politics; [cited 2024 Dec 3]. Available from:* https://www.opensecrets.org/industries/summary?cycle=2004&ind=H4300

112. **OpenSecrets.** *Following the money in politics. [Internet]. Washington (DC): Center for Responsive Politics; [cited 2024 Dec 3]. Available from:* https://www.opensecrets.org/federal-lobbying/industries/summary

CHAPTER 11

113. **Centers for Disease Control and Prevention (CDC).** *Selecting viruses for flu vaccines. [Internet]. Atlanta (GA): Centers for Disease Control and Prevention; [cited 2024 Dec 3]. Available from:* https://www.cdc.gov/flu/vaccine-process/vaccine-selection.html

114. **American Academy of Family Physicians.** *Don't routinely avoid influenza vaccination in egg-allergic patients. Am Fam Physician. [Internet]. 2017 [cited 2024 Dec 3]. Available from:* https://www.aafp.org/pubs/afp/collections/choosing-wisely/201.html

115. **World Health Organization (WHO).** *The WHO manual on animal influenza diagnosis and surveillance. Geneva: World Health Organization; 2002 [cited 2024 Dec 31]. Available from:* https://iris.who.int/bitstream/10665/68026/1/WHO_CDS_CSR_NCS_2002.5.pdf

116. **American Cancer Society.** *Formaldehyde and cancer risk. [Internet]. Atlanta (GA): American Cancer Society; [cited 2024 Dec 31]. Available from:* https://www.cancer.org/cancer/risk-prevention/chemicals/formaldehyde.html

117. *Herman S, et al. The hidden allergen: Triton X-100, a derivative of polyethylene glycol. J Allergy Clin Immunol Pract. 2021 Jul 7;9(7):2941. [cited 2024 Dec 3]. Available from:* https://pmc.ncbi.nlm.nih.gov/articles/PMC8261041/

118. **Sigma-Aldrich.** *Triton X-100 MSDS sheet. [Internet]. St. Louis (MO): Sigma-Aldrich; [cited 2024 Dec 3]. Available from:* https://www.sigmaaldrich.com/deepweb/assets/sigmaaldrich/product/documents/160/855/t8532pis.pdf

119. **Cochrane.** *Influenza vaccine review suite updated. [Internet]. [cited 2024 Dec 3]. Available from:* https://ari.cochrane.org/news/influenza-vaccine-review-suite-updated

120. *Laupacis A, Sackett DL, Roberts RS. An assessment of clinically useful measures of the consequences of treatment. N Engl J Med. 1988;318(26):1728–33. [cited 2024 Dec 3]. Available from:* https://pubmed.ncbi.nlm.nih.gov/3374545/

121. Feng S, et al. *Number needed to vaccinate for COVID-19 booster doses: a valuable metric to inform vaccination strategies.* Lancet Reg Health Am. 2023 Jun 28;23:100548. *[cited 2024 Dec 3]. Available from:* https://www.ncbi.nlm.nih.gov/pmc/articles/PMC10304837

122. Demicheli V, et al. *Vaccines for preventing influenza in healthy adults.* Cochrane Database Syst Rev. 2018 Feb 1;2018(2):CD001269. *[cited 2024 Dec 3]. Available from:* https://www.ncbi.nlm.nih.gov/pmc/articles/PMC6491184/

123. **Institute of Medicine.** *Federal guidelines needed to ensure safety in animal-to-human organ transplants.* Press release. 1996 Jul 17. *[cited 2024 Dec 13]. Available from:* https://pmc.ncbi.nlm.nih.gov/articles/PMC1381830/

124. **NIH Office of Research Facilities.** *Specific pathogen-free animal research facilities.* Tech Bull NIH Off Res Facilities. 2021 May;112. *[cited 2024 Dec 13]. Available from:* https://orf.od.nih.gov/TechnicalResources/Documents/Technical%20Bulletins/21TB/Specific%20Pathogen-Free%20Animal%20Research%20Facilities-May%202021%20Technical%20Bulletin_508.pdf

125. Norman JE, Gilbert WB, Jay HH, Leonard BS. *Mortality follow-up of the 1942 epidemic of hepatitis B in the US Army.* Hepatology. 1993;18(4):790–797. *[cited 2024 Dec 13]. Available from:* https://aasldpubs.onlinelibrary.wiley.com/doi/pdf/10.1002/hep.1840180407

126. Bookchin D, Schumacher J. *The virus and the vaccine: The true story of a cancer-causing monkey virus, contaminated polio vaccine, and the millions of Americans exposed.* New York: St. Martin's Press; 2004.

127. Zhubi B, et al. *Transfusion-transmitted infections in haemophilia patients.* Bosn J Basic Med Sci. 2009 Nov;9(4):271-7. *[cited 2024 Dec 13]. Available from:* https://www.ncbi.nlm.nih.gov/pmc/articles/PMC5603681/

128. Felder MP, et al. *Steps and mechanisms of oncogene transduction by retroviruses.* Folia Biol (Praba). 1994;40:225-35. *[cited 2024 Dec 13]. Available from:* https://www.researchgate.net/publication/15303084_Steps_and_mechanisms_of_oncogene_transduction_by_retroviruses

129. **Food and Drug Administration, Center for Biologics Evaluation and Research.** *Evolving scientific and regulatory perspectives on cell substrates for vaccine development.* 1999 Sep 10.

130. Weissmahr RN, et al. *Reverse transcriptase activity in chicken embryo fibroblast culture supernatants is associated with particles containing endogenous avian retrovirus EAV-0 RNA.* J Virol. 1997 Apr;71(4):3005-12. *[cited 2024 Dec 13]. Available from:* https://journals.asm.org/doi/10.1128/jvi.71.4.3005-3012.1997

131. Tsang SX, et al. *Evidence of avian leukosis virus subgroup E and endogenous avian virus in measles and mumps vaccines derived from chicken cells: Investigation of transmission to vaccine recipients.* J Virol. 1999 Jul;73(7):5843–51. *[cited 2024 Dec 13]. Available from:* https://www.ncbi.nlm.nih.gov/pmc/articles/PMC112645/

132. Johnson ES. *Poultry oncogenic retroviruses and humans. Cancer Detect Prev. 1994;18(1):9-30. [cited 2024 Dec 13]. Available from:* https://pubmed.ncbi.nlm.nih.gov/8162609/

133. McReardon B. *What is coming through that needle? The problem of pathogenic vaccine contamination. [cited 2024 Dec 13]. Available from:* https://www.researchgate.net/publication/253371948_What_Is_Coming_Through_That_Needle_The_Problem_of_Pathogenic_Vaccine_Contamination

134. Speicher DJ, Rose J, Gutschi LM, et al. *DNA fragments detected in monovalent and bivalent Pfizer/BioNTech and Moderna modRNA COVID-19 vaccines from Ontario, Canada: Exploratory dose response relationship with serious adverse events. OSF Preprints. 2023. [cited 2024 Dec 13]. Available from:* https://osf.io/preprints/osf/mjc97

135. Dean DA, Dean BS, Muller S, et al. *Sequence requirements for plasmid nuclear import. Exp Cell Res. 1999;253(2):713-22. [cited 2024 Dec 13]. Available from:* https://pmc.ncbi.nlm.nih.gov/articles/PMC4152905/

136. McKernan K, et al. *Sequencing of bivalent Moderna and Pfizer mRNA vaccines reveals nanogram to microgram quantities of expression vector dsDNA per dose. [cited 2024 Dec 13]. Available from:* https://osf.io/preprints/osf/b9t7m

137. Weissmahr RN, Schupbach J, Boni J. *Reverse transcriptase activity in chicken embryo fibroblast culture supernatants is associated with particles containing endogenous avian retrovirus EAV-0 RNA. J Virol. 1997;71(4):3005–12. [cited 2024 Dec 13]. Available from:* https://hero.epa.gov/hero/index.cfm/reference/details/reference_id/6985035

CHAPTER 12

138. **The Writing Committee of the World Health Organization (WHO) Consultation on Human Influenza A/H5.** *Avian influenza A (H5N1) infection in humans. N Engl J Med. 2005 Sep 29;353(13):1374-138. doi: 10.1056/NEJMra052211. [cited 2024 Dec 13]. Available from:* https://www.nejm.org/doi/10.1056/NEJMra052211

139. Mattes B. *293 and PER C6 cell lines using AD5. Life Issues Institute. 2012 Apr 10. [cited 2024 Dec 13]. Available from:* https://lifeissues.org/article/293-per-c6-cell-lines-using-ad5/

140. **FDA and Vaccines and Related Biological Products Advisory Committee Meeting.** *Designer cell substrates. 2001 May 16. [cited 2024 Dec 13]. Available from:* https://web.archive.org/web/20170516050447/https://www.fda.gov/ohrms/dockets/ac/01/transcripts/3750t1_01.pdf

141. Austricao N. *Moral guidance on using COVID-19 vaccines developed with human fetal cell lines. The Journal of the Witherspoon Institute. 2020 May 26. [cited 2024 Dec 13]. Available from:* https://www.thepublicdiscourse.com/2020/05/63752/

142. Govorkova EA, et al. Replication of influenza A viruses in a green monkey kidney continuous cell line (Vero). J Infect Dis. 1995 Jul;172(1):250-3. Available from: https://academic.oup.com/jid/article-abstract/172/1/250/853500

143. Macnab JCM, Onions D. Tumor viruses. In: Baron S, editor. Medical microbiology. 4th ed. Galveston (TX): University of Texas Medical Branch at Galveston; 1996. Chapter 47. Available from: https://www.ncbi.nlm.nih.gov/books/NBK7998

144. **Center for Biologics Evaluation and Research (CBER).** About CBER. U.S. Food and Drug Administration. [cited 2024 Dec 13]. Available from: https://www.fda.gov/about-fda/center-biologics-evaluation-and-research-cber/about-cber

145. **Midthun K, MD.** Letter to sponsors using Vero cells as a cell substrate for investigational vaccines. U.S. Food and Drug Administration, Center for Biologics Evaluation and Research. 2001 Mar 12.

146. **European Commission.** Scientific conclusions and grounds for maintenance of the marketing authorisations subject to conditions. 2011 Dec 9. Available from: https://ec.europa.eu/health/documents/community-register/2012/20121206124429/anx_1244

147. Cox MM, et al. FluBlok, a recombinant hemagglutinin influenza vaccine. Influenza Other Respir Viruses. 2008 Nov;2(6):211-9. Available from: https://www.ncbi.nlm.nih.gov/pmc/articles/PMC4634115

148. McKenna M. Plant cancellation shows problems in flu vaccine business. CIDRAP News. 2008 Oct 2. Available from: https://www.cidrap.umn.edu/business-preparedness/plant-cancellation-shows-problems-flu-vaccine-business

149. **U.S. Department of Health and Human Services, Food and Drug Administration, Center for Biologics Evaluation and Research (FDA CBER).** Guidance for Industry: Characterization and qualification of cell substrates and other biological materials used in the production of viral vaccines for infectious disease indications. February 2010. Available from: https://www.fda.gov/media/78428/download

150. Vorberg I, Ziegler U, Weiland F, et al. Susceptibility of common fibroblast cell lines to transmissible spongiform encephalopathy agents. J Infect Dis. 2004 Feb 1;189(3):431-9. doi: 10.1086/381544.

151. Piccardo P, Zhen Y, Lamothe C, et al. Candidate cell substrates, vaccine production, and transmissible spongiform encephalopathies. Emerg Infect Dis. 2011 Dec;17(12):2262-9. doi: 10.3201/eid1712.110505.

152. Larsson J, et al. SARS-CoV-2 spike amyloid fibrils specifically and selectively accelerate amyloid fibril formation of human prion protein and the amyloid β peptide. bioRxiv. 2023 Sep 1:555834. doi: 10.1101/2023.09.01.555834v1.

153. Roh JH, et al. A potential association between COVID-19 vaccination and development of Alzheimer's disease. QJM: Monthly Journal of the Association of Physicians. 2024 Oct;117(10):709-716. doi: 10.1093/qjmed/hcaa399.

154. Boros LG, et al. Long-lasting, biochemically modified mRNA, and its frameshifted recombinant spike proteins in human tissues and circulation after COVID-19 vaccination. Pharmacol Res Perspect. 2024 Mar;12(3):e1218. doi: 10.1002/prp2.1218.

155. Lalani H, et al. US public investment in development of mRNA COVID-19 vaccines: Retrospective cohort study. BMJ. 2023 Jun 12;380:e073747. doi: 10.1136/bmj-2023-073747.

156. Siri A. Judge orders FDA to expedite Pfizer's COVID-19 vaccine data. Fierce Pharma. Jan 7, 2022. Available from: https://www.sirillp.com/fierce-pharma-judge-orders-fda-expedite-pfizers-covid-19-vaccine-data-aaron-siri/

157. **Public Health and Medical Professionals for Transparency v. FDA.** Court order. Dec 6, 2024. Available from: https://fingfx.thomsonreuters.com/gfx/legaldocs/lgpdjabmbpo/Public%20Health%20and%20Medical%20Professionals%20for%20Transparency%20v%20FDA%20-%20order%20-%2020241206.pdf

158. **Cumulative Analysis of Adverse Event Reports.** Nov 2021. Available from: https://phmpt.org/wp-content/uploads/2021/11/5.3.6-postmarketing-experience.pdf

159. **Centers for Disease Control and Prevention (CDC).** CDC Recommends Updated 2024-2025 COVID-19 and Flu Vaccines for Fall/Winter Virus Season. June 27, 2024. Available from: https://www.cdc.gov/media/releases/2024/s-t0627-vaccine-recommendations.html

CHAPTER 13

160. Del Giudice G, Rappuoli R, Lopalco L, et al. What are the limits of adjuvanticity? Vaccine. 2001 Oct 15;20 Suppl 1:S38-41. doi: 10.1016/S0264-410X(01)00295-7.

161. Tomljenovic L, Shaw CA. Aluminum vaccine adjuvants: are they safe? Curr Med Chem. 2011;18(17):2630-7. doi: 10.2174/092986711797631485.

162. FDA. 21 CFR 610.15 - Test requirements for biologics. Accessed December 2024. Available from: https://www.accessdata.fda.gov/scripts/cdrh/cfdocs/cfcfr/cfrsearch.cfm?fr=610.15

163. Simmer K. Aluminium in infancy. In: Zatta PF, Alfrey AC, editors. Aluminium toxicity in infants' health and disease. Singapore: World Scientific Publishing; 1997. p. 203-15.

164. Kenny T, Edelman, R. (2003). Survey of human-use adjuvants. Expert Review of Vaccines, 2(2), 2003. pg 180.

165. Weibel RE, et al. Ten-year follow-up study for safety of adjuvant 65 influenza vaccine in man. Proc Soc Exp Biol Med. 1973 Sep;143(4):1053-6.

166. Tanner, P., Edwards, J., & Finkelstein, J. (2001). Adjuvant formulation comprising a submicron oil droplet emulsion. U.S. Patent 6,299,884. Retrieved from https://patents.google.com/patent/US6299884B1/en

167. Holm B, Svelander L, Bucht A, et al. Adjuvant-induced arthritis: the disease-triggering adjuvant squalene accumulates in draining lymph nodes but not affected joints. Arthritis Res Ther. 2001;3(Suppl 2):P051.

168. Matsumoto G. Vaccine A: The covert government experiment that's killing our soldiers and why GIs are only the first victims. 1st ed. p. 54-55.

169. Gajkowska B, et al. The experimental squalene encephaloneuropathy in the rat. Exp Toxicol Pathol. 1999;51(1):75-80.

170. Coors EA, et al. Polysorbate 80 in medical products and non-immunologic anaphylactoid reactions. Ann Allergy Asthma Immunol. 2005 Dec;95(6):593-9. doi: 10.1016/S1081-1206(10)61106-7.

171. Garçon N, Di Pasquale A. From discovery to licensure, the Adjuvant System story. Hum Vaccin Immunother. 2017 Jan 2;13(1):19-33. doi: 10.1080/21645515.2016.1247756.

172. Kenny T, Edelman R. Survey of human-use adjuvants. Expert Rev Vaccines. 2003;2(2):167-170. doi: 10.1586/14760584.2.2.167.

173. Zhang H, et al. Serum IgG subclasses in autoimmune diseases. Medicine (Baltimore). 2015 Jan;94(2):e387. doi: 10.1097/MD.0000000000000387.

174. Cui M, et al. Immunoglobulin expression in cancer cells and its critical roles in tumorigenesis. Front Immunol. 2021 Mar 24;12:613530. doi: 10.3389/fimmu.2021.613530.

175. Perez Duque, M., et al. "Mumps Outbreak Among Fully Vaccinated School-Age Children and Young Adults, Portugal 2019/2020." Epidemiology & Infection, vol. 149, 2021, e205. PubMed Central, https://www.ncbi.nlm.nih.gov/pmc/articles/PMC8447046.

176. Nuwer R. Fully vaccinated woman contracted and then spread measles. Smithsonian Magazine. 2014 Apr 15. Available from: https://www.smithsonianmag.com/smart-news/fully-vaccinated-woman-contracted-and-then-spread-measles-180951114/

177. Narkeviciute I, et al. Clinical presentation of pertussis in fully immunized children in Lithuania. BMC Infect Dis. 2005 May 27;5:40. Available from: https://www.ncbi.nlm.nih.gov/pmc/articles/PMC1177947/

178. Ko L, et al. COVID-19 infection rates in vaccinated and unvaccinated inmates: A retrospective cohort study. Cureus. 2023 Sep 4;15(9):e44684. Available from: https://pmc.ncbi.nlm.nih.gov/articles/PMC10482361/

179. Haru B, et al. An unusual case of evolving localized tetanus despite prior immunization and protective antibody titer. Cureus. 2020 Jul 31;12(7):e9498. Available from: https://www.ncbi.nlm.nih.gov/pmc/articles/PMC7466034/

CHAPTER 14

180. Markel H. *Quarantine! Eastern European Jewish Immigrants and the New York City Epidemics of 1892*. Baltimore: Johns Hopkins University Press; 1997. p. 141.

181. Novick L, Morrow CB. *Defining Public Health: Historical and Contemporary Developments*. Sudbury (MA): Jones and Bartlett Publishers; p. 11. Available from: http://www.jblearning.com/samples/0763738425/38425_CH01_001_034.pdf

182. Cutler D, Miller G. *The Role of Public Health Improvements in Health Advances: The 20th Century United States*. National Bureau of Economic Research; May 2004. p. 5-6. Available from: https://www.nber.org/system/files/working_papers/w10511/w10511.pdf

183. *Documentary History of American Water Works*. Jersey City, NJ. Available from: http://www.waterworkshistory.us/NJ/Jersey_City/

184. Cutler D, Miller G. *The Role of Public Health Improvements in Health Advances: The 20th Century United States*. Harvard University; Feb 2004. PMID: 15782893, DOI: 10.1353/dem.2005.0002.

185. McGuire MJ. *The Chlorine Revolution: Water Disinfection and the Fight to Save Lives*. American Water Works Association; 2014.

186. National Academy of Sciences. *Summary Report: Drinking Water and Health*. 1977. p. 68-72.

187. Bonner TN. *Medicine in Chicago 1850–1950: A Chapter in the Social and Scientific Development of a City*. Madison (WI): American History Research Center; 1957. p. 182.

188. *The American Presidency Project*. Available from: https://www.presidency.ucsb.edu

189. Newman RK. *Hill-Burton Act (1946)*. In: *Major Acts of Congress*. 2004. Available from: https://www.encyclopedia.com/history/encyclopedias-almanacs-transcripts-and-maps/hill-burton-act-1946

190. HRSA. *Hill-Burton Free and Reduced-Cost Health Care Act of 1946*. Available from: https://www.hrsa.gov/get-health-care/affordable/hill-burton

191. Blumenthal D, et al. *Mirror, Mirror 2024: A Portrait of the Failing US Health System. Comparing Performance in 10 Nations*. Sept 9, 2024. Available from: https://www.commonwealthfund.org/publications/fund-reports/2024/sep/mirror-mirror-2024

192. US Congress. *Congressional Record, 111th Congress, 1st session*. 19 Dec. 2009. p. 14-15. Available from: https://www.congress.gov/111/crec/2009/12/19/CREC-2009-12-19.pdf

193. *Improper payments*, GAO-24-106927. Available from: https://www.gao.gov/products/gao-24-106927

CHAPTER 15

194. *Eligible Professional Meaningful Use Table of Contents Core and Menu Set Objectives Stage 1 (2014 Definition). Last updated May 2014. Available from:* https://www.cms.gov/Regulations-and-Guidance/Legislation/ EHRIncentivePrograms/Downloads/EP_MU_TableOfContents.pdf

195. *Seh AH, et al. Healthcare Data Breaches: Insights and Implications. Healthcare (Basel). 2020 May 13;8(2):133. Available from:* https://pmc.ncbi.nlm.nih.gov/ articles/PMC7349636/

196. *CDC.gov. Executive Summary of IIS Strategic Plan, v1.3., finalized on November 30, 2013. Available from:* http://www.cdc.gov/vaccines/programs/iis/downloads/ strategic-summary.pdf

197. *CDC.gov. Public Health Law. State Immunization Information System Laws— Demographic Data Collection. Available from:* https://www.cdc.gov/phlp/docs/ IIS_Sociodemo.pdf

198. *CDC.gov. Immunization Information Systems Resources. Privacy and Confidentiality. Available from:* https://www.cdc.gov/iis/about/index.html

199. *Bill & Melinda Gates Foundation. Press release. Bill and Melinda Gates Pledge $10 Billion in Call for Decade of Vaccines. Available from:* https:// www.gatesfoundation.org/ideas/media-center/press-releases/2010/01/ bill-and-melinda-gates-pledge-$10-billion-in-call-for-decade-of-vaccines

200. *US Department of Health & Human Services. Protecting the Nation's Health through Immunization. National Vaccine Plan Implementation. Available from:* https://www.hhs.gov/sites/default/files/nvpo/vacc_plan/2010-2015-Plan/ implementationplan.pdf

201. *Gallagher A. Study: 88.9% of US Population Lives Within 5 Miles of a Community Pharmacy. Pharmacy Times. 2022 Aug 4. Available from:* https://www.pharmacytimes.com/view/ study-88-9-of-us-population-lives-within-5-miles-of-a-community-pharmacy

202. *US Department of Health and Human Services. National Adult Immunization Plan. 2015. Available from:* https://www.hhs.gov/sites/default/files/national- adult-immunization-plan.pdf

203. *WHO. Decade of Vaccines - Global Vaccine Action Plan 2011-2020. p. 40-41. Available from:* http://www.9789241504980_eng.pdf

204. *IFFIm. Press release. World Leaders Describe IFFIm as 'Catalytic Success.' May 22, 2012. Available from:* http://www.iffim.org/library/news/press-releases/2012/ world-leaders-describe-iffim-as-a-catalytic-success/

205. *IFFIm. List of Additional IFFIm Donors and Pledge Rate. Available from:* http:// www.iffim.org/donors/

206. GIVS - Global Immunization Vision and Strategy 2006-2015. p. 6. Available from: http://apps.who.int/iris/bitstream/10665/69146/1/WHO_IVB_05.05.pdf

207. Flynn T. Hope of the Wicked, The Master Plan for the World. MaxKol Communications, Inc.; 2000. p. 22-23, 172.

CHAPTER 16

208. World Economic Forum. "'My Carbon': An Approach for Inclusive and Sustainable Cities." Sept 12, 2022. Available from: https://www.weforum.org/stories/2022/09/my-carbon-an-approach-for-inclusive-and-sustainable-cities/

209. US Department of Health, Education, and Welfare. Healthy People: The Surgeon General's Report on Health Promotion and Disease Prevention. 1979. Available from: https://files.eric.ed.gov/fulltext/ED186357.pdf

210. US Department of Health and Human Services. Promoting Health/Preventing Disease: Objectives for the Nation. 1984. Available from: https://files.eric.ed.gov/fulltext/ED209206.pdf

211. Gostin L. The Model State Emergency Health Powers Act. Oct 23, 2001. Available from: https://biotech.law.lsu.edu/blaw/bt/MSEHPA.pdf

212. Gostin L. The Model State Emergency Health Powers Act. Dec 21, 2001. Available from: https://publichealth.jhu.edu/sites/default/files/2023-06/msehpa.pdf

213. Gostin LO, et al. The Model State Emergency Health Powers Act: Planning for and Response to Bioterrorism and Naturally Occurring Infectious Diseases. JAMA. 2002 Aug 7;288(5):622-8. Available from: https://pubmed.ncbi.nlm.nih.gov/12150674/

214. Platt E, et al. Trends in US State Public Health Emergency Laws, 2021–2022. Am J Public Health. 2023 Mar;113(3):288-296. doi: 10.2105/AJPH.2022.307214. Available from: https://ajph.aphapublications.org/doi/full/10.2105/AJPH.2022.307214

215. Mello MM, Gostin LO. Public Health Law Modernization 2.0: Rebalancing Public Health Powers and Individual Liberty in the Age of COVID-19. Health Aff (Millwood). 2023 Mar;42(3):318-327. doi: 10.1377/hlthaff.2023.00185. Available from: https://pubmed.ncbi.nlm.nih.gov/36877897/

216. Office of the Press Secretary. President Details Project BioShield. The White House. January 28, 2003. Available from: https://georgewbush-whitehouse.archives.gov/news/releases/2003/01/20030128-19.html

217. Institute of Medicine (US) and National Research Council (US) Committee on Accelerating the Research, Development, and Acquisition of Medical Countermeasures Against Biological Warfare Agents; Joellenbeck LM, Durch JS, Benet LZ, editors. Giving Full Measure to Countermeasures: Addressing Problems in the DoD Program to Develop Medical Countermeasures Against Biological Warfare Agents. Washington (DC): National Academies Press (US); 2004. Available from: https://www.ncbi.nlm.nih.gov/books/NBK215954/

218. S.1873, *Biodefense and Pandemic Vaccine and Drug Development Act of 2005*. The Library of Congress, THOMAS. Available from: https://thomas.loc.gov/

219. *Congress Poised to Rush through Sweeping Immunity for Possibly Unsafe Vaccines and Other Drugs – Americans Likely to Become Human Guinea Pigs*. Center for Justice and Democracy. October 17, 2005. Available from: https://www.informationliberation.com

220. *Congressional Record. 109th Congress*. December 22, 2005. Vol 151, No 168, p. 5-6. Rep. Obey's Statement on Defense Appropriations Correction Bill – "A Shameful End to a Shameful Congress." United States House of Representatives. December 22, 2005. Available from: https://www.congress.gov/109/crec/2005/12/22/CREC-2005-12-22.pdf

221. Whelan AM. *The PREP Act and the Countermeasures Injury Compensation Program: Past, Present, and Future*. Depaul Law Rev. Available from: https://via.library.depaul.edu/cgi/viewcontent.cgi?article=4200&context=law-review

222. FederalRegister.gov. *Twelfth Amendment to Declaration Under the Public Readiness and Emergency Preparedness Act for Medical Countermeasures Against COVID-19*. Available from: https://public-inspection.federalregister.gov/2024-29108.pdf

CHAPTER 17

223. Mello MM, Brennan TA. *Legal Concerns and the Influenza Vaccine Shortage*. JAMA. 2005;294:1817-1820. Available from: https://pub.jm.dermavidya.com/journals/jama/articlepdf/201654/jco50028.pdf

224. Gentry RJ. *National Vaccine Injury Compensation Program Needs Modernizing*. Testimony before the Select Subcommittee on the Coronavirus Pandemic. Available from: https://oversight.house.gov/wp-content/uploads/2024/03/Gentry-Testimony.pdf

225. Vaccinelawyers.com. *Compensation for COVID-19 Vaccine Injuries*. Available from: https://vaccinelawyers.com/compensation-for-covid-19-vaccine-injuries

226. *Vaccine Adverse Event Reporting System Summary*. Available from: https://wonder.cdc.gov/wonder/help/vaers.html

227. *VAERS 2.0 Reporting Form*. Available from: https://vaers.hhs.gov/docs/VAERS%202.0_Checklist.pdf

228. *VAERS Wonder*. Available from: https://wonder.cdc.gov/

229. Black J. *Is the US's Vaccine Adverse Event Reporting System broken?* BMJ. 2023;383:p2582. Available from: https://www.bmj.com/content/383/bmj.p2582

230. OpenVAERS.com. *Confirmation Comes That Indeed There Are Two Sets of Books*. Available from: https://openvaers.com/faq/confirmation-comes-that-indeed-there-are-two-sets-of-books

231. React19. React19 Research: VAERS Audit. Dec 3, 2022. Available from: https://react19.org/research-studies-surveys/react19-research-vaers-audit

232. National Childhood Vaccine Injury Act Vaccine Injury Table. United States Department of Health and Human Services. Available from: https://www.hrsa.gov/sites/default/files/hrsa/vicp/pre-march-2017-vaccine-injury-table.pdf

233. HRSA Data and Statistics. Compensation Table. Available from: https://www.hrsa.gov/sites/default/files/hrsa/vicp/vicp-stats-07-01-24.pdf

234. Vaccine List and Abbreviations. Centers for Disease Control and Prevention. Available from: https://www.cdc.gov/vaccines/terms/usvaccines.htm

235. OpenVAERS.com. VAERS COVID Vaccine Adverse Event Reports. Available from: https://www.openvaers.com/covid-data

236. CDC.gov. Vaccine Adverse Event Reporting System (VAERS) Standard Operating Procedures for COVID-19 (as of February 2, 2022). Available from: https://www.cdc.gov/vaccinesafety/pdf/VAERS-COVID19-SOP-02-02-2022-508.pdf

237. Black J. Is the US's Vaccine Adverse Event Reporting System broken? BMJ. 2023;383:p2582. Available from: https://www.bmj.com/content/383/bmj.p2582

238. CDC.gov. V-safe COVID-19 Public Health Surveillance. Available from: https://data.cdc.gov/Public-Health-Surveillance/v-safe-COVID-19/dqgu-gg5d/about_data

239. The Informed Consent Action Network. Available from: https://icandecide.org/

240. EpochTimes.com. Edward Dowd Breaks Down Findings on Excess Death, Disability, and Injury Statistics. April 27, 2024. Available from: https://www.theepochtimes.com/epochtv/edward-dowd-breaks-down-findings-on-excess-death-disability-and-injury-statistics-5633806

241. Countermeasures Injury Compensation Program. Available from: https://www.hrsa.gov/cicp

242. Federal Register. Vaccine Injury Compensation. Section 110.42. Available from: https://www.ecfr.gov/current/title-42/chapter-I/subchapter-J/part-110/subpart-E/section-110.42

243. Congressional Research Service. Compensation for COVID-19 Vaccine Injuries. March 31, 2023. p. 15. Available from: https://crsreports.congress.gov/product/pdf/R/R46982

244. The Federal Register. Countermeasures Injury Compensation Program: Smallpox Countermeasures Injury Table. Aug 16, 2021. Available from: https://www.federalregister.gov/documents/2021/08/16/2021-17216/countermeasures-injury-compensation-program-smallpox-countermeasures-injury-table#citation-8-p45656

245. Congressional Research Service. Compensation for COVID-19 Vaccine Injuries. March 31, 2023. p. 5. Available from: https://crsreports.congress.gov/product/pdf/R/R46982

246. HRSA.gov. Table 1. Alleged COVID-19 Countermeasure Claims Filed. Nov 1, 2024. Available from: https://www.hrsa.gov/cicp/cicp-data/table-1

247. Wolf N. The Pfizer Papers. 1st ed. New York: Post Hill Press; 2023.

248. 42 USC Chapter 6A, Subchapter II, Part G: Quarantine and Inspection. Available from: https://uscode.house.gov/view.xhtml?path=/prelim@title42/chapter6A/subchapter2/partG&edition=prelim

CHAPTER 18

249. H.R.3448 - Public Health Security and Bioterrorism Preparedness and Response Act of 2002. Available from: https://www.congress.gov/bill/107th-congress/house-bill/3448

250. Congressional Budget Office. Pay-As-You-Go Estimate. July 8, 2002. Available from: https://www.cbo.gov/sites/default/files/107th-congress-2001-2002/costestimate/hr344800.pdf

251. 42 U.S. Code § 271 - Penalties for violation of quarantine laws. Available from: https://www.law.cornell.edu/uscode/text/42/271

252. Lee JW. Meeting on avian influenza and pandemic human influenza. World Health Organization; Nov 7, 2005.

253. World Health Organization. Department of Communicable Disease Surveillance and Response Global Influenza Programme. WHO global influenza preparedness plan: The role of WHO and recommendations for national measures before and during pandemics. Available from: https://iris.who.int/bitstream/handle/10665/68998/WHO_CDS_CSR_GIP_2005.5.pdf

CHAPTER 19

254. Hamowy R. The early development of medical licensing laws in the United States, 1875-1900. J Libertarian Stud. 1979;3(1):73-119.

255. Kim T. Goldman Sachs asks in biotech research report: 'Is curing patients a sustainable business model?' CNBC. April 11, 2018. Available from: https://www.cnbc.com/2018/04/11/goldman-asks-is-curing-patients-a-sustainable-business-model.html

256. Smith JM. Seeds of deception. Fairfield: Yes! Books; 2003.

ABOUT THE AUTHOR - DR. SHERRI TENPENNY, DO, AOBNMM, ABIHM

Dr. Sherri Tenpenny is a globally recognized leader in exposing vaccine dangers and medical corruption. With over 50,000 hours of research spanning more than 25 years, she was one of the first medical professionals to sound the alarm on vaccine risks, paving the way for many of today's voices in the medical freedom movement. Her relentless dedication to uncovering the truth behind public health policies, pharmaceutical influence, and vaccine-related injuries has made her one of the most sought-after educators and speakers in the field.

Dr. Tenpenny began her career as an emergency room physician and served as Director of a Level II Trauma Center for 12 years, where she gained firsthand experience in critical care and the failures of conventional medicine. Realizing the limitations of the mainstream medical system, she founded Tenpenny Integrative Medical Center near Cleveland, Ohio, where she helped thousands of patients from all 50 states and more than 20 countries achieve true wellness through natural, holistic approaches.

She was also one of the first doctors in the world to warn about the dangers of the COVID-19 shots. In April 2021, she released the groundbreaking ebook and webinar, "The 20 Mechanisms of Injury," detailing how the shots could cause widespread harm. By July 2021, she expanded her research with "20 MORE Mechanisms of Injury," further exposing the devastating effects of these experimental injections. Her work provided early, critical insights into the long-term consequences of the COVID-19 jab, helping countless people make informed choices—insights that other media sources slowly began to acknowledge long after her early dire warnings.

A dynamic speaker, prolific writer, and fearless advocate, Dr. Tenpenny has appeared on countless media platforms, challenging the medical establishment and exposing the systemic deceptions behind vaccines, public health mandates, and Big Pharma's unchecked power. She continues to educate, empower, and fight for medical freedom, making her one of the most influential and unwavering voices in the movement today.

UNLOCK EXCLUSIVE EDUCATION

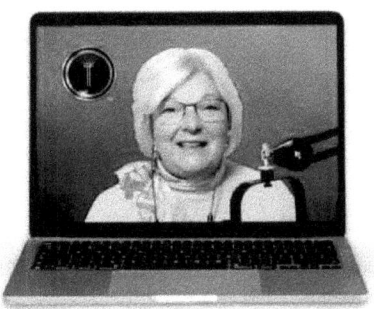

**You've taken the first step toward uncovering the truth.
Now, go even deeper.**

Get exclusive discounts on vaccine education courses and resources that reveal the undeniable facts they don't want you to know.

Explore Essential Topics:

✓ **"Safe and Effective?"** – The biggest myth in vaccine history.
✓ **"Problematic Ingredients – Chemicals"** – What's really inside the shots?
✓ **"The Stork Series"** – Critical vaccine facts for parents.
✓ **"The COVID Series"** – Breaking down the greatest medical experiment.
✓ **"Vaccines and the Law"** – How Big Pharma stays protected, not you.

Take Control of Your Knowledge & Protect Your Health!

Use code **KNOWLEDGE** for your exclusive 10% reader discount!
Visit **ShopTenpenny.net** & **Learning4You.org** to start learning TODAY!

Index

α-tocopherol 235

A

AAFP (American Academy of Family Practice), 172, 379
abandonment, 116
Abbott Labs, 208
AbbVie, 208
abdominal cramping, intense, 253
abdominal surgery, 225
ABIHM, 407
ability, 55, 58, 92, 122, 160, 184, 202, 206, 216, 229, 235, 254, 264, 355, 361, 370
ability to replicate, 55, 58, 184
abnormal buildup, 212
abnormalities, 149
  structural, 371
abolition, 290
abortions, 201, 236
abortogenesis, 236
Abryvso, 196
abscesses, painful, 236
absentee rates, 75
ACAMBUS, 196
acceptable limit, 203
access, 165, 265, 269, 275–78, 280, 282, 284, 287, 301, 303
  better, 270
  ensuring equitable, 284
  equal, 286
  expanding, 264
  health-related organizations, 275
  improving, 300
  long-term, 289

poorest communities lack, 259
  sustainable, 283
  unauthorized, 273
accessibsa.org/mrna, 394
access patient, 276
accident, 163, 276
  cerebral vascular, 131
accidental avian viruses in vaccines, 189
acclaim, 215
  historical, 154
accomplices, 116
accountability, 306, 317, 323, 375, 377
  public, 234
Accountability Act, 275, 382
accumulation, 248, 368
  rapid, 71
accuracy, 73, 278, 301
accusations, 244
ACE-inhibitor, 223
acellular pertussis, 227
aches, 142, 175
  muscle, 233
acid-alkaline ratio, 368
acid-soaked gauze, 102
ACIP (Advisory Committee of Immunization Practices), 172, 298, 330, 393
ACLU (American Civil Liberties Union), 304
acquired exclusive rights, 152
Acquired Immunodeficiency Syndrome HPAI, 382
acquired long term hepatitis, 179
acronym, 13, 237, 379, 381, 383
Acta Neuropathologica, 52, 387

F

FA180/FA180, 387
fabrications, complete, 43
Facebook, 17, 40, 269
facial pockmarks, 153
facial recognition scanners, 293
facilities, 113, 162, 178, 248,
    252, 273
  assisted-living, 319
  bio-containment, 206
  cell-culture manufacturing,
    208
  dining room, 252
  dirty, 317
  existing manufacturing, 194
  existing production, 194
  licensed day care, 299
  line-based manufacturing,
    194
  long-term, 260
  major production, 194
  new medical, 262
  new US-based, 208
  pathogen-free animal
    research, 396
  renovated, 194
  sterile, 178
  vaccine research, 83, 388
factories, new, 193
factoring, 104
fads, 243
FAERS (FDA Adverse Event
    Reporting System), 148,
    380
failed system, 16, 18–20, 22,
    24, 28, 30, 32, 36–282,
    284, 286, 288, 290, 292,
    296–350, 354, 356, 358,
    360, 362, 366–408
failing US Health System, 401
failure of Congress to update,
    327

failures, 108, 164, 259, 305,
    327, 407
  congestive heart, 77
  organ, 35
  renal, 16, 236
  respiratory, 72, 97
  widespread bank, 270
Fairfield, 406
fair to poor job, 305
fallacies, 106, 243
Falls, Ashley, 86
Fall/Winter Virus Season, 399
False Claims Act, 151–52
falsified scientific conclusions,
    151
families, 53, 84, 95, 117, 140,
    149, 165, 179, 245, 251,
    271, 276, 344, 375
  aristocratic, 288
  coronavirus, 113
  triazine, 373
  viral, 116
family birds, 60
family farmers, 38
family loyalty, 290
Fam Physician, 395
families, 53, 84, 95, 117, 140,
    149, 165, 179, 245, 251,
    271, 276, 344, 375
  aristocratic, 288
  coronavirus, 113
  triazine, 373
  viral, 116
family birds, 60
family farmers, 38
family loyalty, 290
family members, 101
family outings, 84
Family Physicians, 395
family's neighbors, 37
Family Support
    Administration, 262
fan, 53, 100, 351

O

Q

V

www.ingramcontent.com/pod-product-compliance
Ingram Content Group UK Ltd.
Pitfield, Milton Keynes, MK11 3LW, UK
UKHW021720220925
8017UKWH00044B/1366